Long Term Care

Story of the Cover Artwork

The picture on the cover is of Margaret Blaschko in her christening gown framed by a memory quilt by joan burlingame, her daughter-in-law. Margaret Blaschko was born in 1910 into a family of missionaries who served in rural Colorado during the turn of the last century. The women in the small town hand made a christening gown including hand-tatting the lace for the hems and collar. Because the family was poor and could not afford many toys for young Margaret, one of the ladies in the congregation gave young Margaret one of her own, well-loved porcelain-faced dolls as a toy. The ladies in the congregation made a matching christening gown for the doll.

Eighty years later, as Margaret was recovering from an operation, joan sat with her for hours, as company seemed to ease the pain. One of the projects that they worked on were two quilts, one to display the christening gown and one to display the porcelain-faced, sawdust filled doll wearing the matching christening gown. Sewn into these crazy quilts were pieces from Margaret's past; buttons from a relative's Union uniform, lace from a special dress, beads from a favorite, but broken necklace. After Margaret passed away, her daughter-in-law found the old photograph of Margaret in her christening gown in an old hat box. Wanting to display the photograph with the other two quilts, joan burlingame made the crazy quilt frame from more objects of Margaret's past: the lace in the upper right part of the frame is from a dress made in the 1940's, the beads are from beadwork on one of Margaret's "Sunday" dresses from the 1950's, the black buttons on the frame are from Goodyear (where her husband worked after the war) and were some of the first hard rubber buttons, the humming bird was one of Margaret's favorite birds, and the spider web is a traditional symbol used in crazy quilts to symbolize how all the memories are died together by nearly invisible threads.

Long Term Care

for

Activity Professionals, Recreational Therapists, and Social Services Professionals

Fourth Edition

Elizabeth Best Martini, MS, CTRS, ACC
Mary Anne Weeks, MPH, SSC
Priscilla Wirth, MS, RRA

Published and distributed by

Idyll Arbor, Inc.

PO Box 720, Ravensdale, WA 98051 (425-432-3231)

Editors: joan burlingame, CTRS, ABDA, HTR and Thomas M. Blaschko, MA

ISBN 1-882883-50-0

Contents

Table of Forms

Index of Activities

Acknowledgments

This book was created from the many years of combined direct clinical experiences, teaching and consulting expertise of the three authors. It was not only these experiences that melded together in the philosophy of the work, but much more important — the people whom we each have worked with who inspired us and taught us about what one needs to live a life with meaning and purpose.

There are many familiar faces of friends and family throughout these years who have left an imprint on my life and work and I wish to acknowledge them in this book: Thanks and love to my treasured husband John who believes not only in me but also in the importance of my work, Aunt Barbara who encouraged and taught me how to venture into this business, my grandmother who taught me appreciation of the elderly, each of my family members for all their love, and my dear colleague, Ann Argé Nathan who taught me how to truly be a recreational therapist; thanks to Mary Anne and Priscilla for their expertise; all of the activity professionals I have had the honor of teaching and working with and joan and Tom (our editors) for seeing the potential of this book.

— Elizabeth Best Martini, MS, CTRS, ACC

I've always considered myself to be lucky; and now, with the opportunity to write this book, I once again need to say, "Thank you." All of my life experiences have led me up to this point and I hope that I have done justice to the world full of people who have inspired me along the way. Some have left their vision with me, some only a word in passing, I am the sum of all that.

Thank you to all the residents and their families who have taught me my job and given a special meaning to my life; thank you to Betsy and Priscilla: it's been fun; thank you to joan and Tom for having faith in us and thank you always to my family — from the beginning in Holley, New York to the present in Sonoma, California. Thanks, Mom and Dad; thanks Nick, Nick and Lucia.

— Mary Anne Weeks, MPH, SSD

I have been most influenced by the countless staff members in many nursing facilities who constantly remind me that health records reflect peoples' lives and that documentation is much more than recording vital signs. I wish to acknowledge Brenda Huntsinger, ART, who first introduced me to long term care consulting; Sharon Carrier, RN, ART, who made it real and fun; my parents who encourage me always; my husband Tom; and all of the medical records directors who teach me new ways of looking at things every day. My thanks to Elizabeth Best Martini for envisioning this book and asking me to contribute and to joan burlingame and Tom Blaschko for pulling it all together.

— Priscilla Wirth, MS, RRA

We would also like to recognize the authors who contributed to the various sections in this book.

Chapter 2: People We Serve
- Theories on Aging by joan burlingame, CTRS, ABDA, HTR
- Mobility Losses and Multiple Medical Issues by Mary Kathleen Lockett, RPT
- Demographics of the People We Serve by Jane Martin, BS, ACC and joan burlingame, CTRS, ABDA, HTR
- Myths and Realities of Aging by The National Council on Aging.

Chapter 3: The Work We Do
- Our History by Nancy Williams, CTRS; Joy Cornelius; and joan burlingame, CTRS, ABDA, HTR
- Recreational Therapist by joan burlingame, CTRS, ABDA, HTR

Chapter 4: Environment
- Survey Form 19: Signage, Figure 3: Wheelchair Turning Space, Figure 38: Storage Shelves and Closets and Figure 45: Minimum Clearances for Seating and Tables from the United States Government

Chapter 6: Activities
- Leisure Room by Pat Hubbard, AC, SSD and Elizabeth Best Martini, MS, CTRS, ACC.
  - Mountain Theme by Ann Argé Nathan and Elizabeth Best Martini, MS, CTRS, ACC
- Theme Weeks by Mary Anne Clagett, CTRS, ACC
- Intergenerational Programs by Marcia Weldon
- Levels of Participation by joan burlingame, CTRS, ABDA, HTR

Chapter 7: Programming for Low Function
- Sensory Awareness Ideas: Shadow Design, Hair Dryer Bubble Blow, Free Form Ball Toss, Free Form Pillow Toss, Powder and Facial Scrubber Time and Tactile Finger Walk by Lois Herman Friedlander, RMT, MFCC.
- Touch for Individuals with Alzheimer's Disease and Other Types of Dementia by Lorraine Brown, MS, CTRS

Chapter 8: Programming for Moderately Impaired Function
- Let's Talk: Fifty Topics Guaranteed to Get Discussion Started by Harriet Berliner, RN-C, MSN, ARNP.
- Men in a Women's World — Discussion by Michael Watters, CTRS.

Chapter 9: Rehabilitation Focused Groups
- Short Term Rehab Activities by Lauren Newman, OTR
- When the Participant is in Need of Recreational Therapy Services by joan burlingame, CTRS, ABDA, HTR
- Recreational Therapy Services in Community Integration Programming by joan burlingame, CTRS, ABDA, HTR

Chapter 11: Designing the Treatment Plan
- Recreational Therapy Assessment, Standardized Scales and Assessment Tools by joan burlingame, CTRS, ABDA, HTR
- Writing the Discharge Summary by joan burlingame, CTRS, ABDA, HTR

Chapter 16: Quality Assurance, Infection Control and Risk Management
- Infection Control, Risk Management, Immediate Jeopardy and Sentinel Event by joan burlingame, CTRS, ABDA, HTR

Chapter 17: Management
- Behavior Management by Kay Garrick, LCSW
- OBRA Regulations by Centers for Medicare and Medicaid Services, State Operations Manual

Purpose

Long Term Care is a programming and documentation manual for professionals in long term care settings. The book is designed to be a "how to" guide which will discuss the people we serve; the environment we are working in; programs that we can provide; work descriptions for a recreational therapist, an activity professional and a social services professional as members of the health care team; documentation of our programs; and management issues for the positions, including dealing with federal regulations.

All of the authors have been working in the field of aging and long term care since the late 1970's. It has been a time of great change and progress in the provision of services and the types of places we work. One of the greatest changes of all has been the expansion of the types of services provided and where these services are provided. No longer is health care provided only by nursing. Now the focus is much more holistic. In order for an individual to progress, to heal or to accept a new lifestyle with limitations, all services must work together as a team and blend their perspectives and treatment goals. The individuals we serve benefit from the diversity of outlooks and develop new strategies for coping both within and outside the facility.

Because of this new focus, professionals need to have a greater understanding of diagnosis, assessment and team approach. In order to be a vital part of the interdisciplinary team, they need to be both articulate and assertive along with being skilled in documentation and federal and state regulations. They also need to be versed in the varied levels of programming required by the people they serve, from the individual who is very alert and independent to the person who is profoundly regressed.

This book is the joint effort of a Certified Therapeutic Recreation Specialist, a Social Services Coordinator with a Masters in Public Health and a Registered Health Information Consultant who is a Registered Records Administrator.

We dedicate this book to the many individuals who have inspired us with their resilience and wisdom. We also dedicate it to you the reader in the hopes of bringing continued inspiration so that your work improves the quality of life for others.

Publisher's Note:

We have promoted the development and publishing of the fourth edition of this book because we feel that the people we serve deserve the best of care. This book was written for activity professionals, recreational therapists (CTRS), social services professionals, social workers (MSW and LCSW), occupational therapists, occupational therapy assistants and gerontologists.

To the best of our knowledge, the procedures and recommendations of this book reflect currently accepted practice. Nevertheless, they cannot be considered absolute and universal. For individual application, recommendations for therapy for a particular individual must be considered in light of the individual's needs and condition. The authors and publisher disclaim responsibility for any adverse effects resulting directly or indirectly from the suggested procedures, from any undetected errors or from the reader's misunderstanding of the text.

Chapter 1
Introduction

The professional opportunities to care for the growing number of people who will use the supportive assistance offered in day treatment, assisted living and long term care settings are expanding faster than professionals can be trained. These positions can be rewarding, challenging and fulfilling — if the individual feels that s/he is competent because of his/her training and is able to feel like an accepted member of the health care team. The purpose of this book is to provide you with the knowledge and skills you need. There are increasing options for people who need assistance with daily living — from help a few hours a day to 24 hour care. Some of the main choices are home health care/home health aids, adult day programs, assisted living communities, long term care and specialty units. This book covers both what the people you see will need based on what they can do and what the rules (laws and standards) say you need to do. The types of services you provide for the people you serve should remain pretty much the same, regardless of where you provide the services, because you are providing what they need. However, the manner in which you provide the services (e.g., based on formal assessment, care plans, etc.) and how you record the services (and the person's response) can vary significantly. What drives the differences in the manner services are provide is based on regulations (laws) and standards (peer-set expectations of performance). Regulations and standards vary depending on the type of setting where the services are provided.

The New Approach

The reader will find that this book is organized without the clear-cut divisions between the different professions that it had in its two earlier editions. There are three reasons for this. First, there is a trend in health care to have all staff "cross-train" so that they can help fill in gaps in care. The second is the increased emphasis on the continuum of care through all levels of service. The third reason is the changing emphasis on quality of life/quality of care seen in areas such as quality assurance, the rights of individuals who are receiving services and the increased power of the Ombudsman.

Because facilities are now staffing activity, social services and therapy professionals seven days a week instead of the traditional five days a week, staff are expected to be able to provide a wider range of services. The reasoning behind this change is that the individuals who are receiving our services should not have to wait two days (Saturday and Sunday) for the range of motion or other treatment they need. While the physical therapist may work a Monday through Friday schedule, the activity professional or recreational therapist should be able to implement some of the patient's physical therapy goals through activities over the weekend. This way the patient receives the maximum benefit. This is not providing restorative care but encouraging the individual to use some of the same movements when they are part of the regular leisure or activities program.

During the last part of the twentieth century the services provided to the people we serve tended to be fragmented. The individual may have visited his/her personal physician, been admitted to a hospital then discharged to a nursing home that was not connected to either the hospital or to his/her personal physician. Today, many of the services are provided by one company, making continuity of care much easier. The organizations that set standards, such as the Joint Commission on the Accreditation of Healthcare Organizations (JCAHO: www.jcaho.org), have developed standards for health care that emphasize the need for continuity through the entire continuum of care. Both of these situations have not only increased the continuity of care each individual is likely to experience but also provide a broader range of settings where the activity professional, recreational therapist and social services professional may work.

As of October 1990, all nursing homes in the United States were required to comply with the new federal regulations known as OBRA (Omnibus Budget Reconciliation Act). These regulations signaled a shift in federal policy from emphasizing the quality of nursing care to a realization that the quality of every aspect of the resident's life was important.

In July 1995, the "Final Rule" of OBRA was implemented. This modification to the federal regulations changed some of the terminology and F-Tags (specific requirements outlined in federal law) within the regulations. The most significant change has been to the survey process and the interpretation of the regulations.

Surveys are used by governments and accrediting agencies to assure that the individuals receiving care in institutional settings are being provided with appropriate aspects of quality care. The survey process used to focus primarily on how the facility documented the services provided. Now the focus is on the outcome of the service. How well do we, as professionals, assess and then document our findings? How well do we, as a team, provide for the needs and interests of each person receiving our services? We, as a staff, are held accountable for each person's well-being. Everything that we document has the potential for being scrutinized during a survey. We have a responsibility to the people we serve to describe clearly and objectively what we have learned about them and to use this as a springboard for developing a plan of care. If we do this consistently, we will have met our obligations to the people we serve and to the groups that outline what we are to do.

OBRA (nursing home) regulations define three components that combine to create *substantial compliance*. Substantial compliance means that enough of the legal requirements are being met by the facility so that any problems found pose no greater risk to resident health or safety than the potential for causing minimal harm. These three areas are Quality of Care, Resident Practices and Quality of Life.

These new regulations put the emphasis on the individual and how we provide him/her with personal respect, a homelike environment and care so that s/he may "attain or maintain the highest practicable physical, mental and psychosocial well-being.[1]" Significant changes in the work of professionals have resulted from the new OBRA regulations.

In July 1998, an interim final rule was approved and as of January 1999, all skilled nursing facilities were required to be "online" and participating in the new Prospective Payment System. These are the greatest changes yet to the Medicare program and will impact the long term care system tremendously.

---

[1] Omnibus Budget Reconciliation Act, Tag F309.

Quality of Life/Quality of Care

The responsibilities of professionals are based, in part, on the need for quality of life and quality of care for each of the people we serve. The quality of life component includes the services of the recreational therapists, activity professionals and social services professionals and also addresses the emotional and physical environment in which the resident lives.

The people we serve have more power in making decisions concerning various types of activities, treatment and schedules. They are to be a part of the team approach in care conferences, resident council, the survey process and much more. Documents such as the Resident Bill of Rights (in assisted living communities and nursing homes) will be at the forefront of quality of life.

The Ombudsman is a state position established in nursing homes to review resident complaints. The role of the Ombudsman has grown in importance into an integral part of the survey process. With the implementation of the Final Rule of OBRA, the Department of Health, Licensing and Certification has the option to invite the Ombudsman to participate in the survey process and the final exit interview with staff. The Ombudsman can also inform the survey team about any complaints or concerns registered with and/or by the Ombudsman office. It is very important for the professional to develop a good line of communication with the Ombudsman.

The Settings in Which We Work

The way that seniors and people with disabilities live has changed a lot over the last twenty years. They used to have just two choices: living at home (or with a relative) or living in a nursing home. Now the people we serve have many choices including: home health care, hospice, adult day programs, assisted living and nursing homes. As professionals we may find that our services can be provided in any of these settings. Below is a quick overview of each type of setting where you may be providing services.

Home Health Care

Home health care is a program in which the patient receives health care services in his or her own home. The type of services may vary from a one time visit to make sure that the necessary adaptive equipment has been correctly placed (e.g., raised toilet seat, shower chair) to regular, long term visitation for therapy and/or nursing services. Patients may have IVs placed, receive chemotherapy, receive help with range of motion or activities of daily living, wound care, respiratory treatment and many other types of care. There are federal regulations and accreditation standards (Joint Commission) that set minimum levels of quality of care for home health care. The Centers for Medicare and Medicaid Services (CMS) requires that all home health care agencies provide skilled nursing services and at least one of the following other therapeutic services: physical, speech, or occupational therapy; medical social services; or home health aide services. The federal law specifically excludes home-based services whose primary function is to provide for the care and treatment of mental illness. Hospice care is often classified as a specialty of home health care.

Hospice

Hospice is as much a way of thinking as a type of service. The goal is to provide comfort and support to a patient and his/her family/friend support systems when the patient is no longer responding to cure-oriented treatments. The primary goal of hospice is to provide some quality to an individual's last days while neither prolonging nor hastening death. Pain management and other medical treatments are provided to enhance comfort and dignity. Hospice workers, usually a team of health care professionals, volunteers and the patient's support system, try to address the patient's emotional, social and spiritual needs as well as minimizing pain and discomfort.

Dr. Cicely Saunders is credited with starting the first modern hospice program in Great Britain in the 1960's. The first hospice program in the United States was established in 1974 in New Haven, Connecticut. While "hospice" is not a place, like nursing homes or assisted care facilities, there are over 3,100 hospice programs in the United States. The Hospice Foundation of America states that almost 540,000 people in the United States received hospice services in 1998.

The Centers for Medicare and Medicaid Services (CMS) lists specific core services that must be part of a hospice program. These include nursing care; medical social services under the direction of a physician; physician's services; counseling (including dietary and bereavement counseling); physical, occupational and speech therapy; home health aide services; and homemaker services.

Adult Day Programs

Adult day care programs offer daytime assistance for individuals who need the structure and support offered through a formal program. There are two different types of adult day programs: social programs and medical programs. These programs may be free standing (not part of a larger health care system) or be just one part of a larger continuum of care. Adult day care centers may be located in a shopping mall, church, community center, assisted living center or other type of building. Adult day programs do not provide overnight lodging for their participants but may be affiliated with a hospital, assisted care living facility or other respite care type facilities where overnight lodging for short term stays may be arranged when the participant's condition deteriorates.

Socially based adult day programs provide services for seniors who benefit from a structured program and from the opportunity to reduce time spent in isolation. Social adult day programs have no regulations so they tend to be more informal than medically based adult day programs. Due to the lack of regulations and standards, there are no specific staffing requirements, documentation requirements or program/activity requirements.

Medically based adult day programs tend to be a low-cost (about $50 per day per participant), organized day program consisting of health, social and recreational services for adults with physical and mental disabilities. Under the direct supervision of professional staff these programs assist in maintaining or restoring, to the fullest extent possible, an individual's capacity for self-care. These programs usually provide assistance in activities of daily living, cognitive stimulation, leisure activities and at least one meal each day. While regulations vary slightly from state to state, they frequently require the medical adult day program to provide many services, such as transportation to and from the facility, medical monitoring, group activities and medication administration. The types of individuals who use adult day programs have similar medical needs to individuals who are in assisted living facilities or nursing homes. The primary difference between these populations is that adults in adult day programs tend to have very supportive family networks that are committed to keeping their family member at home.

One of the biggest problems facing adult day programs is the provision of safe and reliable transportation to and from the program. Some of the individuals in the program may be able to retain some independence by using public transportation. If this option is to be part of the treatment plan, a therapist may want to assess the individual's level of independence by using both the Environmental Safety and the City Bus assessments found in the *Community Integration Program* by Armstrong and Lauzen (1994) or the *Bus Utilization Skills Assessment* (BUS) by burlingame.

Assisted Living

Assisted living communities are like apartment buildings, only they offer varying levels of assistance to the individuals who reside there. Assisted living is designed for individuals who want companionship, security and assistance with the activities of daily living in a setting that promotes and enhances independence. Individuals who are not ready for the expense and intensive level of care found in a nursing home often chose to live in assisted living facilities.

Assisted Living Resident Profile (from National Center for Assisted Living)[2]

Category	Statistic
Age	The "average" age of residents, women and men combined, is 83 years. The average age of the oldest resident is 97; the youngest is 64.
Sex	Nearly 3/4 of assisted living residents are female; 26 percent are male.
Typical Resident	The "typical" assisted living resident is an 83-year-old woman who is mobile, but needs assistance with one or two activities of daily living.
Number of Residents	Approximately 1.15 million people nationwide live in assisted living settings.
Receive Help with Housework	A full 89 percent of assisted living residents need or accept help with housework.
Medication Assistance	Eighty percent need or accept help with their daily medication.
Average Length of Stay	The typical resident stays three years in an assisted living community.
Activities of Daily Living	Twenty-six percent of all residents need no help taking care of their activities of daily living (ADLs), others did in varying degrees. On average, assisted living residents needed help with 1.7 ADLs. The most common types of ADL assistance (partial or full) are bathing (68%), dressing (47%), transferring (22%), toileting (27%) and eating (13%).

It is interesting to look at where people are moving from when they go into or out of assisted living facilities. Most of the people move toward a more intensive level of care, but a significant number (13 percent) actually move back home after living in an assisted living facility.

Assisted Living Move-In/Move Out Profile[3]

Moved into Assisted Living from:	Type of Residence	Moved from Assisted Living to:
58%	Home	13%
12%	Another Assisted Living[4]	9%
12%	Hospital	11%
13%	Nursing Home	43%
5%	Other Location	3%
—	Funeral Home/Cemetery	22%

Assisted living communities have regulations (governmental laws) and standards (peer-set performance standards) that outline the minimum level and quality of services expected. Assisted

---

[2] This information is from the National Center for Assisted Living's web site on May 28, 2000. http://www.ncal.org/about/resident.htm

[3] This information is from the National Center for Assisted Living's web site on May 28, 2000. http://www.ncal.org/about/resident.htm

[4] The discrepancy in these numbers is because two sample groups were used: One sample consisted of people who moved *into* the communities in the study and the second group consisted of people who moved *out of* the communities in the study.

living communities must provide basic housing and meals, help the individual coordinate his/her personal needs, offer 24-hour supervision and assistance, offer an activities program and health-related services. The staff must design and offer services that allow each individual to remain as independent as possible, for as long as possible, while providing an atmosphere of respect, dignity and autonomy. Supporting and encouraging the involvement of the individual's significant others is an important component of the assisted living community. The level of assistance provided can be minimal to comprehensive. The types of services offered are to be custom-tailored while also providing routine activities. This allows individuals to avoid paying for more care than they need, while enjoying all the advantages of a caring environment.

Long Term Care

In years past, the skilled nursing setting was almost always a facility that provided services to frail elderly people in need of 24 hour nursing attention. This was what defined a skilled nursing facility/long term care facility. Today, this setting is referred to as a long term care facility or a Nursing Facility (NF) according to the OBRA regulations. The people or residents of a nursing setting today vary in age from teenagers to people over 100. There is no "typical" resident.

The need to be admitted is identified not according to age, but according to acuity level (how sick or disabled someone is) in relationship to how much assistance the individual needs. Some of the people we serve can be placed within the general nursing home population on units with residents who have a wide variety of needs. Many facilities also have "special care units" which function as an individual unit providing specialized services and programs to residents with disorders such as Alzheimer's disease and related dementia disorders. These have separate activity and treatment programs designed to meet special needs. Because they have become so common, the Joint Commission on Accreditation of Healthcare Organizations (JCAHO) has created standards for Special Care Units and criteria for accreditation of these units.

The nursing facility can also be a special unit within the framework of an acute care hospital. This may be called a Transitional Care Unit, Subacute Unit, Medicare Unit or Extended Care Unit. In an acute care hospital, a patient can be transferred from the acute to subacute unit while remaining in the same hospital. The subacute care unit provides the patient with continued coverage of services until s/he is discharged. Medicare coverage continues so this unit benefits the hospital financially. It benefits patients because they do not have to go through another transfer or the transitional trauma associated with many moves while trying to recuperate. Because of these factors, many acute care hospitals are reorganizing their beds to create a nursing facility unit.

This unit is under the same licensure as a nursing facility. It must comply with both governmental regulations and voluntary accreditation. The activity and social services programs are required as a service within the bed rate. The uniqueness of the setting and the high level of acuity of these residents create quite a challenge, especially within the context of regulations that were created before the setting was! Most of the residents (who prefer to be called patients as they are focused on short term stay) are too ill and frail to be out of bed and in groups. In a unit such as this the person we serve may also be dependent on machines and equipment that the professional from a more traditional nursing home may be unfamiliar with. The majority of therapeutic activities are provided on a very specialized, one-on-one basis. The greater the acuity level, the more specialized the activity.

As health care reform continues to affect each of us individually in terms of coverage and special services, it will also play a role in determining which professional services will be provided and covered within a managed care system. The long term care facility is required by law to provide an activity program. Because of this, activity programs in this setting (whether it be a separate long term care facility or a transitional care setting) are protected and will become more important both as a service and as a marketing tool. Professionals need to be vocal, goal oriented and clear as to how they play a significant role in the interdisciplinary approach to health care.

Subacute Care

Subacute care is a level of medical or rehabilitation care that is less intense that what would be provided on hospital unit but more than what would normally be provided for a resident admitted to a nursing home for long term placement. "Transitional care" is another term used in place of subacute care. The individual is transitioning from requiring many hours a day of specialized medical or rehabilitation care to needing only about two to five hours of specialized care a day. Much of the emphasis on treatment will be to help the individual improve his/her ability to take care of himself/herself so that discharge to a less restrictive environment is possible.

Subacute care is a comprehensive and relatively cost-effective inpatient program for individuals who have had an acute illness or injury or who have had an exacerbation of their disease. Subacute care units offer these individuals a specific and determined course of treatment geared toward returning them to the community or to transition them to a lower level of care.

What's in this Book

This book is intended to help you meet the challenges of your profession:
- to work with people at their current level of functioning,
- to see how you fit into the larger health care picture,
- to deal with government regulations,
- to provide a safe and stimulating environment for the people you serve and
- to deal with all of the details of your work (surveys, laws, budgets, quality assurance, time management) without going completely crazy.

The book is divided into chapters that focus on the various aspects of your work:

Chapter 2. People We Serve describes the people we serve. Understanding the variety of residents with their range of skills is an important aspect of understanding how to help them lead the best possible lives.

Chapter 3. The Work We Do describes the work involved with being an activity or social services professional or a recreational therapist. This is an overview of these positions. Many of the details of the work are described in later chapters.

Chapter 4. Environment describes the environment as it exists for the people we serve, their families and the health care team.

Chapter 5. Programs for Your Facility has information about taking your participants' requirements for care and devising a program for your facility that meets all of their needs and satisfies regulations.

Chapter 6. Activities gives you the foundation you need to run groups and activity programs. Leisure, therapy programs, using themes and thoughts about participation are all covered in this chapter. You will also be introduced to an eight level system, based on your participant's abilities, to help you fit your program better to your participant's needs.

Chapter 7. Programming for Low Function describes many of the people you serve who are able to do little for themselves. This chapter provides you with information about how to work with this group through sensory integration and sensory awareness. The last part of this chapter covers information about touch for people with dementia.

Chapter 8. Programming for Moderately Impaired Function talks about the people you serve will who still be able to assist in their care and want to engage in meaningful activities that bring them happiness and purpose. This chapter provides you with ideas of how to work with individuals who fall into moderately impaired categories and will provide you with options for activities.

Chapter 9. Rehabilitation Focused Groups helps you understand the differences inherent in people who have a true opportunity to work their way to a less restrictive environment versus people who are appropriately placed and are interested in maintaining the skills they have. This chapter has extensive information on cognitive stimulation and retraining. These cognitive strengthening activities may also be used with participants who are moderately impaired or who are at a lower functioning level.

Chapter 10. Documentation discusses the legal requirements for documenting the care you are providing. It includes information about assessments, care plans and monitoring care plans.

Chapter 11. Designing the Treatment Plan covers the discipline-specific assessment process, including setting discharge goals as part of the participant's admission to the program.

Chapter 12. Resident Assessment Instrument talks about the required assessment and care planning process for nursing homes. We will cover specific information on filling out your part of the interdisciplinary Resident Assessment Instrument, writing a care plan from the assessment information, updating the care plan at appropriate (and legally required) intervals, planning a program based on resident's needs and preparing discharge summaries for residents who are leaving the facility.

Chapter 13. Monitoring the Treatment Plan takes you beyond the assessment and helps you create a care plan. It then goes on to provide information so that you can understand the types of tools you will need to monitor your participant's progress (or regression) on the objectives in the care plan. Specific types of progress notes and updates are discussed at the end of the chapter.

Chapter 14. Councils discusses the OBRA requirement that you give residents (or their guardians) control over their lives, in general and through the specific use of resident and family councils.

Chapter 15. Volunteers talks about using volunteers in your programs.

Chapter 16. Quality Assurance, Infection Control and Risk Management deals with being part of the quality assurance program at your facility, being sure that your environment and your activities meet infection control guidelines and understanding the basic elements of risk management.

Chapter 17. Management gives you help understanding resident rights (especially the right to be free of restraints), writing policies and procedures, complying with laws, dealing constructively with surveys, developing a budget and other topics.

Appendix A. Abbreviations provides you with a short list of the most commonly used health care abbreviations.

Appendix B. MDS and RAPs shows you examples of the Minimum Data Set (MDS 2.0) and Resident Assessment Protocols (RAPs).

Appendix C. Standards of Practice provides you with the standards of practice from the National Association of Activity Professionals along with other information about professional practice.

Appendix D. References and Further Reading gives you places to learn more about long term care.

Terminology

In the first two versions of *Long Term Care* we used the terms "activity professional," "social services professional" and "resident." Health care and residential care provided for seniors (and others needing such care) have changed drastically since the first edition was published in 1994. Two significant changes are, first, the management trend to "cross-train" staff and, second, the trend to offer more options for where one can receive services.

As unemployment dropped and the demand increased to provide services seven days a week instead of five, employers found that it was necessary for each employee to provide a broader range of services. While specialization is still respected, in reality, staff are now required to provide a wider range of services than in the past two decades. Activity professionals may need to occasionally help nursing staff with meal times, offering social events planned around a meal, such as a men's football dinner or a retired teachers' luncheon with a guest speaker on school violence. Social services professionals may need to help the therapist teach a budgeting skills class for individuals recovering from a stroke and getting ready to go back home. This movement toward multiple disciplines being able to fulfill the same task was evident when the Centers for Medicare and Medicaid Services first wrote the current set of nursing home laws a decade ago. An example is the position of "Activity Director." There are five different types of training or professional certification that qualify an individual to work as an activity professional.

Long Term Care Facilities: Regulation F248 and F249:
(2) The activities program must be directed by a qualified professional who —
  (i) Is a qualified therapeutic recreation specialist or an activities professional who
    (A) Is licensed or registered, if applicable, by the State in which practicing: and
    (B) Is eligible for certification as a therapeutic recreation specialist or as an activities professional by a recognized accrediting body on or after October 1, 1990; or
  (ii) Has 2 years of experience in a social or recreational program within the last five years, one of which was full-time in a patient activities program in a health care setting, or
  (iii) Is a qualified occupational therapist or occupational therapy assistant; or
  (iv) Has completed a training course approved by the State.

An activity professional is a person who is responsible for designing and running activity programs for the people we serve. Most of the book is appropriate for all of you who are responsible for programs. In the particular cases where we discuss the activity professional who is responsible for the administration of the activity department, we are referring to an individual who meets the requirements in F248 and F249 above.

A recreational therapist is a person who is responsible for designing and implementing rehabilitation oriented treatment that is prescribed by a physician. This type of treatment is outside the typical services offered by the activity professional. Most of the accreditation standards require the recreational therapist to be nationally credentialed as a Certified Therapeutic Recreation Specialist or hold the equivalent state credential. Much of this book is appropriate for the recreational therapist who is working in a rehabilitation capacity as it provides you with a background in the population served, the federal requirements and specific aspects of treatment.

A social services professional is a person who is responsible for ensuring that the social, psychological and physical needs of each of the people we serve are being met. Most of the book is appropriate for all of you who are responsible for making sure these needs are being met. In the particular cases where we discuss the social services professional who is responsible for the administration of the social services department, we use the term social services director.

The second change is in the wide variety of places that the people we serve can receive these services. Many of the choices have been covered above, including home health care, adult day care, assisted living and long term care. In the first two editions we generally used the term "resident" when we referred to the people we serve. This term is not always appropriate when we are talking about issues that may also impact the delivery of services in adult day programs or home health care. Generally, when we do use the term "resident" in this book, we are talking about issues related to long term care facilities.

We will use the term "patient" for people in subacute settings whose focus is on leaving the facility and going back into the community. In general we will not try to label particular segments of people who receive health care, calling them, instead, the "people we serve."

Chapter 2
People We Serve

The long term care and assisted living settings have no "profile" resident. The types of individuals who find themselves living either for a short time or a long time in these settings span the categories of age, disability, socioeconomic status, cultural background and diagnosis. An 82-year-old man with a fractured hip may share a room with a 19-year-old man suffering from a head injury sustained in a motorcycle accident. In the next room, a 17-year-old woman who is comatose from an overdose of crack cocaine may have as her roommate a 74-year-old woman who is incontinent, suffers from short term memory loss and is blind.

Many people over 65 will spend some time in a long term care facility. Some will live out the rest of their lives there. A much larger percentage of the residents will be admitted for a short period to deal with an acute problem. After their stay they will return to a lesser level of care.

It is important to address the diversity and its consequent impact on programming needs.

This chapter will talk about the people we serve and some of their important issues. We will look at the expectations of these individuals and their families, the kinds of physical and cognitive disabilities that they may have and opportunities for continuing a meaningful lifestyle in a long term care or assisted living setting.

Theories on Aging

A theory is a speculation on why and how something happens. Over the years, biologists, psychologists and anthropologists have all speculated on why and how people react and adjust to growing older. The belief is, if we can understand why common problems and strengths have developed, then we can know what to do to improve the quality of life for the community as a whole. This section will introduce you to the most common theories of aging including biological and psychological theories of aging. We hope that they will help you better understand the people you serve and that you can improve the overall quality of life for the individual and for the larger community.

For thousands of years people have been curious about the aging process, striving to find everlasting youthfulness or immortality. Our history is full of stories such as the Spanish explorer, Ponce de León, and his search for the Fountain of Youth in Florida in the late 1400's. There are many relics from ancient Egyptian and Chinese historic towns that show interest in potions and ceremonies to prolong life or to achieve immortality. While the use of extracts made from tiger testicles and other rituals may seem laughable now, look at our everyday advertising to see all of the products offered. We have products to make one's wrinkles fade, megavitamins to prolong life and the increased used of cosmetic surgery. People study the aging process to help us better understand the body as it ages, to improve our abilities to cope and to improve our interpersonal relationships through the life cycle. Because there is no single action or event that can cause or prevent aging, the complex aging process cannot be described by just one or two theories. Additionally, over the last century there has been a change in how we look at theories that add to the complexity of speculations on the why's and how's of aging. During the early and middle 1900's, the people who studied development and aging focused on descriptions of milestones at each phase of life, asking "what happens" and "when does it happen" questions. As the end of the twentieth century closed, researchers started focusing on the explanations of how the changes occurred by asking "why" and "how" questions. This lead to theories based on both descriptive and explanation-based ideas.

Biological Theories of Aging

Biological theories on aging focus on anticipated changes in the organs of the human body. The aging process is called *senescence*, taken from the Latin word *senescere* meaning to grow old. The aging process usually involves a decline of the body's ability to function in almost all biological systems including respiratory, cardiovascular, endocrine, immune and genitourinary. However, the myth that people experience significant cognitive and physical capacity losses as they age has been shown to generally be false. Many people retain a significant portion of their cognitive and physical abilities as they age.

Developmental (and descriptive) theories focus on life expectancy. Life expectancy has been studied enough that we know that morbidity (illness and disease) and mortality (death) have changed significantly over the last hundred years. For example, there has been a 60% drop in the death rate from cerebrovascular disease in the last 30 years in the United States while at the same time it is anticipated that 50% of the 15 years olds living in southern Africa will die of AIDS before they are 50 years old. There are many different theories that try to help us understand and anticipate how morbidity and mortality will impact aging. Three of the more common biological theories on aging are the Genetic Factors Theory on Aging, the Nutrition Theory on Aging and the Environment Theory on Aging.

The *Genetic Factors Theory on Aging* states that one's DNA plays the primary role in how well one will age and how long one can anticipate living. Both the person's genetic ability to continue normally dividing cells (thus, prolonging life) and the person's genetic ability to reduce the amount of organ decline through avoiding mutations of DNA determine how long the person will live.

Genetic Factor Theory of Aging
DNA Mutates
⬇
Mutations are Perpetuated During On-going Cell Divisions
⬇
Number of Mutant Cells Increase in Body
⬇
Malfunction of Tissues, Organs and Systems in Body
⬇
Loss of Body Functions

The *Nutrition Theory on Aging* stresses the importance of good nutrition (an adequate amount of vitamins and other nutrients and a limited amount of cholesterols and fats). This is one of the older theories on aging and prolonging life, although the sophistication of this theory has increased as more research has gone into it. The relationship between eating in a healthy way and living longer has been documented for thousands of years. Even though we do not understand many of the specifics of nutrition and aging, enough is known to lead to the belief that a good diet may minimize or even eliminate some of the negative effects of aging on the body.

The *Environmental Theory on Aging* focuses on the elements of our environment — toxins in the environment, viruses, density of population, smoking, the effects of the sun and other factors — that are thought to influence how we age. In his book, *The Stress of Life*, Dr. Hans Selye lists elements of the climate and environment that cause the biology of the body (due to stress reactions) to suffer trauma and reduce longevity. They are air and water pollution, social and cultural stressors, crowding, sensory deprivation and boredom, isolation and loneliness, captivity, relocation and travel, urbanization, catastrophes, meteorological factors and neuropsychological stressors. As an example of one of the stressors, Selye says of relocation and travel

> For the aged, the stress of being transferred into "old folks' homes" is exacerbated by the feeling of being useless burdens on their families and of having no further purpose in life. (p. 390)

Because of the complexity of biological factors that impact the body and aging process, it is felt that no one biological theory on aging answers enough of the questions of "what, when, why and how" to be *the* answer to the biological theory on aging.

Psychological Theories on Aging

There are three main psychological theories on aging: the Continuity Theory, the Activity Theory and the Disengagement Theory.

The *Continuity Theory*, often referred to as the Developmental Theory on Aging, is based on the belief that the personality, coping skills and behavior patterns that one used during his/her earlier stages of life will remain basically the same as one ages. This theory recognizes that individuals may choose to react to changes and challenges in the environment and community based on how they chose to react to similar events in their past, bringing in things learned as they move through the change(s). Theorists feel that healthy developmental aging happens when an individual is able to successfully fulfill the developmental tasks of aging, making the necessary changes to be ready for the next developmental challenge. The developmental tasks of aging are adjusting to one's losses (both physical and interpersonal losses), developing a sense of satisfaction with one's accomplishments in life and preparing for death.

Erik Erikson listed eight stages of human development, the last being old age. Erikson felt that the challenge of getting older was to accept and find meaning in one's life. Finding such acceptance would give the individual "ego integrity" allowing coping skills and the ability to adjust to the reality of aging and death. Robert Peck further developed Erikson's developmental level of old age into three specific challenges of old age:

1. Ego differentiation versus role preoccupation: to develop satisfaction from one's self as a person rather than through parental or occupational roles.

2. Body transcendence versus body preoccupation: to find psychological pleasures rather than becoming absorbed with health problems or physical limitations imposed by aging.

3. Ego transcendence versus ego preoccupation: to achieve satisfaction through reflection on one's past life and accomplishments with the finite number of years left to live. (Eliopoulos, 1993)

Aging is a complex process and, of all the psychological theories on aging, the continuity theory considers these dynamics more than others.

The *Activity Theory of Aging* was developed during the 1960's by Robert N. Butler. The basic premise of the activity theory is that as individuals age, they make a choice not to turn inward and be self-absorbed, but instead keep about the work of their lives and remain an active participant in all that brings importance to them. Activity theory includes the use of activity (and adapted activity) to help someone through the multiple losses associated with aging. Some of the adaptations associated with this theory is the elder's use of "brain instead of brawn" to solve problems.

The activity theory suggests that the older individual continues to try to live a middle age lifestyle as long as possible, unlike the continuity theory that emphasizes a continual passage to the next developmental task. The activity theory suggests that just because people age, it does not mean that they change in terms of their emotional and social needs. A dynamic struggle in society between recognizing the abilities of its elders versus perpetuating "ageism" is a key component of the activity theory. Ageism is a problem for people who are older (and not just related to the activity theory). Kaplan, Sadock and Grebb (1994) report:

> … old age is universally associated with loneliness, poor health, senility, and general weakness or infirmity. The experience of aged persons, however, does not consistently support those attitudes. For example, although 50 percent of young adults expect poor health to be a problem for those over 65, only 20 percent of those over 65 report health as a problem. Similarly, although 65 percent of young adults expect loneliness to be a problem for the aged, only 13 percent of old persons actually experience loneliness. (p. 70)

A third theory of aging, which is highly controversial and now generally considered to be discredited, is the *Disengagement Theory of Aging*. This theory suggested that as people got older they slowly withdrew from society and society slowly withdrew from them. A mutual satisfaction with this separation as one prepared for death encouraged health care professionals and family members to allow the elder to isolate himself/herself from activity, social interaction and societal roles. While individual elders may go down the path of increased isolation, this action is considered to be pathological in nature and not an action that should go unexamined.

Demographics of the People We Serve

There are many changes in our lives that affect how (and how long) we live. Some of these changes, such as the computer and information revolution, are currently causing major changes in how we live. One of the greatest changes is the length of time people live. Life expectancy is the term used to describe how long the average newborn infant can be expected to live. During the time of the Roman Empire the average newborn was only expected to live 28 years. From the time Christ was born until the turn of the last century (1900), life expectancy increased three days a year. Such dramatic changes have taken place since the turn of the last century that we are now seeing an increase of life expectancy of 110 days a year. Much of this change is due to better medications, surgery, personal exercise, better eating habits and general prosperity.

As we move further into the twenty-first century we are finding that global migration of cultural groups is changing the dynamics of our communities. Combining this with our increasingly greater life expectancy, we must ask ourselves, "Who is this group of seniors that we serve?" Are we just increasing the number of older people who are sick and in need of care or are we increasing our number of healthier and more active seniors? And how does the blending of cultures impact whom we serve? Row and Kahn (1999) state:

> When you compare 65 to 75-year-old individuals in 1960 with those similarly aged in 1990, you find a dramatic reduction in the prevalence of three important precursors to chronic disease: high blood pressure, high cholesterol levels, and smoking. We also know that between 1982 and 1989, there were significant reductions in the prevalence of arthritis, arteriosclerosis (hardening of the arteries), dementia, hypertension, stroke and emphysema (chronic lung disease), as well as a dramatic decrease in the average number of diseases an older person has. And dental health has improved as well, the proportion of older individuals with dental disease so severe as to result in their having no teeth has dropped form 55 percent in 1957 to 34 percent in 1980, and is currently approaching 20 percent.

But what really matters is not the number or type of disease one has, but how those problems impact on one's ability to function. For example, if you are told that a white male is 75, your ability to predict his functional status is limited. Even if you are given details of his medical history, and learn has had a history of hypertension, diabetes, and has had a heart attack in the past, you still couldn't say whether he is sitting on the Supreme Court of the United States or in a nursing home![5]

This section will cover what we know about the people we serve by looking at numbers such as the number of individuals who experience specific illnesses or other major events at specific ages. We will also look at the numbers of individuals based on cultural and other backgrounds. Next we will look at a health initiative sponsored by the United States Government (and other groups) called Healthy People 2010. This initiative is aimed at improving health and quality of life.

Profile of Older Americans[6]

The American population is getting older. In 1998 over 34 million Americans were 65 years old or older, making up 12.7% of our population. In 1900 only 4% of the population was over 65 years of age. And the number of people over 65 years of age is growing faster than the number of people under the age of 65. Between 1990 and 1998 people over 65 years of age increased 10% compared to 8% for people under the age of 65. Older women outnumber older men by 143 to 100. While that difference, with almost one and a half times as many women as men, is significant, breaking down the numbers further shows that for women between the ages of 65-69 there are 118 women for every 100 men. By the time women reach the over-85 age group, there are 241 women for every 100 men.

Americans are not dying as fast either. In 1998 an average of 5,190 people celebrated their 65th birthdays each day while an average of 4,794 people over the age of 65 died each day. That means that in the United States the number of people over 65 increases by 396 people every day. This increase does not reflect the future rate increase of people over the age of 65. The people who turned 65 during the 1990's were people born during the Great Depression when the birth rate was down. Between the years 2010 and 2030 the "baby boom" generation will reach the age of 65, further swelling the numbers of people over the age of 65. By the year 2030 there should be almost twice as many people over the age of 65 as there were in 1998. It is estimated that one out of every five people in the United States in the year 2030 will be over the age of 65.

In addition to the changes in the age of Americans, the United States is becoming vastly more culturally diverse. In 1998, of the people who were 65 years old or older living in the United States, almost 16% was minorities. The largest minority group were African-Americans (8.0%), followed by persons of Hispanic origin (5.1%), Asian or Pacific Islanders (2.1%) and American Indian or Native Alaskan (less than 1%). This percentage is expected to change dramatically. In the report *Profile of Older Americans: 1999* by the Administration on Aging it states:

> Minority populations are projected to increase to 25% of the elderly population in 2030, up from 16% in 1998. Between 1998 and 2030, the white population 65+ is projected to increase by 79% compared with 226% for older minorities, including Hispanics (341%); African-Americans (130%); American Indians, Eskimos and Aleuts (150%); and Asians and Pacific Islanders (323%).

[5] Rowe, J and Kahn, R. (1999). "The future of aging." In *Contemporary Long Term Care*, Vol. 22, No. 2, pg. 38.
[6] The information from this section comes from the United States Administration on Aging's Web site, www.aoa.dhhs.gov/aoa/stats/profile/default.htm, July 7, 2000. It is from their *Profile of Older Americans: 1999* report.

Of the people over the age of 65 in 1998, 75% of the men and 43% of the women were married. Divorce accounted for only a small percentage of the reasons people over 65 were not married (7%). And the majority of older people who were not institutionalized (67%) lived in a family setting in 1998. Breaking that number down we find that 80% of older men (7% with family members other than spouses) and 58% of older women (17% with family members other than spouses) lived in a family setting. By the time people reached 85 years or older, only 45% lived in a family setting.

Another aspect of diversity among elders is that they tend to be unevenly distributed around the country. Data from the Administration on Aging states:

- In 1998, about half (52%) of persons 65+ lived in nine states. California had over 3.5 million, Florida 2.7 and New York 2.4 million, Texas and Pennsylvania had almost 2 million, and Ohio, Illinois, Michigan and New Jersey each had over 1 million.
- Persons 65+ constituted 14% or more of the total population in 11 states in 1998: Florida (18.3%); Pennsylvania (15.9%); Rhode Island (15.2%); Iowa (15.1%); North Dakota (14.4%); Connecticut, Arkansas, and South Dakota (14.3%); Maine (14.1%); and Massachusetts (14.0%).
- In sixteen states, the 65+ population increased by 13% or more between 1990 and 1998: Nevada (55%); Alaska (49%); Arizona (29%); Hawaii (27%); Utah (22%); Colorado and New Mexico (21%); Delaware (19%); North Carolina and South Carolina (18%); Georgia (14%); West Virginia (13.9%; and Tennessee (13.7%).
- The ten jurisdictions with the highest poverty rates for elderly over the period 1995-1997 were the District of Columbia (20.6%); Arkansas (17.1%); Mississippi (16.6%); Louisiana (16.3%); Texas (15.8%); New Mexico (15.7%); South Carolina (15.6%); Georgia (14.0%); West Virginia (13.9%); and Tennessee (13.7%).
- Persons 65+ were slightly less likely to live in metropolitan areas in 1998 than younger persons (77% of the elderly, 81% of persons under 65). About 28% of older persons lived in central cities and 49% lived in the suburbs.
- The elderly are less likely to change residence than other age groups. In 1997 only 5% of persons 65+ had moved since 1996 (compared to 18% of persons under 65). A large majority of those elderly (81%) had moved to another home in the same state. (Administration on Aging's web site, July 7, 2000)

For individuals over the age of 65 major sources of income are from Social Security (91% of older persons) followed by income from assets accumulated prior to retirement (63%), public and private pensions (43%), income from current employment (21%) and public assistance (6%). When looking at households that had the "head" of the household over 65 years, the median income in 1998 was $31,568 with approximately one out of seven (13.7%) having incomes less than $15,000 and approximately two out of five (44.6%) having incomes more than $35,000. The average median income varied depending on race: whites ($32,398), African-Americans ($22,102), and Hispanics ($21,935). Many of the elderly were from two income families with the average male having a median income of $18,166 and the average female having a median income of $10.504. While the difference in income between males and females is significant, women are closing the gap. Between 1997 and 1998 (adjusting for inflation), women's income increased +2.8% while men's income increased 0.7%. Poverty among the elderly in 1998 was no different than poverty levels for individuals under the age of 65. Both groups had 10.5% living below the poverty line.

One of the biggest changes in demographics of older adults is the amount of education. In 1970 only 28% of people over the age of 65 had graduated from high school. In 1998 that percentage had risen dramatically to 67% of adults over 65 having completed high school with 15% having at least a bachelor's degree.

The Diseases of the People We Serve

As people get older, their health tends to fail, not as fast as they expected when they were young, but the trend is still there. In 1996, 27.0% of older people reported that their health was only fair to poor. In the population as a whole, only 9.2% said that they were experiencing only fair to poor health. If we look at cultural and ethnic difference, we see a different story. While 26% of people who were over 65 years of age reported that their health was only fair to poor, a far greater percentage of minorities reported their health to be only fair to poor. Among African-Americans, 41.6% said their health was only fair to poor. People of Hispanic origin reported 35.1%. Poor health does not just mean more visits to the doctor. Over one third (36.3%) of people over 65 reported that they had limitations on their activities because of chronic conditions. A full 10.5% said that the limitations were significant enough to make them unable to complete a major activity. For individuals under the age of 65, only 3.5% reported such a significant limitation.

In 1997 the Health Care Financing Administration (now called the Centers for Medicare and Medicaid Services) reported that there were a total of 14,852 nursing homes in the United States, which had a total of 684,656 beds. In the previous year 1,325,993 people were admitted to a nursing home with 1,423,224 discharged in the same year. The larger number of people being discharged than admitted reflects a national trend to shorten the length of stay in a nursing home.

While the national trend is to shorten the length of stay in nursing homes, lengths of stay were not uniform throughout the United States. It can be reasonably assumed that the diseases (and the severity of diseases) seen in nursing homes around the United States is relatively the same regardless of the region of the country and, yet, the average length of stay in a nursing home varies significantly. Some of the states had average stays of over 45 days: Connecticut (52 days), Hawaii (46 days), Michigan (56 days), Minnesota (46 days) and North Carolina (46 days). Other states had average stays of under 25 days: Arkansas (21 days), California (23 days), Illinois (23 days), Iowa (18 days), Kansas (21 days), Louisiana (19 days), Missouri (23 days), New York (24 days), Oklahoma (20 days), Oregon (22 days), and Vermont (24 days). (Health Care Financing Administration/OIS August 1998 Report).

A study conducted by Spector, Jackson and Rabins (1997)[7] showed that more than half of all nursing home residents had behavior problems. Their study looked at four different types of behaviors: delusions/hallucinations, aggressive behaviors, collecting behaviors (hoarding and stealing) and wandering or inability to avoid dangers. The data showed that 54% of the residents in nursing homes in 1987 cried for long spells, had hallucinations or delusions, stole things from others, got lost or wandered the halls, yelled or physically hurt others. There were noticeable factors that impacted whether an individual would have a behavior problem. If an individual was non-ambulatory, s/he had a decreased likelihood of having behavior problems (probably due to an increased chance of being isolated because s/he couldn't walk). Things that increased the likelihood that behavioral problems would exist included cognitive impairment, inability to independently complete ADLs (eating, dressing, bathing, using the toilet, etc.), a history of psychiatric problems, visual impairment, difficulty understanding what was being said and incontinence.

Often restraints are used with residents who display behavioral problems. However, just as there were significant variations in length of nursing home stay based more on the location of the nursing home than on the severity of illness, the use of restraints varied significantly based on factors other than severity of the behavior. When the 1987 Nursing Home Reform Act required nursing homes to reduce the use of physical and chemical restraints the percentage of nursing homes that used restrains, for discipline or convenience dropped significantly. The number of

---

[7] Spector, D, Jackson, M. and Rabins, P. (1997). "Risk of behavior problems among nursing home residents in the United States. " *Journal of Aging and Health* 9(4), pp. 451-472.

restraint-free nursing homes went from 1% in 1989 to 8% by 1995 (Castle & Fogel, 1998)[8]. The authors listed six reasons not directly related to the behavior of the residents for decreased use of restraints. A facility was less likely to use restraints if (not listed in order of importance):

- The facility had a high ratio of registered nurses to residents.
- The facility had an occupancy rate of less than 68 percent (the facilities with occupancy rates of over 87% had the greatest restraint use).
- The facility was a not-for-profit nursing home.
- The facility was located in more competitive urban areas.
- The facility was not a member of a chain of nursing homes.
- The facility had special care units (other than Alzheimer's units).

Individuals from different cultural groups are also less likely to be admitted to nursing homes. Wallace et al (1998)[9] found that individuals of African-American backgrounds were less likely to be admitted to a nursing home than if they were white. African-American elderly were more likely to use paid home care, unpaid home care or no care at all. Forty-five percent of blacks and 32 percent of whites used unpaid community care. The study determined that older blacks had a higher need for long term care than whites when measured by inability of complete ADLs and/or

Deaths and Death Rates for the Leading Causes of Death for People Over 65 Years in the United States 1997

	All Races, Sexes	All Races, Male	All Races, Female	White, Male	White, Female	Black, Male
All causes	5,073.6	5,620.6	4,691.7	5,614.1	4,727.3	6,385.2
Diseases of heart	1,781.1	1,944.4	1,667.1	1,959.1	1,679.8	2,044.8
Malignant neoplasms, including neoplasms of lymphatic and hematopoietic tissues	1,123.7	1,424.9	913.5	1,407.3	915.7	1,818.7
Cerebrovascular diseases	411.9	371.0	440.5	365.5	443.5	448.2
Chronic obstructive pulmonary diseases and allied conditions	277.1	345.6	229.2	357.5	244.2	262.7
Pneumonia and influenza	227.6	242.8	217.0	243.7	223.1	244.5
Diabetes mellitus	138.8	142.5	136.2	134.8	123.2	231.3
Accidents and adverse effects	92.1	110.8	79.0	110.8	80.6	116.6
• Motor vehicle accidents	23.6	31.9	17.8	31.8	17.9	32.3
• All other accidents and adverse effects	68.6	79.0	61.3	79.1	62.7	84.2
Alzheimer's disease	65.0	49.1	76.1	51.3	81.0	*
Nephritis, nephritic syndrome and nephrosis	63.9	72.5	58.0	69.6	54.1	117.0
Septicemia	53.1	52.6	53.4	48.6	*	106.8
Atherosclerosis	*	*	*	*	50.7	*
Hypertension with or without renal disease	*	*	*	*	*	69.6
All other causes (residual)	839.3	864.4	821.8	865.9	831.5	925.0

Rates per 100,000 population. From the *National Vital Statistics Reports*, Vol. 47, No. 19, June 30, 1999. Center for Disease Control.

---

[8] Castle, N. and Fogel, B. (1998). "Characteristics of nursing homes that are restraint free." *The Gerontologist 38*(2), pp. 181-188.

[9] Wallace, S., Levy-Storms, L, Kington, R., and Andersen, R. (1998). "The persistence of race and ethnicity in the use of long-term care." *Journal of Gerontology: Social Sciences 53B*(2), pp. S104-S112.

by the severity of symptoms from strokes, diabetes and hearing difficulties. Fifty three percent of older whites who required help in three to five ADLs lived in a nursing home whereas only 34% of older blacks with similar functional limitations lived in a nursing home.

While cultural background plays a part in whether someone is admitted to a nursing home, so does loneliness. Over 3,000 individuals over the age of 65 years were interviewed in rural Iowa to determine their degree of loneliness and lack of peer companionship. Four years later, 42% of those individuals who were severely lonely had been admitted to a nursing home, while only 10% of those who score lowest on the loneliness scale had been admitted to a nursing home. (Contemporary Long Term Care, 1998)[10]

The leading causes of death among all elderly in the United States are disease of the heart, followed by malignant neoplasms (cancer) and cerebrovascular diseases. The table on the previous page lists the ten most common causes of death in the United States.

Healthy People 2010

As professionals we need to have an understanding of the population we serve. What we do can help increase the quality and length of life for this population. To do this we must understand the diverse nature of the people we serve. There are health inequalities among this diverse population. The federal government has developed a national program called *Healthy People 2010*. Healthy People is a national health promotion and disease prevention initiative that brings together national, state and local government agencies; nonprofit, voluntary and professional organizations; businesses; communities; and individuals to improve the health of all Americans, eliminate disparities in health and improve years and quality of healthy life.

Healthy People 2010 reflects the scientific advances that have taken place over the past twenty years in preventive medicine, disease surveillance, vaccine and therapeutic development and information technology. The changing demographics of our country, the changes that have taken place in health care and the growing impact on our national health status are areas that need in-depth analysis. There are twenty-eight areas that have been chosen as focus areas to improve the health and well-being of the residents of the United States[11]. They are

1. Access to Quality Health Services
2. Arthritis, Osteoporosis, and Chronic Back Conditions
3. Cancer
4. Chronic Kidney Disease
5. Diabetes
6. Disability and Secondary Conditions
7. Educational and Community-Based Programs
8. Environmental Health
9. Family Planning
10. Food Safety
11. Health Communication
12. Heart Disease and Stroke
13. HIV
14. Immunization and Infectious Diseases
15. Injury and Violence Prevention
16. Maternal, Infant and Child Health
17. Medical Product Safety
18. Mental Health and Mental Disorders
19. Nutrition and Overweight
20. Occupational Safety and Health
21. Oral Health
22. Physical Activity and Fitness
23. Public Health Infrastructure
24. Respiratory Diseases
25. Sexually Transmitted Diseases
26. Substance Abuse
27. Tobacco Use
28. Vision and Hearing

---

[10] Newsfronts. *Contemporary Long Term Care 21*(5), p.13.
[11] For more information about Healthy People 2010 or to access Healthy People 2010 documents online, visit: http://www.health.gov/healthypeople/ or call 1-800-367-4725

Trends are important. From them we can learn what works and what falls short of our goals. Putting prevention into our practices and supporting health-promoting policies in our work setting are important. We must make certain that benefits from advancements in quality of life are options for the people we serve regardless of age, gender, educational level, income, race, cultural customs, language, religious beliefs, disability, sexual orientation, geographic location or occupation. This requires the professional to know what is normal and what is culturally appropriate. The following statistics are to help you determine what you can do for the community you represent. This section represents just a small amount of the information that is available. It is just the beginning for you and your understanding of the population with which you will be working.

Each of the focus areas in *Healthy People 2010* have charts that have a specific target for that health category with a baseline, target setting method and data source. These charts are divided by race and ethnicity, gender, family income level, education level and geographical location. The next two pages show charts from Area 6, Disability and Secondary Conditions. In the first chart the objective is to reduce the proportion of adults with disabilities who report feelings (such as sadness, unhappiness or depression) that prevent them from being active to 7%. Currently 28% of adults aged 18 year and older with disabilities report feelings that prevent them from being active. If we have a high population of residents in our programs that have disabilities, this may prevent them from being active. Look at these trends, and analyze whether this is inherent in your population and what is normal for the population that you serve. After looking at this data, you can help people with disabilities and their families face issues of coping, adapting, adjusting and learning to live well with the disability. We are also looking at good mental health, looking at the social stigma of a disability and finding ways to develop a positive attitude and strong self-esteem. Improving health or adjusting to a changed health status enables the people we serve and enhances their participation skills. The information in the following four tables is from National Health Interview Survey (NHIS) conducted in 1997.

Reported Feelings that Prevent Participation in Activities Adults Aged 18 Years and Over

		With Disabilities	Without Disabilities
Target: Reduce the proportion of adults with disabilities who report feelings such as sadness, unhappiness, or depression that prevent them from being active down to 7 percent.			
Total: Baseline: 28 percent of adults aged 18 years and older with disabilities reported feelings that prevented them from being active in 1997 (age-adjusted to the year 2000 standard population).		28%	7%
Race and Ethnicity	American Indian or Alaska Native	22%	15%
	Asian or Pacific Islander	30%	7%
	Asian	—	6%
	Native Hawaiian and other Pacific Islander	—	14%
	Black or African American	31%	8%
	White	28%	7%
	Hispanic or Latino	40%	9%
Gender	Female	30%	8%
	Male	26%	6%
Family Income Level	Poor	38%	13%
	Near Poor	30%	10%
	Middle/High Income	21%	6%
Education Level (25 years and older)	Less than High School	34%	10%
	High School Graduate	29%	7%
	At Least Some College	25%	5%
Geographic Location	Urban	29%	7%
	Rural	26%	6%

Disabilities and Participation in Social Activities Adults Aged 18 Years and Over

		With Disabilities	Without Disabilities
Target: Increase the proportion of adults with disabilities who participate in social activities to 100 percent.			
Total: Baseline: 95.4 percent of adults aged 18 years and older with disabilities participated in social activities in 1997 (age adjusted to the year 2000 standard population).		95.4%	100%
Race and Ethnicity	American Indian or Alaska Native	87.4%	100%
	Asian or Pacific Islander	99.6%	100%
	Asian	99.5%	100%
	Native Hawaiian and other Pacific Islander	100%	100%
	Black or African American	95%	99.8%
	White	95.6%	100%
	Hispanic or Latino	93.9%	100%
Gender	Female	95.2%	99.9%
	Male	95.7%	100%
Family Income Level	Poor	93.1%	99.9%
	Near Poor	95.8%	99.9%
	Middle/High Income	96.5%	100%
Education Level (25 years and older)	Less than High School	94.1%	99.9%
	High School Graduate	94.8%	99.9%
	At Least Some College	96%	100%
Geographic Location	Urban	95.3%	100%
	Rural	95.6%	99.9%

Reported Satisfaction with Life
Adults Aged 18 Years and Over

		With Disabilities	Without Disabilities
Target: Increase the proportion of adults with disabilities reporting satisfaction with life to 96 percent.			
Total: Baseline: 87 percent of adults aged 18 years and older with disabilities reported satisfaction with life in 1998 (data from 10 States and the District of Columbia).		87%	96%
Race and Ethnicity	American Indian or Alaska native	81%	94%
	Asian or Pacific Islander	82%	97%
	Asian	—	—
	Native Hawaiian and other Pacific Islander	—	—
	Black or African American	83%	92%
	White	88%	96%
	Hispanic or Latino	81%	94%
Gender	Female	88%	95%
	Male	87%	96%
Family Income Level	Poor	78%	90%
	Near Poor	81%	93%
	Middle/High Income	93%	96%
Education Level (25 years and older)	Less than High School	83%	94%
	High School Graduate	87%	95%
	At Least Some College	88%	95%

Reported Sufficient Emotional Support
Adults Aged 18 Years and Over

		With Disabilities	Without Disabilities
Target: Increase the proportion of adults with disabilities reporting sufficient emotional support to 79 percent.			
Total: Baseline: 70 percent of adults aged 18 years and older with disabilities reported sufficient emotional support in 1998 (data from 10 States and the District of Columbia).		70%	79%
Race and Ethnicity	American Indian or Alaska Native	56%	73%
	Asian or Pacific Islander	44%	70%
	Asian	—	—
	Native Hawaiian and other Pacific Islander	—	—
	Black or African American	53%	68%
	White	74%	82%
	Hispanic or Latino	43%	69%
Gender	Female	70%	79%
	Male	70%	79%
Family Income Level	Poor	60%	69%
	Near Poor	59%	69%
	Middle/High Income	76%	81%
Education Level (25 years and older)	Less than High School	57%	70%
	High School Graduate	74%	76%
	At Least Some College	72%	80%

Myths and Realities of Aging 2000[12]

March 28, 2000: The National Council on the Aging (NCOA) launched its fiftieth anniversary conference by unveiling the results of *Myths and Realities of Aging 2000*, a wide-ranging survey on Americans' attitudes about aging. For the second time in twenty-five years, a major NCOA study has overturned stereotypes about aging in America. Conducted with the International Longevity Center and supported by Oppenheimer Funds and Pfizer Inc., Myths and Realities of Aging 2000 showed that most Americans would be happy if they lived to be 90. Nearly half of the respondents age 65 and over (44 percent) described the present as the best years of their lives — a 32 percent increase over 1974 results.

The survey of more than 3,000 US adults produced a number of surprises, besides the percentages of elders who considered their current years to be their best. The survey demolished the myth of intergenerational conflict, showing that most Americans favor spending more — not less — on older people. Older people are less worried about their health, their finances and the threat of crime than they were twenty-five years ago. Myths and Realities showed that in the minds of many, old age begins with a decline in physical or mental ability, rather than with the arrival of a specific birthday. The survey also indicated that younger people tend to overstate the financial and social isolation problems of older people.

Myths and Realities 2000 has far-reaching implications, according to a panel of experts who spoke at the March 28 announcement event. Money and health, said survey research director Neal Cutler, PhD, are more likely than chronological age to determine retirement decisions. Only 24 percent of survey respondents cited "reaching a certain age" as a key potential factor in deciding to retire. The relationship of age, work and retirement said Cutler, is undergoing profound change.

Survey results suggest the need to respond with optimism, but not over-confidence, to the present challenges of aging, according to Robert Butler, MD, president of the International Longevity Center in New York City. Although science has dramatically altered aging-related declines in health, stubborn problems remain. Alzheimer's disease remains a formidable challenge that may affect millions of baby boomers as they age.

Although Americans know what they should do to protect their health, they often fail to take steps that could promote their own longevity. The epidemic of obesity in our society, for example, reflects our failure to act on growing knowledge about predictors of longevity. Also, said Butler, we have failed to include long-term care in our Medicare system, or to educate people on the need to plan how to finance their own long-term care.

For the serious health problems that complicate late life, the medical profession and corporate America are actively seeking solutions, said Tom McRae, MD of Pfizer Inc. Physicians now aggressively treat conditions that they used to accept as inevitable complications of old age. Pharmaceutical companies are working on treatments for heart disease, hypertension, cancer, arthritis, osteoporosis and other conditions that affect older people. He stressed the importance of educating people with chronic conditions about the need to take their medication and to assume responsibility for staying healthy.

Wealth, as well as health, greatly determines happiness in old age. Although 60 percent of respondents took responsibility for key financial decisions, many Americans lack the knowledge and confidence such decisions require. As longevity increases — noted Oppenheimer Funds president and CEO Bridget A. Macaskill — the need for careful planning and extensive discussion

---

[12] Used with permission from The National Council on the Aging. (www.ncoa.org)

increases. Yet forty-four percent of married respondents had never discussed with their spouse when they would retire; 40 percent had never discussed where they will live; and 45 percent had never talked about how much money they would need. To guide long-term financial planning, Macaskill recommended professional guidance for individuals, a higher savings rate for Americans and an awareness that the present bull market is an aberration.

Policy makers, like individuals, must plan for the future of retirement. Yet the survey reveals a chasm between individuals' expectations about government programs and current political priorities, according to Humphrey A. Taylor, chairman of Harris Interactive, Inc. The current stress on cutting government programs threatens the benefits people expect from Social Security and Medicare. Few new proposals address the need to alter working conditions for those who must work well beyond "retirement" age to make ends meet. Such tough challenges will intensify as the number of elders increases in future years.

Myths and Realities 2000, then, presented grounds for optimism and careful thought. NCOA's goal, said president and CEO James Firman, is to ensure that within the next decades, all elders can live the "best years of their lives" in old age. To transform the "twilight years" into the "highlight years," added Bridget Macaskill, NCOA's landmark survey should begin to lead the way.

Dealing with Now

People change as they go through their lives. When adults begin to require help for their basic needs, they are different in some way than they were before. They may have slowly become less capable of taking care of themselves as a result of disease or impairment or disability. These changes may have come about slowly, as with Alzheimer's disease or there may have been a sudden event which drastically changed their lives such as a motorcycle accident. We need to understand that *how* they came to need care is a significant aspect of their future expectations. We also need to understand that other people who knew the person we serve before s/he came to the facility may react very strongly to the change they see in the person.

Often a family member or friend cannot relate to their loved one because s/he has changed so much from what s/he was before. But for us, whenever we meet an individual, that is how we will know that person.

As a staff member, you meet the people we serve as the person s/he is today. You may not have a complete understanding of who s/he was, but you can form a realistic vision of what his/her needs are now. You can see the individual without his/her past, which allows you to see a different present and future.

The difference in expectations is not always obvious, but there are some general trends. Typically a sudden event leaves the family and friends with strong memories of the person before the event. Consequently, they often unrealistically hope for a complete recovery. You will need to deal with the reality of the situation and develop a program that takes the changes into account.

In a gradual process, the family and friends may see the move into supported living or into a long term care facility as a final step after which they have no further expectations for the person. In those cases you may expect more from the person when those who knew them before harbor fewer expectations and hopes.

Helen is a good example. She was a regal woman of 82 years. Married twice, both times to high ranking navy officers, she had lived in exotic lands and treasured her possessions that reminded her of adventures and interesting people from those trips. As a widow, Helen had decided to rent out the rooms of her spacious home to artists and musicians so that she could enjoy their company and talents and continue entertaining as she always had.

As Helen became less able to continue this lifestyle with all of its responsibilities, she found herself depending on family more. Her only family was a niece who lived close by. The niece encouraged Helen to seek the care that she felt was needed and to enter a long term care facility. Helen was still fiercely independent, accustomed to attention, good conversation, good books and three shots of whiskey daily. Within a short time at the facility, Helen was experiencing frustration, anger and depression. Her physical strength began to diminish and her memory began to fade. The books that had brought her such joy sat unopened by her bed.

Helen and I still recited her favorite poems and verses during our frequent visits. She shared with me many intimacies, one of which was her unhappiness with her present life. Helen was a frail woman now, but still with the capacity for relationships and friendship.

When Helen died, her niece invited me to attend her memorial service. I found myself alone in a church full of friends and some distant family members, all of whom were wondering how I fit into Helen's life. No one could understand how Helen in her "obvious state" could have developed a friendship with someone. It is understandable, because she was not the woman whom they had known. But I had never known that Helen and I never established expectations of what she could or could not accomplish. Still, I was her friend.

We share this story because of the lesson learned. No one is to blame. The lesson is that at any age and at any specific time in our lives, we may encounter someone whom we do not completely understand. At these times we need to pay close attention to what is happening now. We should expect as much as we can, anticipate change and look for miracles — because one person can make a difference.

The individuals that we are working with are who they are in the present because of the sum total of many rich and varied experiences. We need to help them get in touch with the good feelings associated with pleasurable experiences, sensory experiences, companionship, exercise and success in doing and being alive. At the same time, we need to be sensitive to the fact that they have limits to what they can do and we should not push them beyond those limits. We need to work with the people who are with us as they are now.

Reactions to Illness

People react in different ways to their illnesses and disabilities. And depending on events in their lives, the way they react may change. It may help to be able to identify the manner in which the person is reacting to the illness or disability before determining a treatment plan. (If the person you serve is denying that s/he will need to live in a long term care facility the rest of his/her life, having a goal of adjusting to living in the long term care facility will probably not be very well received.) You will usually see one of these five identifiable responses:

1. The "I Can Live With It" attitude. These people accept their illness or disability and are in the process of going on with their lives in the best way possible. Chances are they will cooperate with therapy as long as it has a meaningful, positive impact on their well-being.

2. The "How Do I Get Out of Here?" attitude. These people are being limited in their ability to express who they are and to do what they have enjoyed in the past because of their illness or disability (e.g., multiple sclerosis (MS) which limits mobility, chronic obstructive pulmonary disease (COPD) which limits the activity level and early dementia which limits the choice of behavior). These individuals may have unrealistic goals for improvement, waver between

anger/depression (about situation) and bargaining/lability (over hoped changes), making a consistent performance during therapy difficult.

3. The "I'm Not Really That Sick" attitude. These people are not able to accept their illness or disability and are therefore denying the severity of their limitations. Engaging these individuals in therapy may be difficult, as they may not recognize that they need to work to improve function.

4. The "Is There Really Any Other Way to Be?" attitude. These individual define their role in life as being "sick" and must have others take care of them and feel sorry for them. Some people define themselves by this role for their entire lives, while others ease into it. In either case, it's the assumption that one has the *right* to be and act ill. These individuals tend to want treatment to be done to them, not to initiate and be self-guided in treatment.

5. "Unable to Comprehend." The last category is not associated with an attitude, but the reality that due to the severity of the illness or disability the person is not able to engage in meaningful thought about his/her problems. This is especially true for residents with advanced dementia, severe head injuries or other significant insults to the brain. These individuals will tend to be guided by the stimulation (noxious or pleasant) in the environment and by internally felt impulses.

When we set goals for the people we serve, we need to take into account how each person is reacting to being in the facility.

Along with the reaction to his/her illness or disability, there is one reaction that we see in almost every person: the need to be in control. The need to control one's life is one of our greatest needs. From the robust to the frail, feeling like we are in control of what happens to us is important.

The Patient or Resident Bill of Rights goes a long way toward guaranteeing this control. We must use good judgment, however, when we offer choices to the people we serve. We must take into account the previous life style, current abilities and the person's health status when deciding how to offer the choices.

The People We Serve and Their Families

One of the most common myths of long term care— perpetrated far and wide — is that the typical long term care facility resident is dumped into an institution by society or by an uncaring family. In truth, it is the rare resident who has *no one* to care for him/her. This fact actually extends whom we serve and requires that we consider not only the needs of the resident but also the needs of his/her family. To a lesser extent, the same considerations apply when someone starts receiving home health care services or is placed in an adult day program.

As a response to loss of function or declining health with the need for assistance and placement in a program, we find some very complicated, yet common, responses by both the person we serve and the family. Reactions to placement and the progression of feelings are actually the same as we see in any situation where loss is involved:

1. Denial that the loss of independence has occurred and that the need for placement really exists;
2. Anger/Hostility about/toward the placement;
3. Searching for alternatives and bargaining to try to change the situation;
4. Sadness/Depression in response to the loss; and
5. Acceptance of the loss of independence and the need for placement.

The question is "What do we do with all of these feelings and the actions and interactions that result from them?" They will all be there and we need to deal with them effectively.

Any satisfactory placement depends on appropriate staff interventions related to these feelings, actions and interactions. We will analyze them to help you prepare to interpret them and work through them when you see them in your facility.

At any given moment, any of these responses may be occurring between one or another resident and family because the facility is dynamic, with new admissions, new adjustments and continuing attempts to cope with the circumstances of placement.

From your side, you will see the same set of problems played out many times. Remember, though, this may be the first time for the person you serve and the family. Even though you have seen the situation many times, each situation will be different. There will be a difference in the intensity of each reaction depending on what has come before. For example, the family that has had previous admissions to a transitional care unit in a hospital resulting in discharge to a lesser level of care will have had the opportunity to think about this (re)placement and will come in with a different set of emotions/reactions based on already having worked through the progression of reactions to loss. Others will need every opportunity to interpret this new set of life circumstances and will then progress naturally from one through five.

What to do? We suggest that you trust your basic instincts. Ask yourself the questions: "What might I need in this (these) situation(s)? How might I wish to be treated if this were my family?"

We do not pretend to know all of the answers, but there are a few things that all of us can do to bring some comfort and reassurance. No matter what else you say or do, be sincere. Your words may not be remembered but your reactions, the way you act, have the potential of forming a lasting impression and may set the tone for further helpful interactions.

Listen to anger and hostility without reacting defensively; offer to seek answers to questions and concerns and then follow up. In any case, genuine warmth and compassion mean the world at times of loss and transition.

In the next five sections, we will identify expected feelings and suggest interventions that will help the person you serve and his/her family progress toward acceptance of the situation.

Denial

"There's no place like home." Who hasn't felt the comfort of returning home after being away for any length of time? How can home, that place where we most belong in the world, become one day a place that is no longer physically or emotionally nurturing? In fact, how can it represent potential harm for us?

The loss of home, warmth and comfort underlie the person's denial, especially for people who have been admitted to a long term care facility for the first time. It is unimaginable to most to give up the place where one not only belongs, but is also independent and safe.

Typical Timing: Admission to two months

Person	Feelings/Thoughts	Interactions
Person We Serve	"I'm really not as ill/needy as everyone is saying; if you let me go home, I will be able to take care of myself."	"My home is so well organized for me; I have a routine there which allows me to function." "Everyone is counting on my leaving, so I have to."
Family	"This is really only a temporary placement; soon, Mom/Dad will be out of bed doing just what s/he has always been able to."	"I wonder if this might be a permanent placement. I hate to bring the subject up because I don't want to discourage Mom/Dad from making progress so I will continue to speak about his/her discharge as a given."

Intervention

False hope is worse than the truth and only postpones facing the facts. But, arriving at the truth is an evolutionary process. For example, 1. ask both the person you serve and the family to describe actual functioning level and then 2. ask them to describe what level of function is necessary, especially related to the return to the previous environment (usually taking care of themselves). This process takes time; the two steps we recommend are not easily or truthfully answered upon admission. We find, in fact, that an individual admitted to a long term care facility is not usually ready to admit that placement may be long term for at least two months from the time of admission. By that time, a sense of security may have set in and, with support from staff and family, the realization that care is required. (We are, of course, speaking only of those needing long term placement.)

We feel that involving the person we serve, continually asking him/her to assess and reassess the reality of his/her level of function will remove the pressure from the family. It is a tremendous burden for the family to feel they are making this decision against someone's will. The decision is seldom crystal clear. All available resources, including the physician and staff, should be called upon to paint the picture of what is and what isn't possible, what can and what can't be.

Anger

We will preface this section by saying that this is often the most difficult reaction to deal with because of its intensity. Most of us shrink from anger and are frightened by it (in ourselves or in others). As a result, we tend to deny its existence or negate its necessity. By becoming aware of this common human frailty, you can be more compassionate, looking beyond the words and actions to find the motivating pain.

Typical Timing: Two weeks to two months

Person	Feelings/Thoughts	Interactions
Person We Serve	"You've put me here; you're dumping me and leaving me to die. I hate this place and I hate these people. I am not like them." "I am terribly disappointed in what you have done to me." "You're treating me like a child. I can still take care of myself most of the time."	**to staff:** "Everything I eat tastes the same! Why?" "Last night instead of helping me, the aide turned my light off. That's no way to treat me!" **to family:** "When will you take me out of here?" "You don't love me any more and are glad that you got rid of me!" "You've rested enough. How can you leave me here?"
Family	"Everything is topsy-turvy in my life now; not only has my parent been taken from me, but you don't know how to take care of him/her the way I do. The food doesn't suit him/her, no one comes when s/he calls."	"I know I come early in the morning, but I like to see that Mom/Dad eats breakfast, has his/her dentures cleaned properly and is dressed warmly. That's the way we did it at home and I want to continue doing it that way."

Intervention

The family's frustrations often are seen as anger toward the staff. They need our help to understand what has happened and where they need to go from here.

Think about what makes a family angry. It may be caused by a lack of control over what is happening to both the individual and the family. It may be guilt about making the placement, the inconvenience of visiting during perceived visiting hours, driving mom or dad to the center or the stress of needing to deal with others who have different cultural values. It may be that at home everything was always neatly in place and easy to find while now the person can't even be sure that his/her socks will get back from the laundry. We need to look at the possibility that the anger is justified and deal as best we can with concrete and correctable complaints.

In addition to problems that can be fixed, we also need to consider whether the role reversal — parent to child, child to parent — doesn't somehow produce a tremendous sense of responsibility, which shows up as an increase in anger related to expected levels of care. That is, the idea of becoming the parent to our parent may be so threatening emotionally that we feel fear or grief that manifests itself as anger. How can we ever adequately parent the person who gave us life? How can we ever do enough? And will we ever be old enough to outgrow the need for being parented ourselves?

These are all issues we must learn to deal with. They are important because those of us who work in facilities often greet the mad/angry face. If we return anger, it is a significant deterrent to warm relationships between family and staff. If we can wade through some of this emotion, interpret it to the staff and help the family see ways of getting beyond their fears and anger, we will be further along in meeting resident and family needs.

Allow for healing time so that trust can be developed. Time is needed for both the person we serve and the family. We are entrusted with a great responsibility and it is appropriate that the way we work will be closely scrutinized. Do your best to not return anger by realizing that the anger of the family and the person we serve is an attack against the situation, not an attack against *you*.

Advise and inform all concerned about what can be expected of the facility. Guide them in the choice/style of visiting and encourage families to trust the facility resources and to pursue their own, sometimes abandoned, lives.

Establishing trust in communication is most effective in dissipating anger. Become a familiar, reliable source of information and comfort.

Searching for Alternatives

As a result of recognizing and acting on the anger surrounding the placement, the person we serve may prevail upon the family to get him/her "out of here." Likewise, the family may respond to their own feelings by shopping around in hope of finding a program or facility that will be more suitable. Sometimes there is a clear need to change programs or facilities to find one that is more compatible with their needs. Other times simply altering the location of the placement (even if there are only subtle differences in care) will allow the person we serve and the family to regain some of their lost control. Most of the time, the search for alternatives does not result in the person we serve leaving, but it is still necessary for both the family and the person we serve to know that they have done their best to make the situation as ideal as it possibly can be. When they are sure that the situation can't be improved, they can move on toward accepting the situation.

Typical Timing: 6 weeks to 3 months

Person	Feelings/Thoughts	Interactions
Person We Serve	"I feel abandoned and isolated. I just don't think this is the best place." "If I could just go home, I know it would be so much better." "There must be a better place."	"I think I can walk as well as I did before. You won't have to lift me at home." "I'll work very hard in therapy so I get well enough to go home." "Please, please, find a someplace else. I just don't fit in here."
Family	"I heard of a place that really is good about getting people back on their feet. I want to check it out." "There must be some way we can take care of him/her at home." "There must be a better place."	**to person we serve**: "We're looking for a better place. They are not that easy to find, though." **to staff**: "We're trying to find a way to take care of Mom/Dad at home. Do you know of any resources that can help?"

Intervention

Some families never reach the point where they feel they have found the best alternative and this can be hard on everyone. For many, the weight of responsibility is tremendous; spouses especially may feel guilty whenever they are enjoying themselves and the person we serve can't share it. We find this to be especially true for spouses of persons we serve with Alzheimer's. They have to watch the person slowly dying and feel neither married nor widowed — in limbo as it were — and guilty for thinking of fun or normalcy in life. If you really feel that the current situation is appropriate, help the person and family to accept the situation, too.

Support groups help both the person and family to resolve many of the issues of searching for alternatives. It helps to see how others have dealt with feelings and restructured their lives. Individuals may need to redefine their lives within the confines of a smaller community (the care facility) and family members must re-enter the community at large with a different identity. Advise individuals and their significant others about support groups and use your experience to assist in reshaping roles and responsibilities.

Remember that there is a chance (even a good chance) that the family and the person we serve will find a better alternative. Support them in their search, especially by helping them find resources in the community which will make it possible for the person we serve to return home or to a lesser care setting. Try to remain open to, and applaud, the possibility that the person we serve would be better suited somewhere else and is actively pursuing this goal.

Sadness/Depression

Sadness and depression are very individual responses. The depth and length of this period depend on the person's philosophy of life, the support available from family and staff and the medical problems the person is experiencing. (Some medical problems, such as a stroke, may cause an organically induced depression lasting months.)

Typical Timing: 6 weeks to 1 year

Person	Feelings/Thoughts	Interactions
Person We Serve	"There is nothing, absolutely nothing that appeals to me here." "I really don't feel like getting up and I certainly don't want to do anything as silly as having my hair done."	Sitting, doing nothing, not interacting with staff or others. "I'm sorry. I really don't feel like doing that now." "I suppose we can talk, but this whole thing just makes me want to cry."
Family	"I miss him/her. It just isn't the same at home any more." "I hate to visit — it makes me feel badly when I come in feeling happy with news from home."	"I cry a lot when I'm home; the only time I'm happy is when I'm here with you." "I just can't visit. It makes me too sad." "It's always good to talk with you about how I feel. It just makes me feel better."

Intervention

Once again, time, opportunity to experience control and security of placement will contribute to a change in mood away from sadness. It is essential, however, to acknowledge the feelings, never trying to negate or "soft pedal" sorrow.

In order to encourage ongoing family visiting and to make it a positive experience for everyone involved, you might give some of your favorite ideas for visiting[13]:

1. Come during a meal when you will be assured of having something to focus on; use the meal's beginning (or end) as the beginning (or end) of your visit, a natural breaking point.
2. Come just before the person's normal bedtime to offer pleasant good night wishes.
3. Bring in a special treat — a milk shake, a spring bouquet from your garden or some homemade soup.
4. Bring in a special friend or a new great-grandchild; encourage friends to visit, even for a moment.
5. Personalize the room with a picture from home, family pictures, a favorite vase. Not only will this trigger happy memories, but these objects will also be icebreakers for conservation when facility staff are in the room.
6. If the person is enrolled in an adult day program, develop a special routine that is enjoyable to the person either before or after each time s/he attends the program.

The important thing is to work toward accepting the sadness at the loss of independence and to start looking for the good things that are still possible in the new situation.

---

[13] An excellent reference on visiting someone in a long term care facility is available, Gayle Allen-Burket, 1988, *Time Well-Spent: A Manual for Visiting Older Adults*, BiFolkal Productions, Inc., Madison, WI.

Acceptance

There are those who appear to acknowledge the need for placement from the time of admission — immediate acceptance, you feel. Don't be fooled!! Almost everyone who starts out seeming to accept the placement will still go through the previously described reactions. Even a person who is being readmitted is back again because something has changed (and probably something has been lost).

We have seen almost everyone work his/her way through all four of the previous stages. Once those stages have been experienced, you can look for true acceptance.

Typical Timing: May start at 2 months

Person	Feelings/Thoughts	Interactions
Person We Serve	"I am enjoying the activities here, especially cards and BINGO. I have chosen Saturday for one of my shower days so that I can feel good about myself for church on Sunday. My room looks so comfy with my TV and chair and all those family photos. Best of all my son goes to the bank and tends to all of my affairs for me."	You will observe relaxed body language and warm relationships with others. "I've made so many friends here, residents and staff. I trust that they do care about me, maybe not as much as my family, but I can still complain and express my true feelings without worrying about what will happen. I know you can't really make me get a lot better, but I certainly appreciate your help making me comfortable."
Family	"I enjoy visiting a lot more now. It's so nice to see Mom/Dad smiling again. It's fun to bring in flowers from the garden for the room and for the staff. It's nice to have Mom/Dad in a place where s/he feels comfortable. It's nice to be able to get out of the house and do things without worrying all the time if Mom/Dad is all right."	You will see an easygoing relationship with staff; warm and friendly attitude; freely seeking to resolve grievances as they occur. "Everyone is friendly here. You are always willing to listen when I have a concern and you usually take care of it right away."

Intervention

Acceptance comes after much hard work and usually some emotional stress. It is welcome as a time for appreciating relationships and enjoying the time left. At this point, everyone involved (the person we serve, family, staff) is visibly satisfied with the quality and quantity of interactions. An easy camaraderie exists between individual and family and the feeling generates goodwill with the staff. There is usually free give and take and consistent involvement in all aspects of care. During this period, you may find individuals and families needing more encouragement to attend resident care conferences because they will say, "We're here so often."; "We speak with you regularly."; "I trust you to phone if there is a new problem."; "I know you take good care of me."

A final note: The five reactions we have described here are a continuum and people generally go through them step by step. However, residents and families will often seem to drop back several levels. When this happens, look for some additional loss that has occurred. We go through the stages with each loss and there is no guarantee that it gets any easier with time. But our struggles and our eventual acceptance show the lifelong potential for growth and change that all of us carry within ourselves.

Diagnosis

Diagnosis refers to the reason or reasons why the individual is in a care setting. A diagnosis is important to you for two reasons. It helps identify known risk factors during activities (what you can expect of the person now). It gives you some indication of prognosis (what you can expect of the person in the future). There are other factors that interact with the diagnosed condition to affect what the person is capable of doing. The two most significant factors are the acuity of the condition and the excess disability resulting from the person's environment.

Acuity refers to the severity or the level of intensity of the diagnosed illness or condition at the present time. Perhaps this condition represents a crisis (acute) situation as opposed to a chronic condition that is more stable and long lasting. People on an intensive care unit represent a higher level of acuity than an individual who is recuperating from a broken leg. The acuity of the condition can have a significant influence on the types of activity that the person can successfully participate in. Knowing the level of acuity also helps professionals know how quickly they can expect a change.

Excess disability refers to a "decline of functional abilities, alertness, cognitive status, orientation, communication, physical status and socialization attributed to the environment and not specifically attributable to a disease process."[14] This decline is greater than, or in excess of, the decline expected from the illness or disability. Something besides the illness or disability is making the person worse than expected. One of the jobs of the professional is to help identify what this "something" is.

Excessive disability refers to all potential factors that can impact an individual's cognitive and functional level more profoundly than their diagnosis. One set of reasons for this excess disability comes from the environment: the physical environment, social issues and attitudes exhibited by staff and family. Other reasons for excess disability are found in individual beliefs and attitudes including problem solving skills, life skills and the ability to be resilient during stressful experiences. Many of these factors causing excess disability can be improved through changes in the facility environment, group activities and one-on-one interactions between the professional and the individual or family. One other contributing factor is medication, which may be increasing memory loss, depression, lethargy and balance problems. You can often provide information to the health care team about effects of medication that may not be obvious in other settings.

You are often the member of the interdisciplinary team who assesses how a person's diagnosis, acuity and excess disability influence his/her leisure needs, interests and quality of life. Goals need to specifically correlate to the individual's present functional level. Federal law (OBRA) mandates that the nursing home facility provide quality of life experiences to all individuals residing in a long term care setting. (When the quality of life component is out of compliance, the facility is deemed to be in substandard compliance.) As with other determinants, you should understand all of the limitations a person is experiencing related to his/her diagnosis and use that knowledge to find and focus on abilities, rather than disabilities, a holistic rather than medical model approach for planning the activity program.

---

[14] Katsinas, René, 1995, *Excess Disability: Recognizing the Hidden Problem in Long Term Care*, presented at the American Therapeutic Recreation Association Conference, October, 1995.

The Therapeutic Intervention Grid

This Therapeutic Intervention Grid was designed to provide professionals with a quick overview of specific disorders that may affect the people they serve. It also summarizes what the individual may be experiencing and the consequent implications for programming and communications for those individuals.

The Therapeutic Intervention Grid is a quick reference to diagnostic groups and corresponding therapeutic programming needs and psychosocial needs. You need to work with the rest of the health care team to coordinate the specific guidelines and treatment plans. In addition, you have much to offer in terms of continued training and understanding of the people we serve.

This form cannot cover all the people we serve or all situations, but it will help explain many of the diagnoses seen. It is also useful as a training tool and has been successfully shared with staff and volunteers alike who work with you. After becoming acquainted with this chart and its underlying ideas, they will better understand how and why specific activities are designed to meet specific needs.

How to Use the Therapeutic Intervention Grid

The grid is designed to give you important information about specific disorders and what this individual may be experiencing. After you have met and begun your assessment of the person, use this grid as a reference to determine what type of activity may be both appropriate and therapeutic.

Health Issue (Column One):
This column defines some of the categories and health issues that may be found in the populations we serve.

Health Implications (Column Two):
This column describes some of the implications of the health issues found in column one. A review of these issues will help you understand the disorder more clearly by observing common effects and responses.

Psychosocial Implications (Column Three):
This column deals with the psychosocial aspects that may be related to the health issue. Some of these may be perceptions of an individual's condition that his/her family members and other visitors may also experience. In order to better understand the diagnosis and current needs of the individual, you must be sensitive to all of the emotional and psychological aspects that affect not only the individual but also his/her significant others' ability to cope with the diagnosis or illness and suggested interventions.

Programming Ideas (Column Four):
This column suggests a variety of therapeutic programming ideas specific to the health issues in column one. Which activities are appropriate depends partly on the diagnosis and partly on the cognitive functioning of the individual.

Therapeutic Intervention Grid

Health Issue	Health Implications	Psychosocial Implications	Programming Ideas
Dementia Progressive and degenerative organic disorders such as Alzheimer's disease, multi-infarct (vascular) dementia and alcohol-related dementia **Cognitive losses** **Disorientation** **Delirium** **Periods of confusion**	Short attention span Anxiety Wandering, restlessness Catastrophic responses Possible decrease in activity levels and physical fitness Lost compensatory skills Memory loss Disorientation Difficulty with directions (path finding) Negative response to over-stimulation Combativeness Decrease in ability to learn new material	Depression based on realization of loss No longer treated as an intelligent person by others due to loss of ability to communicate well in conversation The need for structure increases with confusion & disorientation Decreased ability to interact appropriately in community settings Feelings of helplessness/hopelessness Personal awareness of cognitive losses during more alert periods Decreased safety awareness Inability to perceive physical threats within the environment	Reality awareness Validation therapy Sensory stimulation Music activities Theme activities Object identification, sorting Reading Breathing exercises Remotivation, reminiscing Exercise/movement Flash cards, Etch-A-Sketch Velcro activities Compensatory skills training Promote outings and contact with family and the community Decrease the stress and fear the individual may be experiencing by using structured & relaxing activities
Sensory Deficits (vision, hearing, touch, taste, smell)	Partial to total loss of one or more of the senses Great potential for isolation Potential limited hand strength Potential pain Stiff and swollen joints Limited dexterity and coordination Lack of color discrimination and/or blurriness	Perceived as mentally impaired or incapable of conversation and/or normal activity Socially isolated related to sensory impairment	Sensory stimulation Weaving Theme activities Exercise/movement Visual cues Auditory cues Activities to learn strategies to compensate for losses Focus on senses still intact
Language Barriers	Inability to make needs known and to communicate in primary language	Perceived as mentally impaired or incapable of conversation and/or normal activity Loss of familiar language, customs and music	Communication cards in primary language Visual cues Communication board Tapes in primary language, music & foreign newspapers

Therapeutic Intervention Grid

Health Issue	Health Implications	Psychosocial Implications	Programming Ideas
Comatose	Non-responsive Limited or no vision Communication deficit Potential for skin integrity problems Possible NG tube (feeding tube)	Isolation Family and friends feel helpless or hopeless about visiting unless able to assist in the rehabilitative process	Music Eye tracking experiences (mobiles, posters if eyes are open) Soft range of motion exercises Hand over hand activities Tactile stimulation Auditory stimulation Reading out loud Pet therapy Pat mat
Head Injury	Need for compensatory skills Impaired memory and judgment Impulsivity Weak problem solving Catastrophic reaction to stress Irritability due to limited cognitive, motor and language abilities Slow processing of information and learning and remembering new information Poor safety skills	If the injury is not visible, expectations are often greater than potential resulting in frustration for the person and caregivers Lack of initiative Decreased ability to structure or manage time Change in social relationships and behavior Decreased ability in work, academic and leisure performance	Sequencing activities Sensory integration Sorting games Word games Body awareness and movement Word search activities Hangman Crossword puzzles Large sectional puzzles Attention to task building activities Pat mat Theme activities Links to community resources
Subacute **IV therapy** **NG tube** **Keosh feed line**	Limited mobility Low level of energy	Loss of control based on limited mobility Feelings of vulnerability Exhaustion due to condition and therapy	Music Talking books Oral history visits Reinforcement of therapy goals Environmental/relaxation tapes Theme activities

Therapeutic Intervention Grid

Health Issue	Health Implications	Psychosocial Implications	Programming Ideas
CVA (stroke) Left-sided brain injury	Right hemiparesis/hemiplegia Language, reading/writing problems Aphasia, word finding problems Attention deficits Decreased verbal learning Difficulty distinguishing left and right Visuospatial neglect Memory deficits Lability, mood swings Low frustration tolerance Sleep disturbances Frustration with group experiences Impaired verbal and math skills Lack of inhibition Behavior is slow, cautious, anxious Good attention span Underestimates ability	Isolation depending on location of CVA and degree of impairment Depression — both physiological and related to loss(es) or expectations beyond potential Impatience, frustration with new functional status and lack of speedy recovery Self-conscious about appearance and language difficulties	Involve in appropriate exercises as soon as possible after stroke Activities which stimulate cognitive functioning Body image activities Retraining cognitive and perceptual abilities Repetitive tasks and movements to achieve mastery and therefore transfer skills to other activities Sensory integration activities Sequencing activities Communication group experiences Working with significant others to identify leisure interests and opportunities Exercise activities Opportunities for community reintegration as part of rehabilitation Life skills training Focus on strengths vs. limitations Memory enhancement exercises Word and trivia games
CVA (stroke) — Right-sided brain injury	Left hemiparesis/hemiplegia Perceptual problems Poor spatial orientation and concepts of direction Gets lost easily Decrease or increase in sensation Change in vision Seizures Decreased eye-hand coordination Impaired concrete thinking Sleep disturbances Left side neglect Behavior is fast, impulsive, with lack of inhibition and verbal outbursts Short attention span Constant talking Overestimates ability		

Therapeutic Intervention Grid

Health Issue	Health Implications	Psychosocial Implications	Programming Ideas
Short term rehab Pre-discharge/post therapy rehab residents (i.e. hip fracture, etc.)	Limited energy & easily fatigued Primary focus on therapy goals Disinterest in group activities Self-consciousness	Relationships may be strained due to pain and due to the resident needing to adjust to new (usually lower) ability Impatience with the current situation Fantasies about home and about the ability to care for him/herself Lack of information about home health care and unreasonable expectations can cause anxiety for individual and family	Reading Relaxation tapes Exercise/movement Bird watching Outdoor social activities Work/service oriented activities Community integration Reinforcing therapy goals Resident council Volunteering Memory book
Huntington's Chorea	Severe mood swings Involuntary movements Twitching Nervous behavior Depression Communication problems Aggression Hallucinations Difficulty swallowing	Hopelessness, isolation and feelings of anger and abandonment Guilt based on the genetic component of this disease Inability to feel independent due to tremors Difficulty communicating related to slurred speech Intoxicated appearance which can overwhelm people around them	Exercise Expressive opportunities Weaving Music for relaxation Ceramics Homemaking activities Adaptive switches Verbal word games Communication groups Theme activities
Parkinson's Disease	Resting tremors Rigidity Brady kinesia (slow movement) Has difficulty with more than two movements at one time Softness of voice Depression Need extra time to respond Unsteady gait Possible limb apraxia Poor coordination Possible dementia & hallucinations	Isolation as communication becomes more difficult Perceived as having dementia when this is not necessarily true Flat affect (disease related) maybe perceived as disinterest or dementia	Exercise Expressive opportunities Weaving Music and relaxing Ceramics Homemaking activities Adaptive switches Verbal word games Communication groups Theme activities

Therapeutic Intervention Grid

Health Issue	Health Implications	Psychosocial Implications	Programming Ideas
Multiple Sclerosis **Amyotrophic Lateral** **Sclerosis (ALS)**	Possible loss of fine and gross motor skills; Possible speech and language disorders; Possible vision impairments; Fluctuation both physically and emotionally; Possible fluid retention; Gastrointestinal problems; Depression; Possible limb apraxia — keep movements large and allow space	Total loss of control is possible; Anger; Attempts to manipulate the environment in order to have needs met; Fantasizing about home and the ability to care for oneself; Lack of participation in activities; Anxiety; Impatience and frustration over situation; Depression	Exercise; Movement; Need for energy conservation techniques; Relaxation; Creative outlets; Opportunities to socialize with peers in age-appropriate activities; Visualization; Empowerment activities; Adaptive switches; Communication activities with yes/no responses
Cardiopulmonary **Problems** **COPD** **Asthma** **Hypotension** **Hypertension**	Anxiety; Coughing; Light headed depending on body positioning; Inability to breathe deeply; Decreased endurance; Low tolerance to dust, odors and crowded spaces; Depression; Activities requiring raising the arms over the head are too taxing; Limited time up; Added stress on heart	Attempts to manipulate the environment and personnel secondary to feelings of anxiety and claustrophobia; Need to feel in control of personal environment as much as possible	Hand work; Breathing exercises; Relaxation; Energy conservation techniques; Need for balance of active and passive activities; Slow-paced activities; Activities which do not require lifting heavy objects; Crossword puzzles; Puzzles; Reading; Creative writing; Theme activities
Critically Ill **Terminally Ill** **Hospice**	Limited energy and time awake; Depression; Potential for pain	Changing moods depending on state of anger, depression and acceptance; Existential issues of life and death; May have unfinished business that needs to be completed including questions of religion and spirituality	Relaxation; Being read to; In room travel slides or environmental tapes; One-on-one volunteers; Memory book; Companionship; Visualization; Opportunity to talk; Light range of motion activities

Therapeutic Intervention Grid

Health Issue	Health Implications	Psychosocial Implications	Programming Ideas
Ventilator Dependent	Potential for sensory deprivation Lack of mobility/freedom of movement Potential for skin integrity issues Communication problems Lack of endurance Potential for significant hours a day in bed Pain related to injuries and condition Cardiopulmonary issues Partial to total loss of one or more senses May be non-responsive Potential for total care in ADLs May have a tracheostomy May be fed by tube	Inability to move around without equipment = loss of independence Depression related to condition Anxiety related to breathing ability Limited emotional outlets Potential for social isolation Short or long term need for ventilator Potential for embarrassment in groups related to equipment and equipment sounds	Visualization & relaxation tapes Mobiles Music Slide shows Activities related to body awareness and directionality games Opportunities to be outdoors Range of motion activities Pain management techniques Reading and being read to Intellectual activities Pets Theme related decorations Volunteer visitors Small fish bowl in room within visual range Computer games Dot to dot puzzles Wrist bands with bell to enhance movement and auditory stimulation Drinking straw with streamer attached to enhance breathing exercises
Spinal Cord Injury[15]	Loss of mobility Loss of motor strength Loss of Sensory Awareness Depression Change in self-image Change in physical fitness Loss of bowel and bladder control Susceptibility to pressure sores Potential for long term pain	Change in vocational abilities Change in independence Change in self-image Change in social relationships	Assess physical and psychological dysfunction Increase functional abilities through the use of recreation/leisure oriented programs Teach functional skills, recreational skills and provide adaptive equipment Provide opportunities for creative self-expression Teach progressive relaxation techniques Teach stress management skills Build community resources and skills

---

[15].Spinal Cord Injury information from the American Therapeutic Recreation Association, 1992, *Therapeutic Recreation Services*, ATRA, Hattiesburg, MS.

41

Mobility Losses and Multiple Medical Issues[16]

Preventing loss of mobility is a primary goal of physical therapy and is greatly enhanced by exercises in a group setting or on a one-on-one basis provided by other members of the health care team. With the increasing constraints of insurance companies, many individuals are no longer able to receive the extended therapy they need. This is resulting in greater numbers of people who depend on the activity professional and other staff to continue this focus on therapy goals. You need to have not only a basic knowledge of diagnoses but also the ability to blend this understanding with movements and exercises that will help to maintain and enhance functional skills.

Below is a list of the more common conditions encountered, with brief descriptions and suggestions about the best approach to exercise. Every disorder has a basic description but remember that every person you see will present himself or herself in a unique manner.

Medical Groups

Cardiac

Individuals with cardiac disorders may have sustained a myocardial infarction or have undergone open heart surgery for valve replacement, had a coronary artery bypass or even a heart transplant. Clinically, they may present varied appearances from no outward signs to shortness of breath with minimal activity.

Have the individual monitor his/her pulse before, during and after the sessions with caution not to exceed 20–30 beats above his/her resting heart rate. Some medications modify the individual's responsive heart rate so that this target heart rate will not be appropriate. If in doubt, ask the individual's physician or the nursing staff for assistance. Many areas also have a local cardiac rehab group, which can provide the facility's staff with additional good information.

Suggestions for exercise:
* Limit upper extremity activity thus reducing stress on the heart. Do not use arm weights.
* Encourage activities that involve walking.
* Encourage stationary bicycles.
* Encourage dance activities.

Chronic Obstructive Pulmonary Disease — COPD

Chronic Obstructive Pulmonary Disease results in the individual's decreased ability to breath normally. Many of the people with this condition will need portable oxygen.

Suggestions for exercise:
* Sitting exercises.
* Decrease the number of upper extremity/arm exercises.
* Stop all exercises if the individual becomes winded.
* Pacing activities is the key to functional independence for the individual with COPD.

---

[16] This section on Mobility Losses and Multiple Medical Issues was written by Mary Kathleen Lockett, RPT.

Note: The position where the individual will be most comfortable is with the head and shoulders forward. Continue to encourage activities to lengthen the trunk such as one-armed overhead stretches.

Neurological Groups

Cerebral Vascular Accident — CVA

Cerebral Vascular Accident (CVA) is a neurological disorder also known as a stroke. Whether an individual has sustained a right CVA with resulting left-sided weakness or a left CVA with a right-sided weakness will determine the cognitive and physical deficits present. It is important to remember that individuals can be affected very minimally with excellent recovery or have extensive damage with poor recovery.

Left Hemiplegia (Right CVA)

While language is mostly intact, beware of impulsive behavior and neglect of the left side. Encourage the person to keep his/her head centered in midline. Encourage left-sided activities and movements. Be aware that reasoning with an individual with left hemiplegia is often difficult.

Right Hemiplegia (Left CVA)

Language is often affected resulting in aphasia, which may be receptive, expressive or global. Establish a communication task and expect the individual with a right hemiplegia to have fair reasoning skills.

Suggestions for exercise:
- The individual may go from having flaccid extremities to having spastic extremities.
- Be alert to painful shoulder syndromes seen with either condition.
- If the individual is in a wheelchair, make sure that his/her upper body is supported in midline.
- Be sure the affected arm is supported and have the individual use the non-affected leg to propel the chair.
- Lapboards are strongly encouraged by the therapists. Because they are considered to be physical restraints, interdisciplinary team approval in a long term care setting is required.
- If the individual is ambulatory, balance may still be affected so encourage sitting exercises. If standing, have the individual hold on to a secure surface.
- Expect frustration and occasionally inappropriate behavior especially with an individual who is aphasic. Ask his/her therapist for suggestions if you are having difficulty with a particular individual.

Multiple Sclerosis — MS

Multiple Sclerosis is a neurological disorder affecting more women than men. It can be very mild or very severe. There can be remissions for years or no remissions and it can allow a person to remain ambulatory or cause them to be in need of a wheelchair for mobility. Common clinical presentations are tremors and sensory losses of the extremities, visual disturbances, unsteady gait and occasional personality disorders.

Suggestions for exercise:
- It is important for these individuals to exercise with the goal of increasing strength and range of motion.
- Of equal importance is the need to avoid getting overly fatigued.
- Allow frequent rest periods.
- Encourage sitting exercises if balance is affected; otherwise allow standing exercises with support.

Parkinson's

This chronic neurological disorder can present a range from mild rigidity with no cognitive deficits to severe rigidity with cognitive deficits.

Suggestions for exercise:
- Start the exercise session with head rotations to the right and left.
- Follow with reciprocal arm exercises and trunk rotation to the right and the left.
- Marching in place is an excellent activity either standing or sitting.
- Use a metronome for the individual to keep time to.
- It is felt that reciprocal and rotational activities help to decrease rigidity.

Note: Be very alert to these individuals leaning or falling backwards and having trouble initiating movements.

Head Injury

Many individuals who are in their teens, twenties and beyond are being admitted to long term care facilities with head injuries. It is highly recommended that these individuals be screened for appropriateness by their therapist prior to entering your activities. This is due to their variable cognitive status and a decreased ability to tolerate certain levels of stimulation.

Suggestions for exercise:
- Limit auditory and visual stimulation to reduce the possibility of over-stimulation.
- Try and work on a one-on-one basis and gradually incorporate them into a group setting (small first).
- A calm and firm voice works best. Avoid yelling or speaking too loudly.
- Be patient but do not tolerate any aggressive behavior.
- Again, ask the therapist for appropriate interventions.

Orthopedic Groups

Many individuals with THR (total hip replacements) and with TKR (total knee replacements) come for short term rehab and are not always interested in participating in social activities. But many individuals also have to undergo procedures and are quite willing to participate in activities.

Total Hip Replacement

If your individual is between one and eight weeks following a total hip replacement, s/he has some very important precautions.
- S/he cannot bend at the hip greater than 90 degrees. Therefore, s/he must be in a semi-reclining position with a firm seat. (No low seated chairs)
- Keep the knees up in a V-position, with pillows below both knees.
- Do not let the foot on the operated leg turn inward.
- S/he will ambulate either with crutches or a walker. No canes at this point. S/he may not be able to bear full weight on the affected leg, so no standing exercises or leaning forward.

Note: After his/her hip has healed (six to eight weeks post op), s/he may return to full weight bearing ambulation with no bending restrictions.

Total Knee Replacement

An individual with total knee replacement may have restrictions as to his/her weight bearing ability, but many are full weight bearing. S/he will use either a walker or crutches and, depending on his/her physician's request, may or may not be wearing a leg brace. Compared to an individual with a total hip replacement, there are fewer restrictions but s/he may have a bit more pain.

Suggestions for exercise:
- Encourage sitting exercises with the brace removed.
- There is no limit to upper extremity exercises.

Weight Bearing Status

For your information, the following abbreviations are frequently used:

FWB   Full Weight Bearing
NWB   Non Weight Bearing
PWB   Partial Weight Bearing (refers to 25% to 75% of weight on leg)
TTWB   Toe Touch Weight Bearing (allows individual to rest leg on floor, but *no* weight may be put on it.)

As previously recommended, stay in close communication with the therapists working in your facility. Your role as a professional — and a team member — is a very important one.

Cognitive and Psychological Disorders

Many of the people we serve have some form of cognitive impairment or psychological disorder. We need to understand the impairment to understand the possibilities for the individual. There are two ways to divide the impairments:
1. whether the impairment is dementia-like or due to a psychiatric diagnosis
2. whether the impairment is acute or chronic.

Dementia is caused by a physical (usually known) impairment in the brain such as Alzheimer's, vascular disease and other causes. Psychiatric impairments are disturbances related to personality and life experiences, which do not always appear to have an obvious organic cause. Examples include phobias and psychoses.

Acute cognitive impairments include any situation that changes quickly (within hours or days) and has a reasonable chance of returning to normal. Alcohol intoxication and overdoses of medication are acute impairments. Chronic impairments change slowly and usually do not allow the individual to return to normal functioning. Dementia and other damage to the brain such as that resulting from long-term alcohol abuse are chronic.

There are a few diagnoses that cover most of the impairments that we see. Before we look at the list, there is an important point to be made about some of these diagnoses — they don't always give us a clear enough picture. For example, dementia is the most common cognitive impairment seen in individuals of long term care facilities. Of the 1.3 million individuals, approximately 60 per cent are estimated to have some form of dementia. (Dementia means that the individual has "multiple cognitive deficits that include memory impairment and at least one of the following cognitive disturbances: aphasia, apraxia, agnosia or a disturbance in executive functioning."[17])

If you are working with an individual who has "dementia," you need to know more. You need to know why the individual has been diagnosed as having dementia:
- Is it because s/he drank a fifth of whiskey every day and destroyed too many of his/her brain cells? (Provide appropriate sensory stimulation activities. Don't expect to see significant improvement.)
- Is it because the doctor prescribing the pain medication didn't realize that the dentist prescribed pain medication and the individual is overdosing on medications? (Speak up at

---

[17] American Psychiatric Association, 1994, *Diagnostic and Statistical Manual of Mental Disorders IV*.

team meetings about your medication concerns. Expect the dementia to improve if the medication dosages are more appropriate.)

• Is the individual simply not hearing what is said so s/he can't respond appropriately? (Work on alternate means of communication and expect an improvement.)

There are many more examples, of course, but the idea is to understand that a diagnosis is not always the final answer when you are working with a particular individual.

The chart below shows one method of classifying cognitive impairments.

Classification of Cognitive Impairments

	Organic Impairments (related to impairments in brain and brain tissue, reversibility depends on cause)	Psychiatric Impairments (Related to personality and life experience, may be organic in nature, frequently treatable)
Acute	**caused by trauma, infection, diabetes, chronic heart failure, drugs and alcohol, reversible to some degree** Delirium Medication Overdose Alcohol Intoxication Stroke (acute phase) Traumatic Brain Injury (acute phase)	**caused by events in one's life, his/her perceptions of life and may be organic in origin, can be treated with psychological intervention, reversible although there may be recurrences** Depression Anxiety Panic Attacks Phobias
Chronic	**caused by physiological degeneration or damage to the brain, generally irreversible, some variation in skill level is seen day to day** Dementia (due to Parkinson's Disease, Pick's Disease, HIV Disease, Creutzfeldt-Jakob Disease, etc.) Alzheimer's Disease Substance Induced Persisting Dementia Stroke (chronic phase, psychosis is a possible result) Traumatic Brain Injury (chronic phase)	**caused by events in one's life, has not been helped by psychological intervention, probably irreversible** Pseudodementia Depression Psychosis

The cognitive impairments shown above can be divided into eight general categories:

1. **Dementia** is not a disease but rather a cluster of symptoms. These symptoms significantly limit a person's ability to perform normal, complex tasks associated with taking care of him/herself. Dementia means a loss of memory (newly learned information and, later, previously learned information) and at least one of the following:

   a. deterioration of the ability to communicate. This includes: Aphasia, the ability to recognize an object or a person but the inability to find the right word to describe the object or person resulting in the excessive use of words such as "thing" or "it." Apraxia, the inability to remember how to move your mouth and tongue to correctly pronounce words. Agnosia, the inability to recognize what an object is or who a person is.

   b. deterioration of executive function. This is a significant impairment in the ability to think through problems, to initiate purposeful activity, to decide in what order actions should be done (as in dressing), to appreciate the significance of one's actions (picking up the unit's cat by the tail may make the cat angry) and to be able to stop what one is doing (to stop pouring milk when the glass is full).

Approximate 50-60 per cent of dementia cases are irreversible. This means that anywhere from 650,000 to nearly one million people with dementia are being cared for with no hope of significant improvement. Dementia may be chronic or acute. It is organic.

The types of dementia are
- Dementia of the Alzheimer's type
- Vascular dementia
- Dementia due to HIV disease
- Dementia due to a head trauma
- Dementia due to Pick's disease
- Dementia due to Huntington's disease
- Dementia due to Parkinson's disease
- Dementia due to Creutzfeldt-Jakob disease
- Dementia due to other general medical conditions
- Substance-induced persisting dementia
- Dementia due to multiple etiologies (causes)

Dementia of the Alzheimer's type is the most common type of dementia. It is an incurable neurological disease in which changes in the nerve cells of the outer layer of the brain result in the death of a large number of cells. This disease is organic, chronic and irreversible.

2. **Pseudodementia** refers to a condition that resembles dementia but is not the result of an organic factor. Typically depression is the culprit, producing dementia-like symptoms, which include memory problems, confusion and attention disturbances or deficits. Apathy, withdrawal and inability to care for oneself are a part of the picture. Whether the pseudodementia is acute or chronic depends on the underlying cause. (Pseudodementia is not an official *DSM-IV* diagnosis.)

3. **Delirium** involves disorganized thinking and an inability to attend to external stimuli and appropriately shift to new external stimuli. It typically occurs suddenly and lasts a short time. (It's acute.) The causes are organic and include infection, fever, post-op condition, drug-induced states, etc.

4. **Stroke** refers to any damage to the brain resulting from lack of blood supply to the affected part. It usually results in the loss of particular functions that vary greatly depending on the part of the brain that is affected. It is organic and has both an acute phase and a chronic phase. Some recovery is usually seen.

5. **Traumatic Brain Injury** describes damage to the brain caused by physical injury to the brain including car accidents and gunshot wounds. The impairment is organic and has both an acute and chronic phase. Recovery may go on for ten or more years after the accident.

6. **Depression** is characterized by "being down in the dumps" or sad for most of the day for many weeks. Over a period of time, this sadness is present more days than not. An individual who is depressed may also experience a change in eating patterns (poor appetite or overeating), a change in sleeping patterns (insomnia or hypersomnia), a drop in energy (fatigue), a drop in self-esteem, a drop in the ability to concentrate long enough to make decisions or to respond to situations and a decrease in the ability to be hopeful. Between 20% and 25% of individuals with major medical problems (e.g., stroke, heart disorders, cancer, diabetes) will experience a major depression disorder. Depression may be chronic or acute.

7. **Anxiety** is the most common psychiatric disorder experienced by the general population. There are twelve major psychiatric disorders grouped under the heading of Anxiety Disorders including: Panic Disorder, Agoraphobia and Post Traumatic Stress Disorder. Anxiety impairs

the individual's ability to respond to events and people in normally expected manners. Anxiety may be due to a variety of organic and other causes and may be either acute or chronic.

8. **Psychotic Disorders** are psychiatric disorders where the individual may experience hallucinations; have disorganized actions or speech or, as an extreme, catatonic behavior; and/or delusional ways of looking at the world (severe lack of normal insight). Psychotic disorders include schizophrenia, delusional disorders, paranoia and other conditions.

Sensory Loss

Everyone who has ever read about Helen Keller has marveled at her ability to adapt to her sensory losses. Her compensatory skills were incredible; her will and her talent, monumental; her support system, constant. But what happens to everyday people like the individuals we serve when they suffer sensory losses? Do they have the skills and the talent to compensate adequately for their losses? How does loss influence one's adjustment and involvement in the long term care facility?

Sadly, by the time most older people come into supportive care, they have already experienced diminished visual or auditory capacity — or both. Vision and hearing can be a factor in the smooth and complete integration into facility life. Loss of one or the other can create a barrier to adjustment and, frequently, to the ability to socialize. As sensitive health care providers, we must be acutely aware of the potential for isolation inherent in this and make every effort to increase the opportunities for interaction.

Imagine how we become comfortable in new surroundings, such as a hotel. We use our vision to orient ourselves to the placement of doors and windows. We find the bathroom. We learn to identify, by sight if not by name, those who might be useful in assisting us with information or problem solving. If we can't see, we depend on our auditory sense to sharpen our awareness of traffic patterns, new or identifiable noises around us and the daily rhythm of activities.

As we age, it is possible that, even if we do not lose total capacity, our senses may diminish enough to make most situations (especially new ones) awkward. In defense, compensatory skills are developed to mask the deprivation and to allow at least the illusion of normalcy. For example, someone with a hearing loss may smile at everything they think they hear in every interaction or s/he may answer yes to all questions. Frequently people are embarrassed to ask us to repeat ourselves; sometimes repeating is to no avail anyway if the hearing loss is significant.

So what is the issue here? That this person may be labeled confused or senile and left to his/her own memories. With the additional loss of social stimulation, memory loss may become an actual problem and we still haven't solved the original problems: a lack of social interaction and the possibility of an incorrect interpretation of the individual's condition.

So what do we do? Look for the problem. If it's there, make sure that others know the problem is with hearing and not cognition, speak clearly, face the person directly, repeat as necessary, use gestures, communication boards, if possible, and in a surprisingly small number of cases, a hearing aid.

As for visual loss, with an individual who is alert, although sight is denied him/her, a vivid word picture can create a colorful image. Of course the individual with a visual impairment is more likely to need assistance to move around the facility and cueing at meals, but coupling this person with a peer as a volunteer can avoid a potential problem.

The really unfortunate thing is that sometimes nothing works well. As a result, we find that people engage in parallel existences. How often family members will say, "My mother has such a nice roommate; I wish they would talk to each other." In actuality, we have attempted on numerous occasions to introduce new roommates to each other only to be thwarted in our efforts by each one's inability to hear the other's voice. What happens? They only coexist, their lives never really touching in a meaningful way; two oriented, interesting and social people unable to fully enjoy the company of the person they live with. This same problem will preclude involvement in many activities. But, all is not bleak as the truly interested individual will (if able) develop a level of involvement s/he is comfortable with and many times this means establishing a relationship with one or more staff members.

It is not uncommon for people to choose staff as kindred spirits. Part of this may be desire; part a refusal to identify with the other residents; but a large part of this may be because these individuals can hear the staff when they are educated to be patient and to repeat as necessary. Staff also have the ability to be heard by projecting their voices, whereas another resident may not have this ability.

Sensory losses pose terrible dilemmas and in many cases frustrate the person, the family and even the staff. Staff should employ a great variety of creative skills and sensory tools to alleviate isolation and communication barriers. If all else proves to be unsuccessful, remember that the sense of touch is likely to remain intact until near death. A kind and gentle touch will almost always be well received.

Letting Go: The Way We Die

What act that we perform in our whole lives is more personal, more private, more self-centered than our death? Many authors have written eloquently about the stages leading up to death. Perhaps the best-known authority on the subject of death and dying is Elizabeth Kübler-Ross. Her five stages of death and dying are well recognized as guideposts in understanding this process for ourselves and others. These stages are *denial, anger, bargaining, depression* and *acceptance*. Of importance to note is that no two people experience grief and death alike. And so, each of us will experience this process in varying stages. If you are working with an individual who is angry and unable to accept his/her situation, do not be quick to judge and do not assume that your role is to help him/her move through these stages. Instead, be a good listener, encourage sharing of feelings and fears and lend emotional strength in any way possible.

If you are not informed about preparing for death, you should read one or more of the books listed below:
- Kübler-Ross, Elizabeth, *On Death and Dying*. Collier Books, 1969.
- Lewis, C. S., *A Grief Observed*. Bantam Books, 1961.
- Manning, Doug, *Comforting Those Who Grieve: A Guide for Helping Others*. Harper and Row, 1985.
- Harris Lord, Janice, *Beyond Sympathy: What to Say and Do for Someone Suffering an Injury, Illness or Loss*. Pathfinder Publishing, 1988.
- Staudacher, Carol, *Men and Grief*. New Harbinger, 1992.
- Caplan, Sandi, *Grief's Courageous Journey: A Workbook*. New Harbinger, 1995
- Lightner, Candy and Nancy Hathaway, *Giving Sorrow Words: How to Cope with Grief and Get on With Your Life*. Warner Books, 1990.

Death is inevitable and we know that it causes the least negative impact on the survivors when the person who is dying has reached an "acceptance" of his/her death. It means that the person understands the inevitability of death and feels prepared to die. We are often fortunate to have a chance to help the people we serve prepare for death and to be a witness to the hopefulness of impending death.

Let's draw a context here. Imagine having lived a full life, having created positive associations and memories. Imagine further having lost close family, then friends, then function and, finally, a physical environment that was supportive of one's illness and disabilities. Having dealt with loss and change, step by step, problem by problem, people will usually arrive at the point of acceptance with a degree of relief. Ongoing love, support and counseling will allow them to find peace in that emotional setting and, instead of mourning what life has been, there is pleasure in one's memories and hope for a peaceful end.

One does not have to have lived a life of comfort and joy to be able to arrive at such a state. In fact, one can still produce a positive face for the future, even without the pleasant memories that we hope will accompany each of us. It is no secret that, as with placement in a long term care facility, it is the resident who frequently accepts the inevitable before the family does. We sense that it relates to the comfort of letting go of all the unnecessary trappings in our lives, of already having made the hard choices and now being stripped to that part of self that is most vulnerable, most human. Without the distractions of the world, there is peace in having our needs met; peace in the assurance that we will be made comfortable to the end of our lives.

Of course, the need to control is still in evidence. In fact, that need is so ingrained in us that many people orchestrate their own dying. It is with pleasure that they cause families to rally round, to feel the power of being responded to, of being capable of living by choice until the end.

This is not true for everyone; but, among us, we often discuss — and believe — that people die the way they wish to. Some wish to die with family nearby; others prefer to be alone (to save family the possible pain of witnessing this final separation?). Most wish to die pain free, which is often our only viable goal as caregivers — comfort for the individual who is dying.

Frequently there is a useful and wonderfully productive time to be lived as people proceed toward death. This can be a more open time, more emotional, more honest, with communication among family members at its best. Reminiscing is appropriate, especially if family members have never taken the time to explore the past with each other. (Amazingly, we find this is often true, as when we ask a resident for a social history and become aware that the family members are hearing life details for the first time, too. "Oh that's how your parents chose your name, Mom.") Sharing memories and stories revives lives led and provides the material for future reminiscing and for creating family legends and folklore.

The caregivers need to pay special attention to changes in health status that may be leading to the terminal state. At such times, it is imperative that you are even more available to the individual and family in order to address any terminal care needs:
- Do they wish clergy to be present?
- Do they wish a private meal with friends and family?
- Are there special arrangements that need to be made (an autopsy)?

Sometimes your presence, sitting with the person and being with the family, is the best you can do. If appropriate, participate in the reminiscence. Help the family interact with the dying resident by modeling: speak to the resident; assure him/her that s/he is not alone and that his/her family is with him/her. Ask if the family wishes to be alone or if they are more comfortable having others in the room. The family may wish you to interpret physical changes; encourage them to speak with nursing as they observe alteration in color, breathing patterns and body temperature.

Finally, determine if anyone in the family wishes to view the resident after death and before the body is removed to the mortuary. Some people draw great comfort in this final good-bye, this private time. Most facilities are able to make accommodation for this.

When there is a death, be certain that the people most involved with the deceased have the opportunity to verbalize feelings of lose or fear. Include them in the dying process. If it seems feasible, allow them to sit with the dying person. Predictably, there is seldom any anxiety displayed by other residents after a death. There is sadness, and a sense of lose and of missing a companion, but the pervasive feeling is of peace with the inevitable. We witness the ability of people to carry on when the natural has occurred.

It often seems to us that when we lose an individual, we lose twice, especially if the person had an active and interested family. The staff misses the spirit and energy of the resident but also the socializing and the communication with the family.

In order to allow all of us to have our final good-byes, to the deceased and to the family and the routine that have become a part of us, we strongly recommend having a memorial service. We are not proposing that you conduct one after each death, but having one monthly or quarterly can be very much of an emotional release. Be sure to invite the families and special friends of all the residents who have died.

The service is simple with perhaps a prayer or a Psalm reading led by a clergyman; this brings the appropriate solemnity to the occasion. These formalities are followed by spontaneous reminiscences, with staff and other individuals at the facility also making their contributions. When the formal service is concluded, there is time for refreshments and informal exchanges. For some, this is the only memorial service they will have had. For others, it is their second, more private one. For everyone, it provides the opportunity for closure.

It never ceases to amaze us how truly uplifting it is to be with someone who is dying. We will qualify this by saying that this is especially true if the death is accepted, anticipated with joy as the natural ending to a life that has been well spent and is essentially pain free at the end. The emotional release is cathartic for all involved and opens our hearts to emotions that keep us most human: compassion, sympathy and, in some cases, empathy.

It is always a privilege for caretakers who witness and ease the way to death; and no matter how one chooses to let go, it is always personal and private and special.

Chapter 3
The Work We Do

This chapter describes the history of our profession and the work done by the various professionals who work with the people we serve. For each of these professions we have included a description of the work that they do, an example of a typical day and a formal position description.

These are rewarding professions, but they can be difficult at times. Significant complications will arise if you are disorganized. We have included some ideas for controlling the chaos of a your setting so that the human needs and the bureaucratic needs can both be met without total loss of sanity. (Some loss of your sanity, some of the time, and the ability to gain it again are part of the informal work description for all of these professions.)

Our History

The use of "leisure time" has changed dramatically over the last 6,000 years. "Emerson declared that all history is biography" (James, 1998, p. 7) so our history is really a retelling of the actions of many individuals. This section will provide you with a short history of leisure, social services, recreational therapy and activity professionals through the actions of individuals.

Origins of Leisure, Activity and Social Services

The concept that leisure time is separate from work time is a relatively new concept. Until about 6,000 years ago mankind wandered the countryside hunting and gathering food and foraging for other elements necessary for survival. This time period is also a time of *preliterate society*. What we know about how people played or aged can only be speculated. However, what we can extrapolate from archeological records is that early man mixed work and leisure. Leisure appeared to be a key element of life involving music, chanting, art and games. As today, it is thought that children played at being hunters or climbed and splashed, practicing skills that would aid survival when they became adults. Adults carried on traditions of music, dance, art and games, often with religious overtones. Life expectancy was not very long, with elders who could no longer travel likely left behind.

Eight thousand years ago in Mesopotamia, and six thousand years ago in Central America mankind domesticated animals and tilled the soil. Thus the *agricultural era* started. This changed life to a more settled and stationary existence. Gathering and storing food, along with the building of more permanent residences allowed increased stability. Life and time became more seasonal with periods of less work. These periods of less work allowed society to pursue the arts, scientific research and to develop religions and governments and to start formal schooling of some of its citizens. A philosopher from Athens, Aristotle, spent many hours discussing the importance of both work and leisure, with leisure being preferable because it allowed the pursuit of intellectual inquiry. The Romans, coming from a society based on military strength, saw many of their leisure pursuits support excellence in military skills. Elders could now be taken care of at home even if they were no longer mobile.

Around the late 1700's in Great Britain (the mid-1800's in the United States) new inventions allowed the mass production of goods, introducing the *industrial era*. The mass production of goods increased the number of individuals who did not toil for work; they hired others to do the work for them. So society went from having leisure time for individuals to pursue artistic, intellectual and religious pursuits to society having an actual leisure class of people. As the numbers in the leisure class grew, many now had more time and resources to follow intellectual pursuits. The invention of the printing press four hundred years previously allowed the mass dissemination of intellectual material. For the first time civilization had both the leisure time and the written material to begin educating large numbers of its citizens. A true middle class was being formed. With larger numbers of people educated and having both leisure time and money to conduct research, medical and other advances occurred faster than any previous time in history. In the 1900's life expectancy increased by three days each year.

During the industrial era the division between work and leisure became more sharply defined. For the individuals working in factories, life was hard. During the agricultural era, children worked alongside of their parents and grandparents. But agriculture allowed for play as well as work. Playfulness and games occurred both in the fields and during the "off" seasons. Children were also required to work during the industrial age, but factory work did not allow leisurely breaks with parents and grandparents. The lower classes were required to have all generations work the long, hard hours in factories just to make ends meet.

Around the same time that the industrial revolution helped emphasize the division between leisure and work, a shift was taking place in health care. In Great Britain, Florence Nightingale pushed for changes to the nursing profession. After she started making significant headway in modernizing the nursing profession, she expanded her vision to the reform of health care as a whole. The following passage by James (1998) in *Perspectives in Recreational Therapy* explains (pg. 8):

> Nightingale protested to all who would listen that the dreary conditions of the hospital were counterproductive and that the monotony endured by the patients adversely affected their recoveries.

> > People say the effect [of a pleasing environment] is only on the mind. It is no such thing. The effect is on the body too. Little as we know about the way in which we are affected by form, by color and light, we do know this, that they have an actual physical effect. (Nightingale, 1859, p. 34)

> Nightingale's observations also led her to conclude:

> > It is a matter of painful wonder to the sick themselves how much painful ideas predominate over pleasurable ones in their impressions; they reason with themselves; they think themselves ungrateful; it is all of no use. The fact is that these painful impressions are far better dismissed by a real laugh, if you can excite one by books or conversation, than by any direct reasoning; or if the patient is too weak to laugh, some impression from nature is what he wants. (Nightingale, 1859, p. 34)

> Nightingale wrote of the benefits that accrued to patients from caring for pets, listening to and performing music, doing needlework and writing. She chastised health care administrators to be more inclusive in their provision of services to patients: "Bearing in

mind that you have all these varieties of employment which the sick cannot have, bear also in mind to obtain them all the varieties which they can enjoy." (Nightingale, 1859, p. 36)

In Great Britain during the fall of 1855 a combination recreation room and coffee house, called the Inkerman Café, was converted from a building on a hospital's grounds. While hobbies, arts and crafts and other leisurely pursuits were offered to help the patients heal, Inkerman Café also offered the convalescing patients a place to pass the time instead of the taverns next to the hospital. Overall, it was a win-win situation. The patients stayed sober while benefiting from leisure activities during convalescing.

Similar changes were taking place in the United States under the guidance of physician Benjamin Rush and the Quakers. The concept of "Moral Treatment," especially of patients with mental illness, was beginning to replace warehouse type hospital facilities with homelike facilities surrounded by gardens. Progress was being made during the first half of the 1800's toward Moral Treatment of patients that included activities run by nurses and others. But this was soon to change. As the 1800's advanced, the United States became a country increasingly populated by interdependent urban dwellers instead of self-sufficient farmers. Work hours in factories were long and few recreation facilities were built in the urban areas. Combined with increased crowding because of immigration and more people in hospitals because of the Civil War, the country's resources were strained trying to accommodate all the unmet needs of the urban dwellers and of the people who over-filled the hospitals.

For the working masses, leisure had become a frivolous pastime. Adults were expected to be productive. At the same time, middle and upper class reformers pushed for changes in child labor laws. By the last quarter of the 1800's many children, no longer allowed to work but having both parents still working the long factory hours, spent many idle hours in the streets of the cities. Between the rampant alcoholism of the adults and the mischief of the children, it became evident to many that further change was needed.

By the 1890's over sixty reform groups had formed, many with the belief that guided recreation experiences would help heal the moral and health problems of a society that were caused, in part, by an imbalance of work and healthy leisure activity. A relatively new field, the field of social work, joined forces with teachers and government reform groups to try to address the problem. The pendulum was swinging back again. Leisure activities moved away from being considered frivolous to being the modality of choice to create morally and physically strong citizens. A graduate of Harvard Law School, Joseph Lee, was so interested in the potential for leisure activities to help cure the social ills of society that he built sand pile play areas, and later, playgrounds in the Boston area. Lee hired and trained activity leaders to run groups and gather data for his research on the benefits of recreation. At the turn of the last century, physician Luther Gulick helped change the YMCA's direction from one of exercise to moral and physical health through recreation. Gulick also proposed that an association of playground professionals be formed. So, in 1906 the first national organization for recreation and activity professionals was formed, called the Playground Association of America (PAA).

That year, United State President Theodore Roosevelt invited eighteen people from around the country to the White House to celebrate the formation of the PAA. Eight of the original eighteen founders of PAA were women. The second national conference was held in Chicago in 1907 with 200 delegates from 30 cities. One of the outcomes of that first conference was the formation of an advisory committee on "play in institutions" aimed at furthering the work of Nightingale, Rush, Gulick and others.

One of PAA's most influential and insightful members was Neva Leona Boyd. She was hired as a social worker at Hull House (a settlement house in Chicago) in 1908 to work with the immigrants who lived there. Her job description was to organize social clubs, play and other small group activities to help Hull House's residents develop appropriate physical, social and intellectual skills. Hull House, originally founded by Jane Addams, provided Neva Boyd with a lab and classroom space to train others. She would accept students who had already completed two years of college to enter her one-year social work/recreation leader program.

> Besides offering extensive technical training in group games, gymnastics, dancing and dramatic arts, the school provided course work in the theory and psychology of play, social behavior problems and "preventive and remedial social efforts" (Simon, 1971, p. 14).[18]

Ms. Boyd called her school the "Chicago Training School for Playground Workers" and termed the work "recreational therapy." In 1927 the school became part of Northwestern University. Similar programs developed at other universities including a Department of Recreation Leadership at the Teachers College, Columbia University.

The United States entered World War I in 1917. The American Red Cross built 52 recreation centers, all using the same design, at military hospitals across the country. The Red Cross hired the Department of Recreation Leadership at Columbia University to help train and staff these centers with professionals who used recreational activities as part of the patient's medical and therapy program.

> The program drew from activity areas consistent with those used by group work services at the time. Among those were music, dance, gardening, community trips, drama, games and social recreation. The military was assigned supervision of physical education. Following the precedents established by the terms social work and group work, the Red Cross titled this new service "Hospital Recreation Work." (Program of Recreation, 1919).[19]

By the 1930's the use of recreational therapy in mental health hospitals was well established. Not only had Boyd promoted the use of recreational therapy in psychiatric hospitals since the early 1900's, but so did the Drs. Menninger (father C. F., brothers Karl and William). The Menningers formed the Menninger Clinic in Topeka, Kansas and used recreational therapy as one of the core treatment specialties at their facility.

The use of activities and recreation as a therapeutic intervention continued to gain recognition. However, the last 70 years of the twentieth century would prove a volatile one for the professionals who used recreation and activities as a means to improve people's health and well-being. Political struggles based on philosophy along with different views on scope and content of professional preparation caused numerous factions to split off, forming new national organizations. At their 1935 National Conference of Social Work, the national organization broke with Boyd's previous group work using recreation so the fields of social work and recreational therapy became distinctly different fields. It was almost forty years later, in 1977, when President Gary Robb of the National Therapeutic Recreation Society, directed a study that lead to the registration of therapeutic recreation specialists (recreational therapists), that a clear split between recreational therapy and activity professionals took place.

---

[18] Simon, P. (1971). *Play and game theory in group work: A collection of papers by Neva Leona Boyd.* Referenced in James, A. "The Conceptual Development of Recreational Therapy" In Brasile, F., Skalko, T. K. and burlingame., j. (1998). *Perspectives in Recreational Therapy: Issues of a Dynamic Profession.* Ravensdale, WA: Idyll Arbor.

[19] Hospital Service (1919, June 30). *The Red Cross Bulletin,* 3(27), 2-3 Referenced in James, A. "The Conceptual Development of Recreational Therapy" In Brasile, F., Skalko, T. K. and burlingame., j. (1998). *Perspectives in Recreational Therapy: Issues of a Dynamic Profession.* Ravensdale, WA: Idyll Arbor.

Recreational Therapy

From the early 1900's until around the 1950's the use of recreational therapy to address social or health ills was well received. But this was not to say that the use of recreation as a therapeutic intervention did not have its distracters. G. Ott Romney, one of the national leaders of the American Recreation Society felt that recreation was a feeling of freedom of choice and not an avenue to be used to change someone else's behavior. He wrote

> Time was when recreation as a social concern was led by the hand of her dignified elders, Character-Building, Physical Education, Delinquency Prevention, Citizenship Education and their ilk, into the living room of social welfare…Now she should be easily distinguished from physical education, occupational therapy, regimented character-building services, and group work…All of which intends to say that recreation is an end unto itself…It does not hide behind the skirts of therapy nor find only group work reflected in its mirror. (Romney, 1945, pg. 35)[20]

By 1949 it was obvious that the newly formed Hospital Section of the American Recreation Society was going to promote Romney's point of view. A group of hospital recreational therapists who supported Boyd's original view of using recreation as therapy formed the Recreational Therapy Section within a different national organization, the American Association for Health, Physical Education and Recreation in 1952. Thus, for the next fifty years recreational therapists would experience numerous national divisions and joinings over the issue of whether recreation belonged within a medical model. At one point, during the formation of the National Recreation and Parks Association in 1965, the groups again tried to merge, using the term "therapeutic recreation" as a compromise term. This group was called the National Therapeutic Recreation Society. This unification lasted only two tumultuous decades with the more medically oriented therapists forming a new national organization in 1985 called the American Therapeutic Recreation Association.

Even with the challenges of internal differences based on philosophy, the field of recreational therapy/therapeutic recreation continued to advance in its knowledge of how leisure time activities impacted the health and well-being of the people they served. One of the most significant events in the field was the publishing of the proceedings of a three-year research project sponsored by the United States Department of Education and Temple University's Program in Therapeutic Recreation. These proceedings, published in a book called *Benefits of Therapeutic Recreation: A Consensus View* (1991) edited by Coyle, Kinney, Riley and Shank, provided over 400 pages of documentation as to the state of the art of recreational therapy using research to document known outcomes. As health care regulations and health care standards were developed during the last third of the twentieth century, recreational therapy was recognized as an important, and often required, element. By the late 1990's it seemed that broader acceptance of the idea that recreation and leisure could be both a state of mind *and* a therapy modality was developing. That, along with outstanding leadership from both Boards of the National Therapeutic Recreation Society and the American Therapeutic Recreation Association, allowed the two national organizations to work collectively. Part of this collective work has been the establishment of Joint Task Forces, one being the Joint Task Force on Long Term Care. This Joint Task Force lists six areas that they intend to address:

- Develop and disseminate a scope of practice statement to delineate the roles and functions of certified therapeutic recreation specialists and paraprofessionals in long term care settings;

---

[20] Romney, G. O. (1945). *Off the job living.* Washington, DC: McGrath Publishing C. and National Recreation and Park Association. Referenced in James, A. "The Conceptual Development of Recreational Therapy" In Brasile, F., Skalko, T. K. and burlingame., j. (1998). *Perspectives in Recreational Therapy: Issues of a Dynamic Profession.* Ravensdale, WA: Idyll Arbor.

- Develop educational materials and presentations targeted towards ATRA and NTRS members;
- Prepare strategies to address regulatory issues in long term care (i.e., PPS, MDS, Nursing Home Initiatives, etc.);
- Develop and implement a marketing and training focus targeted toward administrators of long term care facilities;
- Provide information and resources that are accurate and consistent with current professional practice; and
- Act as a clearinghouse and resource system for the professional organizations related to long term care issues, practices, standards, and funding guidelines.[21]

One of the ongoing discussions since the 1960's had been the type of professional training needed by the professionals using recreation and activities as an intervention. Since the national organizations at that time came from a parks and recreation background, it soon became evident that recreational therapists and activity professionals whose training was not in parks and recreation would not be recognized by these national organizations. Local and state organizations started to form to meet the needs of the professionals who used recreation and activities when they worked with the elderly in our country's nursing homes. After the President of the National Therapeutic Recreation Society, Gary Robb, asked in 1977 for a study on the issue of credentialing for therapeutic recreation specialists, work was done and the National Council for Therapeutic Recreation Certification (NCTRC) was formed in 1981. By 1995 about 45% (13,600) of the estimated number of people calling themselves recreational therapists/therapeutic recreation specialists held a credential issued by NCTRC. The credential, CTRS, required a four-year degree with course work in recreational therapy and related subjects along with a supervised internship before the professional could take the required national exam. NCTRC's action to accept only professionals who met their competency and educational guidelines was taken to help protect the consumer. It also left a lot of professionals (both skilled and unskilled) without a national organization or professional credential.

For years the fields of recreational therapy and activities seemed to be moving away from each other, more because of philosophical differences over how much preparation professionals needed than because of the general services they provided. Both used activities to promote health and well-being. The subsequent separation of recreational therapy and activity directors seemed to be caused, in part, by the credentialing program of the NCTRC.

The National Association of Activity Professionals[22]

To understand the position of activity professional, it is essential that we understand the National Association of Activity Professionals (NAAP). We must recognize the efforts of the activity professionals who had the vision to see what an important role NAAP would have in the lives of our nation's elders. We should value those individuals, applaud their dedication and foresight, and continue to grow.

Activity associations across the nation were surveyed in November 1980 to determine if there was an interest in forming a national association. As a result of the survey, a letter was mailed out on February 2, 1981, and an exploratory meeting was announced. The meeting took place at the Regency Nursing Center in Niles, Illinois, Saturday, March 21, 1981. Attending the meeting were twenty activity professionals from eleven states. With this small but dedicated group, the National Association of Activity Professionals (NAAP) began.

---

[21] National Therapeutic Recreation Society (1998-1999). *NTRS Report 24*(1) p.17.
[22] This portion of the history section is from NAAP newsletters with contributions from Nancy Williams and Joy Cornelius and approval by the NAAP Board of Directors.

A second organizational meeting followed June 26 and 27 of 1981. A Steering Committee accepted draft bylaws, and charter memberships were opened. On October 2 and 3 of that same year, NAAP held its third organizational meeting. The number of states in attendance grew to sixteen. That December saw the publication of the NAAP's first bi-monthly newsletter. It was then called the *UPDATE*.

By February 1982, NAAP began its first political action campaign against threatened federal deregulation of activities and long term care. That same month, the national membership elected a Board of Trustees from a slate chosen at the third organizational meeting. The first President of NAAP was Sister Pat Murphy, who served in her position for the next four years. In March, bylaws and policies were ratified by a charter membership of 254. The first meeting of the NAAP Board of Trustees was held July 9 and 10, 1982, in Des Plaines, Illinois. NAAP established a national office in Illinois, and Marilyn Lamken served as the Executive Director.

The first annual NAAP Convention was held April 29 and 30, 1983, in Cincinnati, Ohio. After that first convention, NAAP began to grow and develop relationships with other organizations. The following March, the State Contact program began; and on September 23, 1983, NAAP was chartered as a nonprofit corporation in Illinois. Two months later, NAAP began liaison with the American Health Care Association (AHCA), the first of its outreach initiatives to other interest groups.

NAAP was off and running, and 1984 was going to be another busy year. To honor activity professionals across the country, the very first National Activity Professionals Day was celebrated January 27, 1984. The fourth Friday in January was designated to celebrate activity professionals annually. The second annual convention was in Denver, Colorado, April 26 through 28. On July 17, 1984, the National Activity Education Organization (NAEO) was chartered. Through the NAEO, NAAP would be able to accept donations earmarked for education use, and the donations would be tax exempt for the donor. Most importantly, NAAP used this money to award scholarships to NAAP members, allowing them to attend the national convention. These scholarships are best known to the members as the Madge Schweinsberg and Gloria Keeti Scholarships. Two $500 scholarships are annual awards in honor of Madge Schweinsberg. This scholarship is awarded jointly between NAAP and National Certification Council for Activity Professionals (NCCAP). The second award is made possible by a bequest from Gloria Keeti. The award is for $200 and the only requirement be that the recipient is a NAAP member. Formal liaison with the National Therapeutic Recreation Society (NTRS) was established in October. On December 12, NAAP submitted a position paper on nursing regulations to the Institute of Medicine. April 25 through 27, 1985 NAAP held its third annual convention in Buffalo, New York.

In 1986, the convention was held in Sacramento, California, on April 24 through 26. It was at the California convention that the first NAAP awards for Distinguished Merit, Service, Excellence and Volunteer of the Year were awarded. Between September and November 1986 the NAAP legislative committee conducted a survey on new long term care survey procedures for input to the Health Care Financing Administration (HCFA). Phyllis Foster was elected to serve as the Association's President for the next four years.

Seeing the need for a certification body designed for activity professionals, the NAAP Board held its first mid-year meeting October 9 and 10, 1986. On October 30, 1986, the National Certification Council for Activity Professionals (NCCAP) was incorporated and a Board of Directors was established. Marilyn Lamken was designated as the Executive Director making her the Executive Director of both NAAP and NCCAP.

Chicago, Illinois hosted the 1987 convention again. It was held April 23 and 24. That year, thanks in part to legislative efforts by NAAP, Congress passed legislation requiring all nursing homes that received federal funds to have an ongoing activities program directed by a qualified professional.

In 1988, the Sixth Annual NAAP Convention was held April 28 through 30 in Minneapolis, Minnesota. During that convention, the Board of Trustees decided to establish a NAAP national office in Washington, DC. Effective June 1, the management firm of Linton, Mields, Reiser and Cottone was retained to manage NAAP affairs. In September, a membership drive was begun that increased membership from about 1,300 to 2,100 by April 1989. The NAAP Newsletter became a monthly publication.

On February 2, 1989, HCFA issued new federal regulations on long term care facilities and NAAP began lobbying to improve the regulations and the interpretive guidelines implementing them. As a result, NCCAP was acknowledged by HCFA as a recognized accrediting body for activity professionals and there were other improvements in the guidelines. The convention that year was held in Charlotte, North Carolina April 26 through 29. In November and December 1989, NAAP was invited by HCFA to participate in national surveyor training.

During 1990, cooperative legislative efforts were launched in partnership with the National Therapeutic Recreation Society (NTRS) and the American Therapeutic Recreation Association (ATRA). NAAP also worked with other interest groups and the film industry to resolve copyright infringement liability for nursing homes and retirement communities that show video movies. NAAP presented written testimony to the House Judiciary Sub-Committee that dealt with copyright laws. The bill would allow residents of nursing homes, assisted living facilities and retirement communities to view video movies in common areas without having to pay a licensing fee. After months of negotiations, Charles Price, Executive Director of NAAP, reported in the September 1990 newsletter that our efforts had paid off. The bill, HR3158 and S1557 had passed.

The 1990 convention was held in Seattle, Washington, April 21 through 23. In October 1990, NAAP co-sponsored a reception on Capitol Hill in Washington, honoring OBRA implementation day; other sponsors included the Senate Special Committee on Aging and the National Citizens Coalition for Nursing Home Reform (NCCNHR). NAAP also helped plan and participated in a special Capitol Hill seminar, also in October, on the resident assessment process, again with the Senate Aging Committee and NCCNHR. NAAP also participated in a case-mix reimbursement demonstration project being conducted by consultants to HCFA.

The 1991 convention was held in Kansas City, Missouri, April 18 through 21. In September 1991, HCFA issued its "final final" regulations governing long term care requirements, which no longer identified NCCAP by name as a recognized credentialing body but left it to each discipline to determine its own accrediting entity. Other changes to the regulations strengthened activity requirements. Just before Christmas 1991, HCFA also released for comment its revised interpretive guidelines. NAAP, NTRS and ATRA again coordinated their comments and presented HCFA a joint submission recommending changes to the activities section.

The 10th anniversary convention was held in Washington, DC, April 22 through 25. During the 1992-1993 year, NAAP commented on HCFA's proposed OBRA enforcement regulations and its final rule on charges to residents' funds. In the latter case, NAAP expressed serious concerns about the equity of the rule and its compliance with OBRA requirements; HCFA pledged to write interpretive guidelines to clarify the rule, and NAAP continued to be involved in that process. NAAP continued its participation in the case-mix reimbursement project and advised HCFA on the content of its Resident Assessment Instrument and a manual on the use of the MDS+. Thanks to a mass mail solicitation, NAAP increased its membership by over 700 members early in 1993, to a total of 3,200. The 11th anniversary convention was held in Milwaukee, Wisconsin, April 14 through 17.

Following up on concerns expressed previously about charges to residents' funds, NAAP provided HCFA written recommendations for revised interpretive guidelines dealing with this issue. NAAP also provided recommendations to HCFA on involvement of activity professionals in surveyor training and on state survey teams. NAAP secured a $10,000 grant from the Unicare Foundation of Milwaukee, Wisconsin, for production of a videotape on the activity profession.

President Jane Carlson was at NAAP's helm as the 12th annual convention was held April 13 through 16, 1994, in Reno, Nevada. The 1994-1995 year was also marked by increased activity in our input to HCFA on interpretive guidelines and survey procedures and by liaison with private accrediting bodies and other professional groups concerned with long term care.

During the 1994-1995 year, NAAP successfully completed the video project and celebrated National Activity Professionals Week with a special premiere showing hosted by The Washington Home in Washington, DC, and by a NAAP member Farlee Wade-Farber, who is featured in the video. The video is entitled, *Activities: Enriching Life's Journey.* This video has come to be used by activity professionals across the country to in-service staff and volunteers, as well as being used in the NAAP/NCCAP 90 Hour Basic Education Course for Activity Professionals.

The 13th annual convention was held March 29 through April 1, 1995, in Nashville, Tennessee. This convention proved to be NAAP's largest with over 600 attendees. The new NAAP video was featured at the convention and was available for the first time to attendees.

During 1996, NAAP was invited to participate in HCFA's Quality of Life Symposium. Surveyors, educators, research analysts, and provider representatives gathered to discuss the survey process and surveyor assessment of a resident's quality of life in long term care facilities. This conference was "by invitation only" for the first day and included several hundred participants. NAAP was asked to serve on one of six responder panels to research presentations made that day. The second day was a much more exclusive session, with approximately 30 participants. Once again, NAAP was included in this session.

NAAP was one of thirteen invited guests to participate in the Surveyor Training for the new interpretive guidelines and enforcement regulations. NAAP's input and expertise were highly recognized by HCFA and other professional organizations. 1996 proved to be a very active year for NAAP. In addition to the many HCFA projects, NAAP played a more active role in the proposal and clarification of Joint Commission standards for nursing facilities. NAAP assisted several state associations and many individual members in defeating certification challenges. Members from across the United States, Canada, and Bermuda attended the 14th annual convention, held April 17 through 20, 1996, in Orlando, Florida, to find out about the changes.

The NAAP Board and members alike had expressed an interest in having its own office one day. With Nancy DeBolt as the NAAP President, along with the NAAP Board of Trustees, this goal was on its way to becoming a reality. In December 1996, NAAP realized the first of many goals involving the association's strategic planning: placing a practitioner in the position of Executive Director. At this time a new management contract was awarded to an independent firm, Selman, McClemore and Associates, and the central office moved from Washington, DC, to Sevierville, Tennessee. The new central office included two activity professionals with over 52 years of combined experience in the health care field: Catherine Selman, Executive Director, and Gail Buckner, Associate Director.

NAAP was not able to hold the annual convention in Canada as planned because at that time because Canadian customary convention charges making it financially unfeasible for NAAP members or vendors. Therefore the convention had to be moved and a new location found. Activity professionals from the upstate New York/Canada area rallied together, and the 15th annual convention was held April 16 through 19, 1997, in Buffalo, New York.

NAAP continued to play important roles with HCFA and Joint Commission projects. NAAP became an active member of Joint Commission's Network Liaison Group and became more involved in field evaluations and other projects. The Alzheimer's Association asked for NAAP's participation and input into the development of a training session for activity professionals working with residents who have Alzheimer's. NAAP also became more visible with its involvement in HCFA's project, Sharing Innovations in Quality.

At the 1997 Fall Board meeting, the management firm informed the NAAP Board of Trustees that they were going to move their office to Jackson, Mississippi. The NAAP Central Office was moved in December 1997.

NAAP geared up for the next conference. The 16th annual convention was held April 15 through 18, 1998, in San Diego, California. During this conference members were able to attend the first workshop on Activity Based Alzheimer's Care, a result of the two association's yearlong hard work. Presently, the workshop is being presented around the country.

The seventeenth annual convention was held April 21 through April 24, 1999, in Louisville, Kentucky, and saw many new Board members take their oath of office. During the summer of 1999, the Board members were busy fulfilling their job duties and responsibilities.

While reviewing the financial status of NAAP, it was noted that NAAP was having a difficult time meeting its financial obligations. The Board agreed that there was an immediate need to meet and develop a plan to ensure that NAAP would be able to survive. Unfortunately, during this time the NAAP President, Phyl Gordon, for personal reasons needed to resign. Vice President, Joy Cornelius, assumed the dual duties of the NAAP President and Vice President.

The Board met in Nashville, Tennessee, over the Labor Day weekend. They all left with very specific projects to accomplish and the hope that when they came together again at the fall Board meeting in Jackson, Mississippi, in November, the future of NAAP would look much brighter. Soon after the meeting was held, Selman, McClemore & Associates tendered their resignation.

On October 1, 1999, Gail Buckner was asked to assume the daily operation of the association. Ms. Buckner agreed to assume the duties of the office and NAAP was back in Sevierville, Tennessee. The membership was notified of these changes via the NAAP News.

NCCAP was also notified of the changes; and understanding what NAAP was facing, they offered their support. Throughout the ordeal, NAAP and NCCAP remained committed to activity professionals and to each other's association

Understanding the importance of the association, NAAP was soon receive the support of many. Among the many that pledged their support were former NAAP Presidents Phyllis Foster and Nancy DeBolt. Many individual members, and local and state activity associations soon joined them.

As the world entered into a new millennium, NAAP was soon to suffer a great, unexpected loss. In January 2000, after attending a meeting of local activity professionals, Phyllis Foster died at her home. As NAAP began rebuilding, the new e-mail address was decided upon based on statements made by Phyllis. She referred to NAAP as The NAAP and so the new address became, <THENAAP@aol.com>.

Government Relations work continued due to the support of the Wisconsin Representatives of Activity Professionals (WRAP). WRAP donated $2,000 to NAAP in order to continue the work with HCFA and Joint Commission.

The Resident Activity Professionals of Ohio (RAP) gave NAAP an interest-free loan to allow the association to continue moving forward. Others lent their support through renewing memberships and giving words of encouragement. Board members were on the road conducting workshops; and membership drives were underway in some states. The NAAP Board was excited to be heading to Colorado.

The 18th annual conference was held April 12-15, 2000, in Colorado Springs, Colorado. During the opening session it was noted that the room held 500 and there was "standing room only." At the annual members' meeting, the members were informed of the current financial status of NAAP. Thanks to the many donations made by individual members, and state and local associations, NAAP's financial future was looking much brighter. During the open forum there were many questions and concerns addressed to the Board, which the board answered. In addition, past Board members, as well as members, echoed support for the association.

NAAP continued its role as a major player in resident issues, networking with like organizations and coalitions. NAAP attended the June 2000, Joint Commission Network Liaison Forum. During the meetings, NAAP stated to Joint Commission that they would support the Public Private Partnership for Assisted Living. NAAP also attended the HCFA Stakeholders Meeting for Measurements, Indicators, & Improvement of Quality of Life in Nursing Homes September 19, 2000.

During the summer and early fall of 2000, the Board received the resignations of several Board members, all citing various reasons for their resignations. The vital office of the Treasurer was immediately filled with past-Treasurer, Rachel Dill, and other vital Board position appointments were made at the Fall Board meeting in November. NAAP members representing 12 states attended the Fall Board meeting that was held in Sevierville, Tennessee. The attending NAAP members were given the opportunity to ask questions about the current status of NAAP as well as it's future. The members also were invited to participate in a number of committee meetings that were held.

The New England States joined together to host the 19th annual NAAP conference April 25-28, 2001, in Burlington, Vermont. During the following year, the NAAP Board remained busy with various projects. Both the NAAP bylaws and Standard of Practice were sent to the membership for approval. Through the efforts of the Special Interest Trustee, reciprocal memberships were made with several associations related to the health care field. The Vice-President solicited the opinions of not only the Government Relations Committee but also the State Contacts and the Board to respond to CMS's (Centers for Medicaid and Medicare Services, formerly HCFA) request regarding Tags 248/249 Interpretative Guidelines of the State Operations Manual. Once again several NAAP members representing four states attended the Fall Board meeting.

The 20th annual NAAP conference was held in Kansas City, Missouri, during the week of April 17-2002. Board members left the conference with several projects to complete during the coming months. NAAP continues its commitment to being a leader in improving the quality of life of our residents in health care related facilities and providing education for those who work within these settings.

Professionalism

Professionalism is a term that we hear used every day. What does it actually mean to you as a recreational therapist, activity or social services professional? Perhaps the easiest way to define professionalism is to identify individuals whom you regard as professionals. What is it about them that creates that feeling of respect and recognition? Is it something concrete about what they do or just a feeling associated with who they are as a person?

You will most likely answer "something concrete" along with a feeling of confidence that the individual carries with him/her in his/her work. The concrete substance that creates a professional is a combination of purpose, vision, goals, skills, hard work, solid ethics and constant upgrading of education and skills. Each professional field has its own purpose, vision, goals, ethics and skills learned through schooling and apprenticeships. While each professional group is unique in many ways, working as a team means that they also need to have much in common.

Professionals share a common goal. That goal is to enhance the quality of life of the people they serve. This creates the vision of how life and programming could be in these settings. It creates a vision of the people we serve coming first and policies being created with considerations of the people we serve coming before concerns about the staff. This sensitivity helps create programs that have a purpose and a goal specific to the quality of life issues we address, regardless of limitations and special needs. We make the positive happen through the use of our skills.

The reality is that this is quite a challenge for the team to meet. Government rules usually mandate that a qualified professional direct these services. This individual needs to be prepared to work hard to educate people about the impact his/her work and programs have and, at the same time, continue to build onto his/her own skills and knowledge.

The position of activity or social services director is a department head position. This means that not only is this individual responsible for all the duties and services provided by the professionals in his/her department, but s/he is also responsible to every other staff member because of the team emphasis.

Being a professional means taking responsibility. In other words, an area of information forgotten, a resident incompletely assessed, documentation past due or a lack of appropriate programs reflects on everyone else on the team. If there is a diagnosis that you do not understand or an individual that you don't know how to care for, you must bring this up and work with other disciplines to seek a solution. This obviously goes both ways in that other departments need to work with you in meeting common goals and understanding your goals and priorities.

One sure way of not only being a professional but feeling that sense of confidence associated with professionalism is to network and be a member of the local, state and national organizations. Not only will you share common issues and concerns, you will also gain important continuing education in the educational meetings, workshops and conventions as well as a tremendous amount of support. So much of our work is done individually and it is easy to feel "out of the mainstream" as pressures at work mount. Keep yourself balanced by taking care of yourself, your own leisure needs and interests and professional development. The people you serve will benefit from a well-balanced professional and a happy team.

Activity Professional

There are many types of facilities where activity professionals work. The position description and list of responsibilities in this section shows what an activity professional would be expected to do in a certified long term care facility. Other facilities, such as assisted living or adult day care, generally have less exacting requirements but the actual work performed to help the people we serve is quite similar.

The professionals who provide activities for residents in long term care facilities play many diverse roles within the care facility, but they are all directed at satisfying the goal of creating a homelike environment where the residents have control of their lives. There are administrative responsibilities and resident care duties and plenty of other tasks that keep the work interesting.

The administrative role is as the director of the Department of Activity Services. In that role the activity professional is responsible for creating policies and procedures that lead to programs that meet the needs of the residents and comply with all appropriate government regulations. One of the major areas of responsibility is the development and analysis of quality indicators. Another major area of responsibility is being the supervisor for all of the activity staff and all activity volunteers within the facility.

The resident care role requires the activity professional to act as a member of the interdisciplinary team in assessing residents, writing and carrying out care plans and updating the plans at appropriate intervals. S/he needs to work with the residents to find out what their capabilities are and to plan activities that maintain and/or enhance those capabilities.

Other tasks like facilitating the Resident Council, publishing a newsletter, coordinating a casino night, helping public relations, conducting community outings and all the rest are part of the work of providing the best possible environment for the residents of the long term care facility.

Position Description

Title: Activity Professional

Purpose of the Position

Under the direction of the Administrator, the Activity Professionals, lead by the Activity Director, are responsible for the planning, coordination and implementation of the activity programs. Activities shall be done on a daily basis and shall make every effort to meet the residents' needs and interests.

Qualifications

A qualified professional who: *"Is a qualified therapeutic recreation specialist or an activities professional who is licensed or registered, if applicable, by the State in which practicing; and is eligible for certification as a therapeutic recreation specialist or as an activities professional by a recognized accrediting body on or after October 1, 1990; or has 2 years of experience in a social or recreational program within the last 5 years, 1 of which was full-time in a patient activities program in a health care setting; or is a qualified occupational therapist or occupational therapy assistant; or has completed a training course approved by the State."*[23]

Duties and Responsibilities

Activity programs are developed within the framework of the facility organizational structure in accordance with federal regulations and the approval of each resident's attending physician. The programs are coordinated in a team effort with related facility services and staff. Programs are to include activities for all residents including residents who are ambulatory, non-ambulatory and on bed rest and the activities are to be planned for both group and individual participation.

With understanding of the adverse effects of institutionalization, which can promote isolation, sensory deprivation and dependence, the activity professional shall build into the program a variety of means to counteract these effects. S/he shall:

1. Evaluate each resident according to his/her background, interest, leisure, previous lifestyle, physical and cognitive abilities, limitations and needs. This shall serve as the base from which the individual activity program shall be developed.

2. Document the individual activity program using the appropriate assessment forms to be placed in the medical record, completing the activity plan within the required time after admission (14 days for federal regulations, 7 days for some states).

3. Attend Resident Care Conferences and record in the resident care plan on a quarterly basis (or sooner, as needed).

4. Maintain timely progress notes specific to the residents' activity plans, recording at least quarterly in the medical record and more frequently when appropriate.

5. Develop appropriate records that indicate resident attendance and participation in the program with reference to residents' response to the program. It is important to note active

---

[23] State Operations Manual, OBRA, Tags F248 and F249.

participation as compared to perimeter participation. These records should also include a bedside log for special programming.

6. Develop, implement, lead and monitor individual and group activities that meet specific needs of the residents.

7. Develop activities providing the opportunity for residents to experience sensory input (touch, smell, taste, etc.), group interaction and personal achievement.

8. Include activities that encourage residents to make decisions, participate in planning and assume a degree of responsibility and independence.

9. Develop a method to implement programs within a designated budget allocated by the Facility Administrator. Keep a ledger and inventory of supplies.

10. Establish an active volunteer program that includes the screening, orientation, training, supervision and evaluation of volunteers.

11. Develop methods for effective utilization of community resources.

12. Serve as a facility liaison to promote positive community support.

13. Interpret to residents, other staff members and the outside community the purpose and achievements of the activity program through at least yearly in-service training and presentations.

14. Attend and participate in staff meetings, department head meetings, designated committee meetings and resident care conferences.

15. Develop a method for obtaining current knowledge of federal and state regulations pertaining to activity programs.

16. Other responsibilities as defined by the administrator.

The Life of an Activity Professional

A typical day at work may look like this:

9:00 – 9:30	Check on census, resident status, new admits Change Reality Orientation board Change arrow on calendar Check with nursing regarding any changes of condition, discharges, etc.
9:30 – 10:00	Announce activities Set up room(s) Assist with transporting residents
10:00 – 12:00	Lead activity groups or supervise other leaders Attend resident care plan meetings Attend department head meetings Attend MDS meetings Take attendance for groups Attend physical and chemical restraint committee meetings Visit one-on-one
12:00 – 1:00	Lunch
1:00 – 1:45	Documentation (new admits, care plans, quarterly notes)

Interview new residents
Coordinate departmental responsibilities
Return phone calls
Volunteer recruitment, interviewing and orienting

1:45 – 2:00   Announce activities
Set up for activities
Assist with transporting residents

2:00 – 4:00   Lead activities or supervise leaders
Visit one-on-one
Take attendance for groups
Documentation (assessments, care plans, etc.)
Special event coordination
Lead a special needs group

4:00 – 5:00   Organize files and office for next day
Write a to do list for tomorrow
Make end of the day farewell visits

OBRA requirements normally mean that there must be some leisure activities in the morning, afternoon and evening, seven days a week, for all residents. This includes activities for residents who are unable to participate in the group activities. The activity department needs to help facilitate evening and weekend activities whether the staff person is there or not.

Some of the specific tasks for activity professionals require them to:
- Assess each resident for individual needs, abilities and interests
- Complete an initial activity assessment for each resident
- Complete the Minimum Data Set (MDS) comprehensive assessment form — Section N (United States) (there may be other areas of the MDS for which the activity professional is assigned by his/her administrator)
- Identify a priority care plan need or problem for each resident if indicated by the assessment to be included in the individual's care plan.
- Develop a monthly calendar of activities to meet the assessed needs of all residents
- Plan, organize and coordinate the activity program
- Schedule and lead activity groups
- Supervise adult education instructors while on site
- Arrange special events and outside entertainers
- Train staff and volunteers
- Establish and develop community contacts and resources
- Manage and supervise the volunteer program
- Be a member of the weekly Resident Care Conference meetings
- Keep a daily record of each resident's involvement in activities
- Keep a bedside log of date, length of visit, type of visit and response to visit for all residents in need of one-on-one visits
- Document the treatment plan in the progress notes at least once a quarter
- Document and address changes in condition
- Assure compliance with federal and state regulations and corporate policies and procedures
- Keep current through national, state and local professional affiliations to update skills and secure continuing education
- Edit the monthly newsletter
- Prepare and keep the budget for the department
- Evaluate programs to assure appropriateness for the current census of residents
- Actively engage in evaluating the care given to all of the residents through a quality improvement program

On a monthly basis the activity professional is responsible for planning and leading activities designed to meet the needs of the residents of the facility. The following pages have samples of activity calendars. The first calendar is for a nursing home, the other for an assisted living facility.

INDEPENDENCE DAY
July 4

Hillside Care Center

July 2000

81 Professional Center Parkway
San Rafael, CA 94903

A Joint Accredited LTC Facility
Lauren Atkinson Administrator

Special programs are offered for Residents uninterested in group activities: room visits, sensory stimulation, pets, Lita volunteer, and religious visits. Personal leisure materials such as daily newspaper, current magazines, library books, new release videos, radio/cassette players, books on tape, playing cards, stationary, crossword puzzles, and board games are provided, in room. Group activity begins each morning at 9:30 with a news chat program called "What's new?," Coffee Social, and light exercise.

Sunday	Monday	Tuesday	Wednesday	Thursday	Friday	Saturday
						1 10:00 Weekend Coffee 10:30 Welcome Visitors 11:00 Piano with Paul 1:05 Baseball on TV 2:00 Outdoor Adventure
2 9:30 Sunday Paper 10:00 Weekend Coffee 1:05 Baseball on TV 2:30 Room Visits 3:30 Marin Christian Life	**3** 9:45 Morning Stretch 11:00 Sizzling Spelling Bee 2:00 Visiting Church 3:30 Bingo 4:00 Summer Sensory	**4** INDEPENDENCE DAY Happy Fourth of July! 11:00 Welcome Visitors 2:30 Ice Cream Social 3:15 Summer Memories	**5** 9:30 What's New? 10:00 Catholic Mass 10:30 Violin Serenade 1:30 Nature Video 3:00 Board Games	**6** 9:30 What's New? 10:30 Strength Training 2:00 Hillside Bar-B-Q 2:30 One Man Band 3:00 Games and Prizes	**7** 9:30 What's New? 10:30 Byron's Music & Song 1:30 Bedside Activity 2:30 In the Garden 3:30 Afternoon Casino	**8** 10:00 Weekend Coffee 10:30 Welcome Visitors 12:30 Men's Hangout 1:05 Baseball on Radio 2:00 Outdoor Adventure
9 9:30 Sunday Paper 10:00 Weekend Coffee 1:05 Baseball on TV 2:30 Room Visits 3:30 Marin Christian Life	**10** 9:45 Balloon Toss 11:00 Crossword Puzzle 2:30 Beauty Boutique 3:30 Bingo 4:00 Beach Sensory	**11** 9:30 Tai Chi with Jack 10:00 Catholic Communion 10:30 Strength Training 1:30 Music Appreciation 3:15 Ice Tea and News	**12** 9:30 What's New? 9:45 Balloon Toss 10:30 Violin Serenade 1:30 Beach Movie 3:00 World News	**13** 10:00 Farmer's Market 10:30 Strength Training 11:30 Tricky Trivia 1:30 You've Got E-mail 3:30 BINGO	**14** 9:30 What's New? 10:30 Byron's Music & Song 1:30 Bedside Activity 2:30 In the Garden 3:30 Afternoon Casino	**15** 9:30 In the News 10:00 Weekend Coffee 10:30 Welcome Visitors 1:05 Baseball on Radio 2:00 Outdoor Adventure
16 9:30 Sunday Paper 10:00 Weekend Coffee 2:30 Room Visits 3:30 Marin Christian Life 5:10 Baseball on Radio	**17** 9:45 Summer Stretch 11:00 Sizzling Spelling Bee 2:00 Fingernail Plan 3:30 Bingo 4:00 Summer Sensory	**18** 9:30 Tai Chi with Jack 10:30 Strength Training 11:00 Movie Outing 1:30 Music Appreciation 3:15 Fruit Smoothie & News	**19** 9:30 What's New? 10:00 Memorial Service 10:30 Violin Serenade 1:30 Nature Video 3:00 Board Games	**20** 10:30 Strength Training 11:00 Summer Songs 12:00 Pic Nic Outing 2:00 Sparking Art 3:30 BINGO	**21** 9:30 What's New? 10:30 Byron's Music & Song 1:30 Bedside Activity 2:30 In the Garden 3:30 Afternoon Casino	**22** 9:30 What's New? 10:00 Weekend Coffee 12:15 Baseball on Radio 12:30 Men's Hangout 2:00 Outdoor Adventure
23 9:30 Sunday Paper 10:00 Weekend Coffee 11:20 Baseball on TV 2:30 Room Visits 3:30 Marin Christian Life	**24** 9:45 Stretch and Smile 11:00 Crossword Puzzle 2:30 Beauty Boutique 3:30 Bingo 4:00 Beach Sensory	**25** 9:30 Tai Chi with Jack 10:00 Catholic Communion 10:30 Strength Training 1:30 Music Appreciation 3:15 Resident Council	**26** 9:30 What's New? 9:34 Smile and Stretch 10:30 Violin Serenade 1:30 Birthday Party 3:00 World News	**27** 10:00 Farmer's Market 10:30 Strength Training 1:30 Making Fruit Salad 2:00 Summer Art 3:30 BINGO	**28** 9:30 What's New? 10:30 Byron's Music & Song 1:30 Bedside Activity 2:30 In the Garden 3:30 Afternoon Casino	**29** 9:30 In the News 10:00 Weekend Coffee 10:30 Welcome Visitors 12:15 Baseball on TV 1:30 Outdoor Adventure
30 9:30 Sunday Paper 10:00 Weekend Coffee 11:30 Baseball on TV 2:30 Room Visits 3:30 Marin Christian Life	**31** 9:45 Balloon Toss 11:00 Summer Songs 2:00 Fingernail Plan 3:30 Bingo 4:00 Summer Sensory					

Hillside Activity Coordinators
Cesar Cabatbat
Sonya Starbird
Connie Hirschmugl

Artwork used with permission from *Creative Forecasting*, Vol. XIII, No. 7, July 2001

Dog Days

Brighton Gardens Assisted Living　　September 2002

300 Fountaingrove Parkway, Santa Rosa, CA 95403　707-566-8600　Maureen Milligan, Director Of Lifestyle & Leisure Services

Sun	Mon	Tue	Wed	Thu	Fri	Sat
1 10:00 Church Service C3; 11:30 Sunday News & Coffee Hour HC; 1:30 Movie Matinee HC; 1:30 Trip: Wine Co. Ride; 3:30 Inspirational Talk: Chicken Soup L; 4:30 Hymn Sing-along HC	**2** Labor Day; 9:00 Trip: Men's Club "I HOP Breakfast" BG Walkers; 10:30 Labor Day Memories & Donut Dollie HC; 2:00 Word Games H; 3:00 Traveling Musician: Rob Sings For Supper! L	**3** 9:00 Exercise Group DR; 10:30 Mental Fitness H; 2:00 Bingo $$$ H; 3:30 Popcorn Social HC; 3:30 Book Club C3; 6:15 Musical Movie HC	**4** 10:00 BG Walkers; 10:30 Coffee Klatch H; 11:00 Lunch Bunch: Sonoma Square; 2:00 Weaving Class H; 3:00 Tina's Sing-along; 4:00 Wine & Cheese HC; 7:00 Bible Study C3 Speaker: Dr. Hample	**5** 9:00 Exercise Group DR; 9:30 Medical Trips; 10:00 Recipe Box H "Alaska ~ Appetizers"; 1:00 Watercolors H; 1:00 Trip: Rosh Hashanah; 2:00 Brain Teasers C3; 6:45 Bingo $$$ H	**6** 9:00 Exercise Group DR; 10:00 Art w/ Cecily H; 1:30 Biography & Trivia H; 2:00 Travel Program~ "Alaska" HC; 3:30 Wine & Cheese L; Port of Call: Alaska & "Birthday Celebrations"; 7:00 Movie Night C3	**7** Rosh Hashanah; 9:30 BG Walkers; 10:00 Cruising w/JudyHC; 10:00 Bingo $$$ H; 1:00 Mind Matters L; 3:00 Rosh Hashanah Celebration H; 7:00 Movie Night C3
8 10:00 Church Service C3; 11:30 Sunday News & Coffee Hour HC; 1:30 Movie Matinee HC; 1:30 Trip: Wine Co. Ride; 3:30 Inspirational Talk: Hour Of Power L; 4:30 Hymn Sing-along HC	**9** 9:30 Shopping Shuttle; 10:30 Music w/ Gary L; 12:30 Quilt Show L; 1:00 Medical Trips; 1:30 Art: Treasure Boxes H; 2:30 Computer Class LB; 3:00 Spirt To Serve H "Volunteer Committee"; 6:45 Travel Program L	**10** 9:00 Exercise Group DR; 10:30 Mental Fitness H; 2:00 Bingo $$$ H; 3:30 Popcorn Social HC & Life Stories; 3:30 Book Club C3; 6:15 Sing w/ Betty HC	**11** 9:15 Trip: Farmers Market; 10:00 BG Walkers; 11:00 Coffee Klatch H; 2:00 Barber Shop Quartet & Icecream Social L; 3:00 Tina's Sing-along L; 4:00 Wine & Cheese HC; 7:00 Bible Study C3	**12** 9:00 Exercise Group DR; 9:30 Medical Trips; 10:00 Recipe Box H "Mexico ~ Appetizers"; 1:00 Watercolors H; 2:00 Brain Teasers C3; 3:00 Karokee Sing L; 6:30 Family Mixer L "Dancing ~ Orderves"	**13** 9:00 Exercise Group DR; 10:00 Art w/ Cecily H; 1:30 Biography & Trivia H; 2:00 Travel Program ~ Mexico HC; 3:30 Wine & Cheese L; Port of Call: Mexico; 7:00 Movie Night C3	**14** 9:30 BG Walkers; 10:00 Cruising ~Judy L; 10:00 Bingo $$$ H; 11:15 Trip: Craft Show; 1:00 Mind Matters L; 1:30-2:30 Nail Clinic HC; 3:00 Cookie Bake Off HC; 7:00 Movie Night C3
15 10:00 Church Service C3; 11:30 Sunday News & Coffee Hour HC; 1:30 Movie Matinee HC; 1:30 Trip: Wine Co. Ride; 3:15 Vespers HC; 4:00 ~ Captains Table ~ Music ~ Appetizers ~ Keepsake Photos	**16** Yom Kippur; 9:30 Shopping Shuttle; 10:00 BG Walkers; 10:30 Music w/ Gary L; 1:00 Medical Trips; 1:30 Art: Treasure Boxes H; 3:00 Spirt To Serve H "Volunteer Committee"; 4:00 Activity Planning H; 7:00 Seminar: HICAP L	**17** 9:00 Exercise Group DR; 10:30 Mental Fitness H; 2:00 Bingo $$$ H; 3:30 Popcorn Social HC & Reminiscing; 3:30 Book Club C3; 6:15 Musical Movie HC	**18** 10:00 BG Walkers; 10:30 Trip: Casino; 11:00 Coffee Klatch HC; 2:00 Weaving Class H; 3:00 Tina's Sing-along L; 4:00 Wine & Cheese HC; 7:00 Bible Study C3 Speaker: Dr. Hample	**19** 9:00 Exercise Group DR; 9:30 Medical Trips; 10:00 Recipe Box H "Italy ~ Appetizers"; 1:00 Watercolors H; 2:00 Brain Teasers C3; 3:00 Karokee Sing L; 6:45 Bingo $$$ H	**20** 9:00 Exercise Group DR; 10:00 Art w/ Cecily H; 1:30 Biography & Trivia H; 2:00 Travel Program~ "Italy" HC; 3:30 Wine & Cheese L; Port of Call: Italy; 7:00 Movie Night C3	**21** 9:30 BG Walkers; 10:00 Cruising ~ Judy HC; 10:00 Bingo $$$ H; 11:15 Whats News? HC; 1:00 Mind Matters L; 1:30 Wellness Seminar: Diabetes Class; 3:00 Cookie Bake Off HC; 7:00 Movie Night C3
22 10:00 Church Service C3; 11:30 Sunday News & Coffee Hour HC; 1:30 Movie Matinee HC; 1:30 Trip: Wine Co. Ride; 3:30 Inspirational Talk: Chicken Soup L; 4:30 Hymn Sing-along HC	**23** 1st Day Of Autumn; 9:30 Shopping Shuttle; 10:00 BG Walkers; 10:30 Music w/ Gary L; 1:00 Medical Trips; 2:00 Seminar: LTC Life Insurance H; 2:30 Computer Class LB; 3:30 Art: Ceramics H; 6:30 Board Games L	**24** 9:00 Exercise Group DR; 10:30 Mental Fitness H; 3:00 Wellness Talk: Living Trust H; 3:30 Popcorn Social HC & Life Stories; 6:15 Sing w/ Betty HC	**25** 10:00 BG Walkers; 10:30 Trip: Snoopy Museum; 11:00 Coffee Klatch HC; 2:00 Weaving Class H; 3:00 Tina's Sing-along L; 4:00 Wine & Cheese HC; 7:00 Bible Study C3; 7:00 Family Support H	**26** 9:00 Execsies Group DR; 9:30 Medical Trips; 10:00 Recipe Box H "South Pacific ~ Appetizers"; 1:00 Watercolors H; 2:00 Brain Teasers C3; 3:00 Karokee Sing L; 6:45 Bingo $$$ H	**27** 9:00 Exercise Group DR; 10:00 Art w/ Cecily H; 1:30 Biography & Trivia H; 2:00 Travel Program~ "South Pacific" HC; 3:30 Wine & Cheese L; Port of Call: South Pacific; 7:00 Movie Night C3	**28** Alzheimers Walk; Trip: 7:30 Shuttles Begin; 10:00 Cruising ~ Judy HC; 1:00 Mind Matters L; 2:00 ~3:00 Nail Clinic HC; 3:00 Cookie Bake Off HC; 7:00 Movie Night C3
29 10:00 Church Service C3; 11:30 Sunday News & Coffee Hour HC; 1:30 Movie Matinee HC; 1:30 Trip: Wine Co. Ride; 3:30 Inspirational Talk: Hour Of Power L; 4:30 Hymn Sing-along HC	**30** 9:30 Shopping Shuttle; 10:00 BG Walkers; 10:30 Music w/ Gary L; 1:00 Medical Trips; 2:00 Town Hall Meeting H "Resident Council"; 3:00 Resident Support C3; 3:15 Art: Ceramics H; 6:30 Board Games L					

Class Locations: Trips & BG Walkers Meet In The AL Lobby

H ~ Hive Activities Room In AL　　L ~ AL Living Room

HC ~ Health Care Center　　C3 ~ Co Kitchen 3rd Floor

LB ~ AL Library　　DR ~ Dining Room　　P ~ Patio

Our Theme For September: Cruising: Ports Of Call: Alaska ~ Mexico ~ Italy & South Pacific. Captains Table Dinner 9/15

Social Services Professional

This section describes the work of a social services professional in a long term care facility. Similar job descriptions would apply to other places where social services professionals work.

While most of the components of the health care team use concrete information (such as a health history) from which to draw their information about a resident, social services is a bit different. We deal with communication and emotion, helping the residents and guardians to express their feelings about what is happening and what is being planned. It makes our perspective different from the others. Social services is a soft science, therefore a bit unpredictable, as is human behavior.

The social services professional's main responsibilities as part of the resident care team can be summarized as follows:
- Assess resident needs
- Update resident status
- Interpret observed behaviors
- Counsel residents and families
- Field grievances from residents and families
- Ensure resolution of grievances
- In-service other staff and members of the community
- Role model professional attributes

Assess Resident Needs

Some of the talents which help in this aspect of a social services professional's work are being naturally curious, genuinely interested, consistently diplomatic and, sometimes, persuasive. During the initial assessment, the resident moves from the one-dimensional, merely charted person to the three-dimensional person with a past, present and future. Background information such as birthplace, siblings, education, marriage, children, occupation, life style, religion, retirement and hobbies emerge to paint a picture of a person in society — his/her past. Next, we find what the circumstances were which brought him/her to needing to use the facility; what series of illnesses, failures in the living situation or changes in health status necessitated placement — his/her present.

By combining past and present, the social services professional should be able to develop an idea of the resident's reaction to illness: how s/he will live with it, be controlled by it or develop the use of a sick role.

In the course of the assessment, it is important to look for and define orientation. Is the resident alert and aware of time, place and events (also referred to as oriented x3) or alert and able to answer simple questions that do not test the memory? Do sensory impairments (especially deafness) impact orientation? Who visits? Who tends to concrete needs? Is the relationship loving or dutiful? What are the special identifying traits? Does the resident always wear hats? Like to wear certain colors? Grab at all passersby?

There are several factors that work in your favor as you approach an assessment interview:
1. Most people like to talk about themselves.
2. Families of residents also enjoy reminiscing about the past and equate your gentle inquiries with caring about the well-being of the resident and about them as well.
3. This is an opportunity to acknowledge the pain of separation (either family from resident or resident from what had been his/her world) and to divide the past from the reality of the "now" and the uncertainty of the future.

A positive experience at this juncture can disarm the resident's anger, as well as the family's depression created by the unnecessary guilt of placing someone in a long term care facility. The assessment can set the tone for all future interactions.

Why should assessment — developing the case history — be so important? Do the "who, what, where, when and why" of a person's past make a difference?

Assessment is important because unless we develop an image of the resident as a complete person, we will always be taking care of faceless "sick folks." We will not ever learn to take care of people. The sadness for social services professionals is that we will never know the residents in the context of their previous lifestyle; we will never see them "well." We can, however, glimpse a person's totality if we ask questions appropriately and use that information to help plan the resident's future.

Once the initial assessment interview has been completed with the help of the resident, family and medical database, it is necessary to complete the Minimum Data Set (MDS) if the resident is in a nursing home. Combing through the information you have gathered should provide the information for the MDS. Essentially the MDS distills what you have learned. But, because it is only a summary of all the facts you have at your finger tips, it would be wise to record the salient data that has not been used for the MDS on another assessment form or as a narrative statement so that nuances of personality and behavior do not become lost to you.

Depending on the information recorded on the MDS and aided by your fact gathering, you will make an entry on the resident care plan. We have sometimes gone into an interview thinking that we know what a person's care entry will be and have been very wrong. One must never assume.

Generally, just rewriting what you have learned will crystallize the problem/need/concern without any need for preconceptions. At the end of this assessment/MDS process, the social services professional will know what follow-up each person requires. For example, is discharge back home or to a lesser level of care of primary concern? Is the resident in the long term care facility for terminal care (i.e., related to illness) as opposed to custodial care? Is the resident having problems adjusting to the change from home to a long term care environment? Or is the resident unable to give you any clues (because of inclination or disease state) and will the social services professional have to use his/her skills to repeatedly assess needs? In any case, there is a job to do.

Update Resident Status

Things change! A resident might suffer a health crisis that impairs orientation. A husband or a child might die. Teeth might get lost. Financial circumstances might be altered. The resident might return to the previous level of function (presumably higher).

A change of condition or social status must be noted so that this information is available to all members of the care team. Never forget that people who are ill in a long term care facility live in a well-controlled balance. Many of their outside influences have been removed from their lives or have been altered or diminished. As a result, changes that are more easily absorbed by a well person can greatly influence the physical and emotional personality of a resident. Obviously, illness will make a difference, but even something as subtle as a change in the visiting pattern of a family member, an argument or the switch from private payment to Medicaid can result in behavior change. Whatever it is, a social services note is important. This will lead to a more accurate interpretation about the resident, as described below.

Interpret Observed Behaviors

We help interpret the psychosocial needs of the resident for other members of the care team. These needs are based on a resident's personality, his/her reaction to illness and his/her reaction to outside influences. Anger, aggression, passivity, and anxiety: these are responses. As a social services professional, you have the information gathered from the database to assist the resident care team with interpretation and determination of why the resident is giving this response to his/her environment. The key to the puzzle is not the response; it is why this response is being used. Use every opportunity (resident care conferences, rehab meetings) to share what you know, especially if it will have a positive effect on resident care.

Counsel Residents and Families

We are in the facility, first and foremost, to tend to the resident. However, most residents come to us with a family and, in many cases, the family also needs our care. The social services professional forms a bridge between community and facility. S/he provides important resource information but, even more importantly, emotional information. If we are successful at interpreting behavior, facility policies and the bureaucracies, the resident and the family will find it easier to accept the placement. If their concerns are not dealt with, they will resist and may never deal with feelings of abandonment, guilt, loss and defeat. This is true for both the resident and the family. Every facility has rules and regulations. We think it is best to give this information to the resident (if well enough) or to the responsible party at the time of admission.

The problem is that so much emotional baggage is being brought into the facility during admission that most of the information cannot be comprehended, no matter how lucidly conveyed or how sincerely received. Therefore, advise family members that they are not expected to know and understand everything. Advise them to observe, make lists and ask questions. There is usually a very good explanation for everything, but one must be in a state of mind that is receptive to understand it. The time of explanations is an excellent opportunity for family/resident/social services professional to become connected initially. From then on, you will often be sought out because you are a constant in an ever-changing environment.

Follow-up on all reasonable requests. One of OBRA's premises is that the residents (and families) have the *right* to make reasonable requests for change and the facility has the *responsibility* to act on the request in a reasonable manner. Get answers for things you don't know. Always be willing to listen to a frustration or a sorrow. You will find that it takes very little to ease a troubled mind — interest and information will do.

Field Grievances from Residents and Families

Never forget that the long term care facility is a new bureaucracy to most people. It is an emotional experience that may create barriers to understanding as well as feelings of impotence. The social services professional has a major role in interpretation: complaints/grievances often are not what they seem to be. Frequently they are a form of communication, a way of entering into conversation and eliciting assistance in a foreign and not always welcoming milieu.

Listen with compassion, not judgment; seek to sort out the real complaint and refer it to the appropriate department unless you are able to deal with it yourself. Listen, write down key words, dates and times, make a list of concerns and tackle them one at a time. Then, return with your follow up information.

You should expect to hear more complaints at the beginning of a placement. This has a great deal to do with personal pain (resident and family) and with misunderstanding or miscommunication. Are clothes being lost in the laundry? Has the family been informed about the facility policy for marking them?

Do not ever assume that someone is simply a chronic complainer. Listen, try not to be defensive and remember that any attempt at a solution goes a long way toward establishing good relationships.

Sometimes, in order to diffuse a volatile situation, we will listen, try to relate to all concerns and ask, near the end of the interview, if the family feels the resident is cared for, liked and responded to. We feel that putting things at this very basic level will sometimes produce a more satisfying outcome — especially if the response is yes. We don't forget about the lost slippers, but their importance will assume the appropriate place in the hierarchy of "what comes first."

Occasionally when we ask a resident if all is going well, s/he won't want to say that it is not for fear of getting someone in trouble. The same is true of families. Both resident and family may feel very vulnerable in these instances and are afraid of reprisal: physical or emotional abuse heaped onto the resident by a vengeful employee. It is important to describe the grievance procedure early in the new resident/family relationship and to impress upon them the importance of the correct process.

To summarize the grievance procedure:
1.   establish this avenue of communication with residents and families early in the relationship,
2.   reassure the timid that you will take action and there will be no reprisal,
3.   follow-up on all concerns, and
4.   report back to the individual who initiated the grievance.

Ensure Resolution of Grievances

Most facilities post the grievance procedure. In cases when the consumer is not satisfied with your response, s/he should be instructed and encouraged to see your administrator. If this is still not satisfactory, the state ombudsman should become involved. An ombudsman is a representative of a government (usually state) program who is appointed to receive and investigate complaints of abuse made by individuals in licensed and certified facilities. The ombudsman program was mandated and funded by the Older Americans Act amendments of 1975. Acting as an advocate for the patient, s/he assesses and verifies each complaint and then seeks a way to resolve it. An ombudsman must report findings to the appropriate agencies (law enforcement and Department of Health Services) and help to achieve equitable settlements to issues. Originally, the concept of ombudsman programs originated in Scandinavia in the 1800's. The ombudsman is often looked on as an enforcer but, actually, they are meant to be neutral and available to assist both residents/families and the facilities. Because of their increasing involvement in the survey process, it behooves us to educate ourselves about who they are and what they can do to help us.

If you have not already established a relationship with your area's or state's ombudsman office and your facility ombudsman, do it now. You will find that familiarity will break down barriers of mistrust and fear of the ombudsman.

Inservice Other Staff and Members of the Community

Although there is no actual mandate which says what or how many inservices social services professionals are responsible for, it makes sense that we focus on those topics that we know best. The reason that social services professionals are reluctant to give inservices is that often we don't have confidence in what we know. Yet, our perspective is unique in the facility and we have a special feeling about residents and their feelings.

An inservice about your role in the facility is a good start! Or, there may be a particular topic you have learned a great deal about and feel comfortable sharing. (Alzheimer's disease and its impact on resident and family interest us a great deal.) Talk about Resident Rights and our responsibilities toward meeting them. Discuss the psychosocial needs of the elderly; demystify the needs of the dying resident; speak of resident dignity and privacy and the right of confidentiality. If you still feel stumped for a topic of interest, examine the elements of communication and what a difference it can make to communicate efficiently.

Prepare three to four topics for discussion so that when you are asked to present, you will be ready and confident. It will be invigorating to share your knowledge and elicit responses from the group, especially if you are speaking about something with which you are very comfortable.

Role Model Professional Attributes

This is the social services professional's most subtle activity in the facility. If you are doing it well, some things you normally do will get done even when you are not there.

Nothing that a social services professional does is either secret or magic — it only seems that way. By being open and friendly with other staff members at all levels (from the administrator to the certified nursing assistants to the housekeeping staff) you are modeling, teaching, being an example of how to do your work so that your absence does not create a void — as it shouldn't.

Always answer questions honestly; discuss such things as how to talk with residents who are dying or how to respond to bereaved family members. Your example may give courage to others to offer solace and support.

Be proud of your professional approach to your work and you will be role modeling and influencing behavior. And even though you will not always be in the facility, your social services skills, your being-there-for-people skills should pervade the entire facility and create a positive atmosphere.

You will know you have succeeded when a staff member comes up to you and says, "When you weren't here the other day, I remembered that you always take Lucy to a quiet spot and speak calmly to her when she is upset. I tried it and it worked for me, too."

Position Description

Title: Social Services Professional

Purpose of the Position

Under the direction of the Administrator, the social services professionals, lead by the Social Services Director, are responsible for assuring that quality social services are provided to residents and their families, assisting them with the social and emotional aspects of illness and disability; also, to promote a therapeutic community including residents, families and the entire staff so that supportive relationships will be developed, thus enhancing the care given.

Qualifications

A qualified social services professional (required by OBRA law in a facility with more than 120 beds) is an individual with "*a bachelor's degree in social work or a bachelor's degree in a human service field including but not limited to sociology, special education, rehabilitation counseling and psychology; and one year of supervised social work experience in a health care setting working directly with individuals.*"[24]

Duties and Responsibilities

Provide social services to attain or maintain the highest practicable physical, mental and psychosocial well-being of the resident as discussed below:

1. Complete a psychosocial assessment and a social history within the required time after admission (14 days for federal regulations, 7 days for some states). This is to include the MDS and appropriate follow-up to that documentation.

2. Process all social services paperwork required by managed care systems in a timely manner.

---

[24] OBRA Tag F251.

3. Begin a discharge plan.

4. Enter on the resident care plan if there is an identified social services problem.

5. Always chart when a social services intervention has been indicated.

6. Complete a quarterly social services progress note.

7. Update the discharge plan annually for long term care residents and at least quarterly for residents who display a potential for discharge to a lesser level of care.

8. Reassess the social services entry on the resident care plan at least quarterly, updating problems, goals and approaches as appropriate.

9. Interpret psychosocial needs, strengths, goals and plans to appropriate staff.

10. Counsel residents and families during orientation and adjustment to the facility and during other times of crisis or trauma.

11. Participate with the interdisciplinary team in resident care conferences, presenting the psychosocial components of the resident's needs and formulating a coordinated plan.

12. Identify changes in responses, behavior or personality, such as depression, anxiety, withdrawal or aggressiveness and discuss this with the interdisciplinary team; chart to this.

13. Maintain a file of community resources including community social and mental health agencies; appropriate referrals are made when necessary.

14. Maintain knowledge of current facility, state and federal regulations, policies and procedures as they apply to social services.

15. Facilitate and convene a Family Council as indicated by facility need.

16. Attend and participate in staff meetings, department head meetings, designated committee meetings and resident care conferences.

17. Participate in the facility inservice education program, especially as it applies to the psychosocial needs of the resident; this is coordinated with the Staff Development Director.

18. Other responsibilities as defined by the administrator.

The Life of a Social Services Professional

We'd like to think when we go to work in the morning that our day will end up the way we had imagined it would. This almost never happens. Chores we had expected to tackle first may remain undone, sometimes until tomorrow or the next day. People we needed to phone may have been unavailable, so our task is incomplete. Paperwork finished — well, that rarely happens.

By its very nature, the work of a social services professional is full of distractions and unanticipated emergencies. It is rare to go from Resident A to Resident B in a straight line! Some days it will feel that your feet don't even touch the floor and that nothing has really been accomplished. This actually means that you abandoned your game plan sometime in the first hour of the day and never returned to it. Remember, though, that unanticipated work is still work!

It is best to begin with a plan of action. This can actually be broken down into segments. Having the full picture, specifying a month's worth of responsibilities, will bring focus to each day.

Daily

Upon arrival in the morning, check in with the Director of Nursing or the Nursing Supervisor. Ask about:
- Anticipated admissions
- Room changes
- Emergency discharges
- Deaths

Check with the staff nurses and aides about:
- Behavior changes
- Change of condition
- Resident needs
- Lost dentures or glasses

Make a list and decide how you will follow up.

Weekly

- Do new resident assessments
- Write quarterly and annual updates for the week
- Chart on new residents, checking for adjustment or progress toward discharge
- Attend resident care plan meetings
- Attend rehabilitation meetings
- Attend behavior management/chemical restraint review committee meetings
- Attend physical restraint review committee meetings
- Attend weight management committee meetings
- Attend falls prevention committee meetings

Monthly (if applicable)

Send out notices for next month's resident care conferences to family members, guardians and other appropriate individuals.

Ongoing

Family and resident contact: the real reason we go to work every day.

Every day is a new day. Remain hopeful that you will "finish," but accept the challenge of a changing environment, while trying not to become too frustrated.

Recreational Therapist

All nursing homes in the United States are required to have an activity director to provide activities for residents. Being credentialed as a recreational therapist (CTRS) is one of the five educational backgrounds approved for the position of activity professional. The recreational therapist who is certified through the National Council for Therapeutic Recreation Certification is able to fill one additional position that is different from that of the activity professional. The recreational therapist may also fill a position as one of the therapists on the rehabilitation treatment team. Unlike the position of activity professional, nursing homes are not required to have a "recreational therapy" position.

This section contains a sample job description for a recreational therapist who is working as a member of the rehabilitation team. The types of services provided by the recreational therapist, separate from the activity professional position, are limited and covered under only one section on the multi-disciplinary MDS ("Section T"). Following the sample job description is an article on the types of services that a recreational therapist might provide in a nursing home setting.

Position Description

Title: Recreational Therapist

Purpose of the Position

Under the direction of the Director of Rehabilitation Services, the recreational therapist is responsible for implementing recreational therapy interventions as part of the treatment team.

Qualifications

Credentialed as a Certified Therapeutic Recreation Specialist (CTRS) through the National Council for Therapeutic Recreation Certification (or equivalent state licensure); has experience working as a member of a rehabilitation treatment team; and has an understanding of the needs of geriatric populations.

Duties and Responsibilities

The recreational therapist is responsible for providing the necessary rehabilitation treatment interventions required by residents and within the therapist's training and credential. Treatment will be provided in both groups and one-on-one sessions. Regular and ongoing communication with the rest of the treatment team and adherence to all local, state, and federal laws and standards of practice is expected.

1.   Provide diagnostic and resident management services in the following areas: community integration, Advanced Activities of Daily Living (AADL), aquatic therapy, adaptive equipment and cognitive rehabilitation.

2.   Participate in the multidisciplinary team in the development, implementation and evaluation of the care plan.

3.   Monitor resident response to treatment. Modify care plan or approach to treatment as indicated by resident needs.

4.   Demonstrate good communication skills in documentation in the medical chart, in working with the other team members and family members, and in other required areas of communication.

5.   Maintain regular, on-going and timely records of contacts with residents; documentation is expected to be per occurrence.

6.   Other responsibilities as defined by the administrator.

Recreational Therapy Services Separate from the Activity Director Position[25]

A Certified Therapeutic Recreation Specialist (CTRS) is sometimes hired as a member of the rehabilitation treatment team (along with the physical therapist, occupational therapist and speech pathologist) and is not hired to be the activity professional. In this case the recreational therapist's (CTRS's) job description would be different than if s/he were working in the position of activity professional.

Community integration is more than taking a resident out into the community to enjoy community resources, even if this involves teaching the resident some new skills in the process. Moving back into the community, even if it is just for a few hours instead of permanently, requires many complex skills. Often, after acquiring a new disability, an individual will need training in the use of adapted techniques and equipment to successfully make the transition. The recreational therapist works on advanced activities of daily living to help the individual return to a less restrictive environment.

Aquatic therapy is more than just exercising or playing in the water (although these activities are very beneficial in and of themselves). For recreational therapists who have specialized training in aquatic therapy, using techniques such as Bad Ragaz in pools with the appropriate water temperature for the resident's diagnosis, should clearly be seen as specialized treatment and procedures.

Adaptive computer equipment (assistive technology) may only be a specialized treatment and procedure if the recreational therapist is evaluating the resident for specialized computer devices that will be used exclusively by that resident to improve function. The following are considered conventional equipment and are not likely to be considered specialized devices: cable, CD-ROM drives, computer or central processing units (CPUs), disk drives, disk operating software (or system software), keyboards, microphones, modems, scanners, monitors, mice, printers, software programs (or application programs), and trackballs. Assistive technology usually includes the following equipment: abbreviation expansion and macro programs, access utilities, arm and wrist supports, Braille embossers, electronic pointing devices, interface devices, joysticks, keyboard additions, menu management programs, monitor additions, optical character recognition and scanners, pointing and typing aids, reading comprehension programs, refreshable Braille displays, screen enlargement programs, screen readers, speech synthesizers, switches and switch software, talking and large-print word processors, touch screens, voice recognition, and writing composition programs. Once the equipment is available, the recreational therapist would provide treatment sessions to help the resident learn how to use the equipment.

Cognitive therapy is the therapist's use of words to teach and counsel the resident to bring about the desired change. Of all four types of specialized treatment and procedures, this may be the most difficult to truly separate out from required and expected activities. The primary difference here is the scope (usually more limited in nature than reality orientation) and intensity (greater intensity). For example, interventions related to increasing executive functions (initiation; self-monitoring/awareness; planning and organization; problem solving; mental flexibility and abstraction; and generalization and transfer) using the assessment process and intervention strategies as presented in *Vision, Perception, and Cognition, Third Edition* (Zoltan, 1996) may well qualify as specialized treatment and procedures because of their scope and intensity.

---

[25] Reprint from Idyll Arbor's *Journal of Recreational Therapy Practice.* www.Idyllarbor.com April 1999 by joan burlingame, CTRS, ABDA, HTR

Teamwork

The moment you walk into a facility, you have joined a team. It is not just you, the residents and the families; the team also includes all of the other workers in your facility:

- nursing (including aides)
- activity staff
- social services staff
- therapists
- dietary workers

- administration
- business office staff
- physicians
- housekeeping staff

Using the data presented to the health care team by each member of the team and input from the resident and his/her family, we develop a resident profile. We are working together to figure out what is best for the resident. Mutual goal setting is a powerful tool for finding the best care plan. It involves give and take of ideas and is stimulating for everyone. With the resident's good in mind and with the resident and/or responsible party being involved to the maximum extent possible, we find that the plans we make usually work well when we implement them.

Sometimes there is a tendency to be elitist in health care settings. It is a mistake. We find the certified nursing assistants (CNAs) to be invaluable sources of information. They are with the residents in a much more intimate way than we are (except perhaps at death) and are sometimes in a far better position to recognize and describe mood changes. CNAs see a lot of visitors, view interactions, share confidences. They know when a resident needs new clothing, is upset by a roommate or just doesn't seem the same. All disciplines can profit from information the CNAs have. Make sure you solicit information, pay attention and then follow up. Make the CNAs your allies. Respect and respond to their inquiries and their requests.

With the new emphasis of the survey process of OBRA's Final Rule, it is more important than ever that we use all available sources to assess the residents' needs. It is essential that we either know or can anticipate what a resident is capable of and of his/her frailties and needs. Using this information, we must have a plan that everyone knows and, to an extent, in which they all participate.

Chapter 4
Environment

How the environment should be designed depends somewhat on the type of facility in which you work. Long term care facilities need to take great care to make sure that the residents' rooms are personalized. Assisted living facilities can rely more on the people living there to bring in personal items. Day care facilities are, of course, not concerned with living space but other ideas about the physical environment discussed in the chapter still apply. Most of the rest of the ideas about making the people we serve comfortable and developing a supportive working environment apply to all types of programs and facilities.

This chapter will look at two aspects of the environment: the environment as it is perceived by the people we serve and the environment in which you will be working. If a professional is not aware of the profound importance and significance of a person's personal environment, s/he needs only look around his/her own home or room. Objects and mementos that could be easily overlooked by the rest of the world have special meaning. They give comfort and joy. They help create a place where a person enjoys spending time. Friendships and feeling like part of the community are important aspects of our lives. Our friends and our culture help us know who we are. Our ability to express our spiritual feelings is vital for understanding the purpose of our lives. This chapter talks about designing an environment so that each of the people we serve will have the best possible opportunity for a high quality of life.

Physical Environment

The physical plants of most long term care facilities were originally designed in the early 1960's when the philosophy for long term care facilities was focused on the bedroom and not the living space or environment. It was believed that, since most long term care residents would be spending most of the day in bed in frail health and eventually die, they did not need a living space or larger environment. This was a damaging myth. Unfortunately for those resilient individuals who helped prove this myth false, there were no areas designated for resident activities and the places in which residents did congregate had to be shared with at least two other services in the long term care facility.

With many adaptations and remodeling over the years, the industry has tried to work within the original structure of the long term care facility while being sensitive to personal needs for space. The goal is not to remodel the long term care facility, but rather to affect change within the existing structure.

Luckily, most other facilities have been designed with more appropriate concern for the people we serve. However, it is still important to ask the questions: How do we create an environment around the people we serve to stimulate them? Here are some answers.

Begin with all of the orientation tools available. Ideally each room should have a clock, a calendar and large-print room numbers. The room itself should have aesthetically pleasing pictures or mobiles. For an individual who enjoys pets, provide animal visits, or, at least, opportunities to see and read or look at books and posters about animals.

For someone who is restricted to bed, have the bulletin board within visual range. If they can only focus up towards the ceiling, place an easy to see poster on the ceiling. Mobiles are also effective for residents who are restricted to bed. (Before placing any object on the ceiling, be sure that it is allowed by local fire codes.)

When there is a special event occurring in the facility, bring theme props to the room so that everyone has the opportunity to feel a part of the community.

Remember that as people age, they require more light to see clearly. Be sure that there is enough light for the resident to see all of the things in his/her room.

Give the residents the opportunity to request and be involved in changes that will enhance further independence and involvement (bookshelves for reading, opening doors or windows, reading lights, calendars, clocks) in accordance with OBRA or other appropriate standards. (OBRA Tag F246, Accommodation of Needs: "*A resident has the right to reside and receive services in the facility with reasonable accommodations of individual needs and preferences, except when the health or safety of the individual or other residents would be endangered …*").

In the United States there are laws that outline minimum measurements for objects and structures in the resident's environment (The Americans with Disabilities Act or ADA). The next four pages provide you with a sample of the requirements. The first two pages are a checklist for permanent signage — those signs that would stay up year after year. The sign for the activity room, residents' lounge and potentially the sign for the bulletin board used for the monthly calendar would all fall into this category.

The other two pages show diagrams for minimum clearance for rooms and hallways. Remember, any object placed in the hallway reduces the space available. Minimum clearances do not mean from wall to wall but the actual space available. Fish tanks and wheelchairs "parked" along the wall make it harder for residents to get around. Chairs and couches, while homelike, may place the facility in violation of the ADA.

Remember that the ADA is a civil rights law. Any violation of this law is a violation of someone's civil rights and civil rights laws are considered more important and more significant than Medicare or Medicaid laws.

Survey Form 19: Signage

Facility Name: _____ **Facility Location:** _____

From: _____ **To:** _____

Section	Item	Technical Requirements	Comments	Yes	No
4.1.2(7) 4.1.3(16) 4.30.1	**Directional and Information Signs**	Do signs which provide direction to or information about, functional spaces of the building comply with 4.30.2, 4.30.3 and 4.30.5 (See below)? **EXCEPTION: Building directories, menus and all other signs which are temporary are not required to comply.**			
4.30.2	Character Proportion	Do the letters and numbers on such signs have a width to height ratio between 3:5 and 1:1; and a stroke width-to-height ratio between 1:5 and 1:10?			
4.30.3	Character Size	Are the characters on such signs sized according to viewing distance with characters on overhead signs at least 3 inches high?			
4.30.5	Finish	Do the characters and backgrounds on such signs have a non-glare finish?			
	Contrast	Do the characters contrast with their background (light-on-dark or dark-on-light)?			
4.1.2(7) 4.1.3(16) 4.30.1	**Room and Space Identification Signs**	Do signs which designate permanent rooms and spaces comply with 4.30.4, 4.30.5 and 4.30.6 (See below)?			
4.30.4	Raised and Braille Characters	Are the characters on such signs raised and accompanied by Grade II Braille?			

Section	Item	Technical Requirements	Comments	Yes	No
	Pictograms	If a pictorial symbol (pictogram) is used to designate permanent rooms and spaces, is the pictogram accompanied by the equivalent verbal description placed directly below the pictogram? (The verbal description must be in raised letters and accompanied by Grade II Braille.) (If the International Symbol of Accessibility or other information in addition to room and space designation is included on the sign, it does not have to be raised and accompanied by Grade II Braille.)			
		Is the border dimension of the pictogram at least 6 inches high?			
	Character Size	Are the raised characters on such signs between 5/8 inch and 2 inches high and raised at least 1/32 inch?			
	Upper Case	Are the raised characters on such signs upper case and sans serif or simple serif?			
4.30.5	Finish	Do the characters and background on such signs have a non-glare finish?			
	Contrast	Do the characters on such signs contrast with their background (light-on-dark or dark-on-light)?			
4.30.6	Mounting Location	Are such signs mounted on the wall adjacent to the latch side of the door? (At double leaf doors, are the signs placed on the nearest adjacent wall?)			
	Mounting Height	Are such signs mounted with their centerline 60 inches above the ground surface?			
	Approach	Can a person approach to within 3 inches of such signs without encountering protruding objects or standing within the swing of the door?			

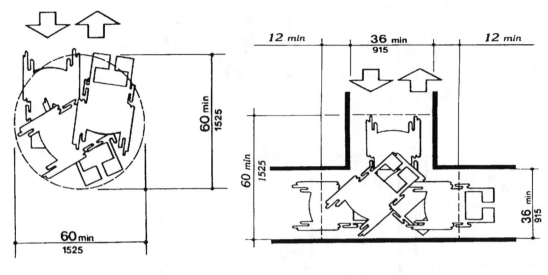

(a) 60-in (1525 mm) Diameter Space   (b) T-Shaped Space for 180° turns

Figure 3: Wheelchair Turning Space

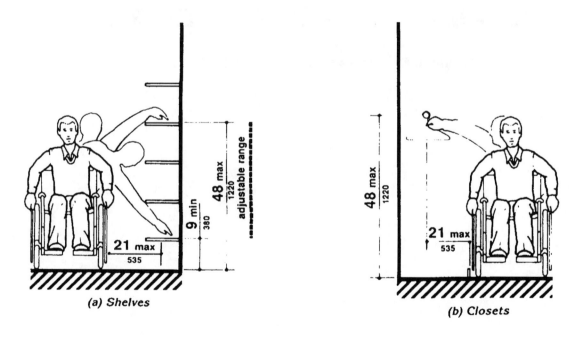

Figure 38: Storage Shelves and Closets

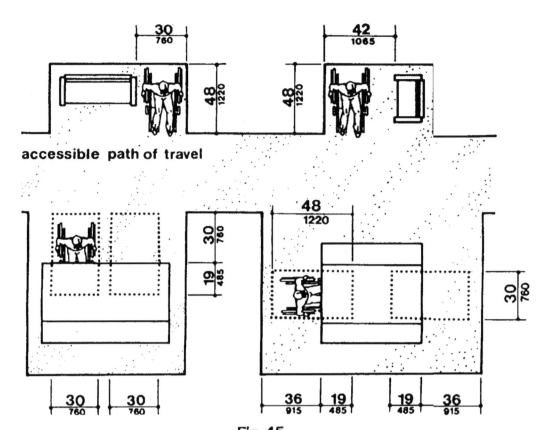

accessible path of travel

Fig. 45
Minimum Clearances for Seating and Tables

Personal Environment

One of the most important elements of our personal environment is the space around us. The facilities we work in do not have much space, usually providing less personal space than the people we work with had in their own homes. The lack of space makes personal space all the more important. This space is one's territory; the amount of territory a person believes to be his/her own is defined by him/her alone. We need to respect the individual's concerns about that space, his/her territory and guard it as s/he does. It may be one of the few things left in the world that remains personal. This space is territory and must be respected with vigor so as to give dignity to each individual.

For example, you are sitting and talking to one of the participants in your adult day care program and suddenly you hear someone yelling out, terrified. You look up and see nothing unusual. The individual who is yelling remains in her wheelchair, holding her book. She is surrounded by others in their wheelchairs and all of them seem to be oblivious to her. However, if you know her well, you have learned to identify, through ongoing interactions with her, what triggers her yelling. In this case, someone in one of those wheelchairs is just a little too close to her!

How will you know that this is true? By asking her and using her verbalization (which you have already heard) and her nonverbal cues (panic in her face) to verify what she is telling you. She needs more personal space. It is your responsibility to see that she gets it.

All people establish their own definition of personal space. The more disabled they are, the more vulnerable they may feel and the wider the personal space they are likely to need. The people we serve have little enough left that is personal; losses abound. But our person, our body, always belongs to us despite the physical and emotional insults it has incurred. We always need to control our physical space.

Culturally, we define this space, these invisible boundary lines. Intrusion into them is a violation of us personally. In the United States, we serve people from many different cultures, some who desire a relatively wide personal space so that even allowing others in to touch or hug can cause emotional flinching.

Personal space must be respected wherever it exists. Meeting the personal space needs of each individual is a requirement for a good personal environment.

The personal environment also includes the things we put in the space around us and in our rooms. Within the interpretive guidelines for environment in long term care settings is the mention of Individuality and Autonomy (OBRA Tags F240 to F245). We can improve a resident's personal environment by seeking out ways to celebrate the resident, his/her life, family accomplishments and interests. Any touch from home that adds a personal touch to the environment is important. Self-expression enhances quality of life. This expression can change one's residence from an institutional setting to a warm environment.

Being surrounded by familiar possessions serves another function — the stirring of memories. For those who have very limited access to the physical environment, memories provide a safe and comfortable dwelling place. Even a resident with dementia may be refreshed and reminded of family and events if given photos or memorabilia that provide entrance into a long-ago past.

Spiritual Environment

The spiritual aspects of the environment involve the questions of purpose and meaning in one's life. This involves personal values and belief systems. For many, it also involves a special routine and religious social contacts. For some residents the day of worship was different from the other six days of the week. The pace was different and frequently offered extra time for family and friends.

Another aspect of spiritual environment has to do with a feeling of reverence toward God. Staff or other residents who make fun of another person's beliefs or who use swear words decrease the quality of a resident's spiritual environment. Empowerment of, and respect for, the resident increases it. Making a better spiritual environment for each resident is one of your responsibilities.

As Joseph Campbell[26] says:

> People say that what we're all seeking is a meaning for life. I don't think that is what we're really seeking. I think that what we are seeking is an experience of being alive, so that our life experiences on the purely physical plane will have resonance within our own innermost being and reality, so that we actually feel the rapture of being alive.

Cultural Environment

Developing an awareness of the unique needs, beliefs and practices of individuals from a different culture is an ongoing process. Culture refers to a sense of belonging to a group or community that holds significance and value for its members. In order to provide a sense of belonging and meaningful life, it is imperative to create and enhance a sense of culture. Culture, in this context, can go a long ways toward giving purpose to the people we serve, employees and volunteers within a specific setting. The feeling of being part of a larger whole can be empowering, particularly for individuals who may feel wrenched from familiar settings, values or capabilities.

Culture contributes to the sensation of life in the environment. It can create:
- A sense of belonging
- A feeling of security and safety
- An affirmation of individuality, autonomy and personal accomplishments
- Respect for diversity
- A sense of purpose and involvement
- Enhanced independence as opposed to learned helplessness
- Opportunities for new and pleasantly surprising experiences
- Growth
- Enjoyment
- A nurturing community

The professional can nurture the creation of a setting that celebrates the various cultures from which the people we serve come by:
- Encouraging all of the people we serve, employees (professional, non-professional and volunteers) to think about and evaluate ideas about lifestyle, leisure and potential
- Encouraging innovation
- Adding the element of appropriate risk-taking for both staff and the people we serve
- Looking for the uniqueness of each person and promoting that quality
- Encouraging leadership
- Becoming a facilitator in as many situations as possible
- Finding the child within ourselves and recognizing that playfulness is a necessary component of growth
- Listening well and communicating clearly
- Lending support in as many ways as possible

---

[26] Campbell, Joseph with Moyer, Bill, 1988, *The Power of Myth*, p. 3, Doubleday, New York, NY.

- Sharing the control
- Giving everyone responsibility for a positive environment

Working Environment

The working environment involves at least four different groups of people who are concerned about a resident's health and well-being. If we could view these interactions from above, this is what we might see:

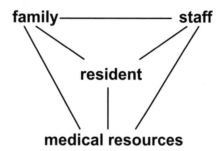

These interactions are complicated and complex and if all parties involved are not scrupulously careful, they will shortly resemble a game of gossip, with a "he said/she said" mode of communication leading to misinterpretation of facts and volatile situations. No one wants to lose control and no one — from the people we serve to family to medical staff — wants to be the last to know! We cannot state clearly enough that communication between all of the interested parties is one of the most important component in quality care.

Environmental Assessment Form

The **Environmental Assessment Form** is designed to encourage us to not only assess the environment of our facility, but to then act to remedy situations that need improvement.

Part 1 — "Psychosocial/Supportive" presents specific beneficial characteristics of a positive environment. Commonly found obstacles are included to help sharpen the focus on problems and point to interventions.

Part II — "Physical Factors" presents physical characteristics of the facility and obstacles in the same format as Part 1.

Part III — "Department Environment" looks at some of the requirements of the work environment for professionals.

This form represents a generic version of an instrument that, hopefully, will become individualized and specific to the setting in which it's used. Use of this form on a regular basis can serve as an on-going progress report on the environmental state of the facility and the level of cooperation among staff members and residents for the benefit of all.

How to use the form:

Step One: Read first characteristic in column one.

Step Two: Read "obstacles" in column to the right. Do these obstacles exist? Are there others?

Step Three: Use this blank column to identify solutions that work for both the people we serve and staff. Think about human and physical resources needed. Think about what is on hand and how it can be used. Be creative.

Step Four: Repeat steps one through three until all items have been covered.

Step Five: Add concerns not noted on the form and continue the process until all items have been addressed.

Environmental Assessment Form

Psychosocial/Supportive

Stimulating Environment	Obstacles	Interventions
Reality Awareness Objects	No clocks. No calendars.	
Sense of Surprise/Newness	No change in schedule or activities offered — every day is the same.	
Variety/Diversity	Lacking programs that meet individual needs.	
Promotes Independence	No opportunity to engage in individual leisure interests. No opportunity for decision making.	
Curiosity	No build-up to an event. No one seems to care.	
Communication	No feeling of inclusion. Confusion as to changes without being informed first.	
Meaningfulness	Feeling of being disenfranchised. No individualization. No feeling of being needed or of a sense of purpose.	
Normal Schedule	Schedule changes with little notice. Canceled activities.	
Motivation	No desire to try something new. Lack of stimulating curiosity. Preferred activities not offered.	
Education	Too advanced/intimidating. Too basic.	
Welcoming	Lack of social interaction between staff and the people we serve or between the people we serve.	
Attitudes	Staff fail to see the individual and his/her potential. Unrealistic expectations.	
Community	Sense of isolation.	
Involvement	Lack of intergenerational programs. Lack of opportunities to help.	
Normal Life Setting	Lack of plants/animals. Lack of normal structure of the daily routine.	
Cohort Factors	No provision of design appropriate to the familiar themes of past lives.	
Multi-Cultural	No diversity in cultural beliefs, customs and environment.	

Environmental Assessment Form

Physical Factors

Factors	Obstacles	Intervention
Light	Privacy curtains pulled near window — no light. Dining room too bright. Bedroom too dark — want to read at night. Amount of light in hallway significantly different than light in rooms.	
Sound	Roommate's TV too loud. Radio on all day — wrong station.	
Available Space	Can't maneuver with chair in room. Too much furniture in living room or dining room.	
Accessibility	Controls out of reach. Bulletin boards behind bed. Can't get to clothes in cupboard.	
Decor	Beautifully decorated, BUT not functional for daily use. Lack of contrast in colors and design. No personal belongings in the room.	
Quiet Spaces	No place to go for privacy.	
Orientation Objects	Disorientation due to lack of clocks and calendars for individual use. Poor signage — not appropriate size or placement. Facility name not available.	
Color	Light shades of color hard to discern if visually impaired. Too bright — hard to relax.	
Visibility	Calendar too small. Room numbers unavailable.	
Adaptability	Need board lower on wall. Light above bed hard to reach. Light switch too small.	
Odors	Always smells. Soiled linen containers.	
Activity Space	Lack of small areas for individuals to sit and watch activities with opportunity for physical distancing from others to avoid over-stimulation.	
Technology	Inappropriate level of technology. Too high tech or too antiquated for age group of resident.	

Environmental Assessment Form

Department Environment

Factors	Obstacles	Intervention
Supply Space	No space for supplies and materials needed to run programs.	
Meeting Space	Inadequate private space to meet with the people we serve for assessments and/or discussions.	
Meeting Space	Inadequate space for meetings with volunteers. Lack of space for other community integration activities.	
Meeting Space	Inadequate space or privacy for meetings with families.	
Work Areas	Private areas for each staff member to keep his/her work materials.	
Work Areas	Quiet areas for making phone calls, doing planning and conducting interviews.	
Quality of Life Services	Department doesn't reflect the facility philosophy for quality of life.	

Plan of action to improve environment:

Chapter 5
Programs for Your Facility

This chapter looks at the specifics of matching the assessed needs of the people we serve with activities and other care program ideas so that you can provide the most appropriate care to each person. Assessment is the process of discovering who the individual is and what their physical and psychosocial needs are in terms of optimum care and functional status. After the assessment, care plans are created for each person that outlines the path the staff will take to meet the individual's needs. Every goal listed on the care plan should be able to be traced back to a need identified on the individual's assessments.

After assessing individual needs, you take a more global view of the population of the people you serve as a whole. This is done by summarizing the individual programming needs of each person and finding individual and group activities which help meet all the needs. While doing this, you can evaluate your current program offerings and make changes to meet the needs of your current population.

Some of the basic ideas that you will want to keep in mind as you assess and design your activity program include:
- Look at the entire population and its diversity. This is the framework of your program.
- Have a philosophy written for your department and program.
- Form a committee of the people being served to give input into the program. This is their program and should be designed around their interests — not your own.
- Identify the talents and leaders in your community and draw them out.
- Wellness, prevention and creativity should be reflected in all activities.
- Find opportunities to give to the community outside of your own.
- Provide social opportunities that include and invite everyone.
- Offer specialized groups that do not include everyone so that there is a balance.
- Create an environment of respect, dignity and accessibility.
- What would you want if you lived in this community?
- Identify percentage of population with varying levels of dementia. Add memory enhancement programs and memory aids to your cognitive programs. These should be included in the program and not as an additional service.
- Each resident's life is a story to be told and celebrated.

Programming Levels for Activities

If the programs are to truly meet the diversity of needs of the current population, the professionals must design and provide programs that meet all levels of functional and cognitive needs.

Following is a table that gives you a visual reference from which to gauge the levels and programming categories. The levels are from one to eight, one being the most severely limited or regressed group of individuals to eight being the most independent group of individuals.

Levels of Therapeutic Programming

The levels are:

1.	Sensory Integration	Basic stimulation of multiple senses. These techniques can be incorporated into all levels.
2.	Sensory Awareness Sensory Stimulation	Basic stimulation to elicit response and focus outside of self.
3.	Validation Therapy	For a person who is very disoriented, whose goals are not focused on orientation. Validate where they are in their thoughts and feelings.
4.	Remotivation/Reminiscing	Stepping-stone phase to and from sensory awareness. The individual is aware of self and motivated to seek out others.
5.	Resocialization	Resident is socializing and is more oriented to person, time and place. Involvement with others is in a structured group and is crucial to maintain the current functional level.
6.	Cognitive Stimulation Cognitive Retraining	Techniques used with an individual suffering from trauma to the brain and showing cognitive disorganization. These are rehab-oriented groups.
7.	Short Term Rehab	Programming which enhances personal goals worked on in physical therapy, occupational therapy, recreational therapy and speech therapy. Team approach involving use of leisure time.
8.	Community Integration	Individuals who are preparing for discharge; focus on skills, resources and independence when back in the community.

1 ----------**2**----------- **3** ----------**4**----------- **5** -----------**6**----------- **7** ------------**8**
Long Term Stay   **Assisted Living**   **Short Term Stay**   **Discharge**

Each level will have varying types of groups and goals. An individual may move from one level to another on an upward or downward path and consequently require different and specialized therapeutic programs to meet his/her current needs.

This chapter provides you with a general overview of these eight levels of programming. After we also discuss other important aspects of running programs we will return again to these eight levels of service. Chapter 7: Programming for Low Function will review ideas on how to work with individual with significant impairments. Because this group tends to be so challenging to work with we will also provide you with many activity ideas.

Chapter 8: Programming for Moderately Impaired Function, covering three levels of function, will talk about working with individuals who are more capable. Again, you will be given many activity ideas to use with this group. This chapter has a special section on working with men and also an extensive section on cognitive stimulation.

The majority of individuals you will work with will fall into these first five levels. Chapter 9: Rehabilitation Focused Groups discusses working with and providing activities for individual who may have the option to regain function and move to a less restrictive environment.

Some individuals will move from level to level. Use this with the Activity Needs Assessment (below) to be sure that you have programming which is appropriate for all of the people you serve.

Activity Needs Assessment

After you have assessed each of the people you serve to find out what needs each one has, you must design a program for your facility that meets the needs of all of them. To do that you need to know the current needs, interests, cognitive and functional levels of the individuals here today. Perhaps the activity program was designed for last year's needs and many of those people are no longer here. Federal law mandates that activity programs in long term care facilities must be *"designed to meet, in accordance with the comprehensive assessment, the interests and the physical, mental and psychosocial well-being of each resident."*[27] Even without the mandate of the federal law, it still makes sense to be sure your program meets the needs of the people you serve.

Ask yourself how many of the people you serve benefit from the activity program. Does the program seem to cater to those able to attend large groups and classes? Are there a good percentage of the people you serve uninterested in attending? Are there a good percentage of residents in need of "supportive" activities (special needs and one-on-one programming)? Why do the alert, short-term rehab residents refuse to go to group activities? What do we offer to them as alternatives? Review the guidelines for the *Needs Assessment Form*, take a current census sheet and complete this form.

---

[27] *State Operations Manual*, OBRA Tag F248.

Guidelines for Completing the Needs Assessment Form, Step 1

Each of the people we serve needs to be listed in a single group. The group selected represents the level where the individual functions most of the time. For example, if an individual is *mostly* active but occasionally passively involved, s/he goes under "actively involved." Place an asterisk (*) next to each man's name, as they also need to be addressed for specialized programs. Add the cognitive level after the name so you can be sure your mix of activities matches the cognitive functioning level of the people you serve.

This assessment form needs to be updated with names of newly admitted individuals so every individual is reflected on the assessment. The form itself should be updated as often as the admission and discharge schedule demands it. (Keeping this form on your department's computer will help make updates easier.)

- Individuals in **GROUP 1** are active **to their own abilities** in group activities.

- Individuals in **GROUP 2** are present at group activities but passive observers — "fringe participants." (Ask yourself why.)

- Individuals in **GROUP 3A** have cognitive impairments.

- Individuals in **GROUP 3B** have cognitive impairments and are unable to tolerate group experiences (place a pound sign "#" next to those individuals with potential for orientation).

- Individuals in **GROUP 4** are alert and independent in both individual and group leisure pursuits. They do not attend activities on a regular basis (at least 2 to 4 times a week). They do keep involved in individual leisure interests, have families and friends visiting and on occasion, attend events or special presentations.

- Individuals in **GROUP 5** refuse all activities. These individuals are alert but do not involve themselves in any individual or group leisure interests. They spend their days in their rooms or in the hall. They do not seek out companionship or activities.

- Individuals in **GROUP 6** have profound multiple and singular sensory losses. Be specific as to type and severity of individual sensory losses.

- Individuals in **GROUP 7** are individuals in short-term rehab. These individuals are receiving therapy with the intent of being discharged as soon as possible. For the most part, they do not wish to enter into the world of a "resident" and avoid social settings and contact with most of the other individuals who will be staying in your program for an indefinite period of time. Their needs and goals are very different from those of an individual on long term care. Many of these individuals are being served through Medicare or an HMO for whom the PPS system of reimbursement applies.

- Individuals in **GROUP 8** may be young people, have naso-gastric (NG) enteral feeding tubes, have IVs or have a critical illness. Each facility varies greatly, so use this column as needed to keep track of individuals who require mostly one-on-one activities.

- Individuals in **GROUP 9** have traumatic head injuries or are comatose. These two categories have separate needs but are grouped together in this form.

- Individuals in **GROUP 10** include other identifiable subgroups that have special needs including smokers, younger participants and individuals dependent on ventilators. They generally have a low attendance at group activities. They are usually alert and social within their own subgroups. These groups are under the same column but obviously have nothing in common in terms of disabilities and program needs.

Activity Needs Assessment Form

Activity Professional _____ Date _____

List the name of each individual in one column only.

1	2	3a 3b	4	5	6	7	8	9	10
Individuals actively involved in group activities and individual leisure interests	Individuals passively involved in groups with limited individual leisure interests	a. Cognitive impairments b. Unable to tolerate group experiences Place "#" next to those with potential for orientation	Alert and independent in both individual and group leisure interests	Refuse all activities and are not involved in leisure interests	Profound multiple and singular sensory losses Be specific with type and severity of sensory loss	Short term rehab	Critically ill, comfort care IV, NG Wound care Dialysis	Head injury Comatose	Other categories: Younger individuals Ventilator dependent

Guidelines for Completing the Needs Assessment Form, Step 2

After the activity professional completes the needs assessment form, s/he must now take a closer look at each category to further assess the population's programming needs.

Group 1: Actively Involved

Individuals in this group attend and participate in leisure activities. Do they need to be better connected to functions out of the facility? Are they physically overexerting themselves by this high level of participation? (MDS 2.0 Section N)

Group 2: Passively Involved

Individuals in this group choose not to initiate interactions and/or engage in leisure activities that require more skills or energy than they may possess. Determine why these individuals are passively involved. Is it due to sensory losses or because they cannot tolerate a large group setting and shut down due to sensory overload? Is this passivity a long standing personality trait, which would not be appropriate to change?

If these or other reasons make them poor candidates for group activities, their needs may be better met in Group 3. If they can be more actively involved, the ideal is to find ways to make that possible and therefore include them in Group 1. Individuals experiencing cognitive losses may be disoriented, but respond successfully to reality awareness and remotivation groups. Help facilitate their involvement to their maximum level of function and ability.

Group 3a: Cognitive Impairments

Individuals in this group are assessed with moderate to severe inability to make decisions and make themselves understood. (Review MDS, Section B4). The types of programs appropriate to this level are listed in Chapter 9: Rehabilitation Focused Groups.

Group 3b: Unable to Tolerate Group Experiences

Individuals in this group cannot tolerate the stimulation, noise and confusion associated with a group event. They appear to escalate in behaviors and anxiety and consequently should not be brought to groups and instead should be provided a one-on-one or a small group experience.

Group 4: Alert and Independent in Leisure Interests

Individuals in this group are able to and do participate in leisure activities of their own. If there is an activity of interest to them, they will usually join in, although this is usually not daily. These individuals are making choices about their leisure time. Be sure to clearly document their involvement in the activities that do not show up on the standard activity list so you can show that their leisure needs are being met.

Group 5: Refuse All Activities

Individuals in this group consistently refuse to engage in any leisure activity either facility sponsored or of their own choosing. These individuals may be involved in the same lifestyle they were accustomed to before admission. If so, be sure to document this and define how you came to this determination. Other causes could be depression, fear of groups, distrust, lack of a culturally appropriate "fit" to the activities or just plain lack of motivation. Obviously these people need a clear assessment to determine why they are making the choices that they are making. They may eventually become more involved in the development of a trusting relationship. They may be in need of specialized one-on-one programs. Or they may simply be making a personal choice not to be involved — which is their right. Be sure that programs are available for them and document their choice not to go.

Group 6: Profound Multiple and Singular Sensory Losses
Individuals in this group have individual needs according to the level and severity of the sensory loss. Many of the individuals in other categories are also dealing with these types of losses so be sure that individuals listed here are those with a profound sensory loss.

Group 7: Short Term Rehab
Individuals in this group are hopeful about receiving necessary therapy and then discharge to a lesser care setting. Many of these individuals are too fatigued from intensive therapy sessions to attend groups. Others choose not to get involved because of the stigma attached to being a long term "resident" in a long term care facility. The professional's role with these individuals will be more along the lines of a resource person or an adjunct therapist to enhance the rehab goals. Separate groups of activities designed for rehab residents may be very appropriate.

Group 8: Subacute, Critically Ill
Individuals in this group have a very high level of acuity. Many are unable to leave their rooms and/or become engaged in activity groups. These individuals' needs are very diverse and personalized. Many or most will be provided with services on a one-on-one basis. For professionals working in units in an acute care hospital, this is the major resident profile. The challenge is in creating a theme-oriented and individualized program that can be offered on a one-on-one basis or small group basis if there are a few individuals up in the day room.

Group 9: Comatose, Traumatic Brain Injury
Individuals in this group may eventually progress to leisure groups, but primarily will be in specialized one-on-one experiences. The individuals with head injury and in a semi- to full-comatose state, are quite a challenge and demand a special understanding of what they can and cannot tolerate in terms of activity programming. Remember that these two groups are very separate with extremely different needs in programming. As with all individuals, be familiar with the interdisciplinary approach and always feel comfortable asking questions of other team members to increase your understanding of the diagnosis.

For the individual in a comatose state, your interactions will vary according to his/her level of consciousness. Individuals with head injuries will usually be much younger people. According to the length of time since the injury and the physical healing of the injured area, this individual will need different types of programming interventions. Be sure to read the therapy notes and talk to the physical, recreational, occupational and speech therapists. They will be happy to help you link your time with the individuals to specific therapy goals.

Cognitive retraining and cognitive stimulation are appropriate during progressive therapy and, again, need the team approach in identifying what is needed. In terms of group activities, be cautious with these individuals. A group may be over-stimulating for them, may cause agitation and combativeness or even seizure activity. It is normal for individuals with head injuries to have fluctuations in their tolerance level. Observe them closely and be aware of their reactions and tolerance to the stimulation. Keep them at a safe distance from commotion and other residents until they have been fully assessed and evaluated for this level of involvement.

Group 10: Others
Individuals in this group choose not to attend most or any of the groups but do spend most of their leisure time in a social network with others they feel comfortable with. (This may be especially true of smokers.) These individuals may not attend most or any of the other groups. Their attendance does not reflect specifics about them. Be sure to document their social skills demonstrated within the group and other information regarding interests, strengths and lifestyle.

When you have identified the needs of the people you serve from the list above, plan a set of activities that meets the needs of all of the individuals. Some ideas for activities are included in the chapters that follow. If you work in a nursing home, it is a good idea to check the activity plan against the OBRA Review forms on the following pages to see if it meets the OBRA requirements for activities.

Activity Review Forms

The purpose of these forms is to assure program compliance with the interpretations and terminology of the OBRA (long term care) regulations. All of the following areas are within the regulations and should be a part of your activity program. While this form was developed for use in long term care settings, it is appropriate for assisted living and other types of settings. After reviewing how to use the form for your department, take your monthly calendar and write down each activity in the most appropriate section. This is a quality review exercise to evaluate the programs you currently offer. (If you want to practice this evaluation on someone else's schedule, you can use the schedule in the section on *The Life of an Activity Professional* in Chapter 3: The Work We Do.)

Stimulation Activities: Activities designed with the goal of offering input and stimulation to one or more of the senses. Examples: music, tactile activities such as pet visits, and multi-sensory experiences such as themes that incorporate touching, tasting, smelling, seeing and hearing within the activity.

Solace Activities: Activities that by their nature provide solace. These are offered to residents who are critically ill, dealing with pain, have limited endurance and are spending most of the time in bed or in their room. Examples: relaxation tapes, pain management tapes, slides and videos, being read to, pet visits, memory book writing, creative and expressive opportunities.

Physical Health: Activities that promote physical well-being. These should be offered to every resident. Examples: exercise class, movement to music, reinforcement of therapy goals, obstacle courses, wheelchair management, breathing exercises, walking and relaxation exercises.

Cognitive Health: Activities that provide intellectual stimulation to maintain and enhance awareness and cognition. Cognitive activities should be provided for all levels of ability. Examples: current events, discussion groups, values clarification discussions, problem solving scenarios, life management skills, trivia, reminiscing, reality awareness, stress management techniques and orientation.

Emotional Health: Activities that promote a sense of self, life review and empowerment. Examples: all activities that bring out the individual either in a group or one-on-one situation, reminiscing, "this is your life" games, opportunities to discuss emotional concerns and needs in a supportive environment, socialization activities which assist in helping individual residents feel a part of a community or group.

Self-Respect: Activities that support individual views and beliefs. Activities that promote respect in content and participation and at all levels of needs and abilities. Examples: cultural activities which introduce different customs and beliefs, all activities which focus on the individual and previous lifestyle and accomplishments, Resident Council.

Male-Oriented Activities: Activities that are designed to meet the special interests and needs of the men at your facility. These groups and activities are offered according to the percentage of men in the facility. Examples: see the *Resocialization* section of Chapter 8: Programming for Moderately Impaired Function for program ideas.

Task-Segmentation: Activities that take into account a resident's need to have the task broken down into subtasks in order to successfully engage in and complete the activity. Task segmentation is addressed on the MDS form and should be reviewed by everyone who supervises activities. Examples: art projects, breaking the tasks down step by step: pick up the brush, dip brush into the paint, place brush onto the paper that is taped to the table, etc.

Seasonal/Special Events: In order to enhance quality of life, staff need to be very aware of the normalization concept. Because many individuals cannot easily continue their previous lifestyle and routines after being admitted your setting, it is the responsibility of all staff members to assist in keeping life as normal as possible. Seasonal celebrations and acknowledgments of special events must be offered and reinforced in activities. Examples: birthdays, holidays, religious occasions, voting issues and elections, national, state, community and facility events.

Indoor/Outdoor: Activities which are offered outdoors, weather permitting or indoors in different locations for variety. Examples: picnics and barbecues, outdoor walks, outings, opportunities for individuals to be outdoors in a safe and secured area.

Community Based: Activities that help connect the resident with the surrounding community so they still feel a part of their community. Examples: outings into the community to the library, lectures, restaurants, fairs, stores. It is also important to provide the reverse so that community members, organizations and groups come into the facility to visit the residents.

Cultural: Activities that identify and honor all cultures. These include activities that bring culture to the resident. Examples: museum docent visits, slide shows of famous painters and artists, painters coming into the facility to paint while residents watch or lead an art class for residents, special activities which honor other cultures and traditions.

Religious: There should be a special group or presentation for all identified religious beliefs. These can be services, presentations, individualized room decorations which are theme specific, family involvement in sharing the event and beliefs.

Adaptations/Special Needs: Activities that are adapted as required so that all residents can participate according to their individual needs and abilities. This could be an adaptive device, special seating arrangement, visual cues, an interpreter, etc.

Activities for All Ages: Assurance that all age groups identified in the population have meaningful and age-appropriate activities available to them. Examples: special outings for young residents to concerts, restaurants, and parks; intergenerational programs; staff involvement with activities so that there are people of all ages involved. This also refers to activities that are familiar to an individual according to his/her age, not the age of the staff designing the program. Involve the residents in identifying what would be appropriate.

In-Room Activities: Activities that are brought to the individual if they are not able or interested in joining a group. Examples: bringing in a seasonal theme to the room along with decorations, providing specialized sensory programs to those in a semi-comatose state, including residents in their rooms on the Resident Council by discussing topics individually in the room after the meeting.

Activity Program Review Form

Facility _____ **Date** _____

Requirement	Activities Offered	Requirement Met
Stimulation Activities		
Solace Activities		
Physical Health		
Cognitive Health		
Emotional Health		
Self-Respect		
Male-Oriented Activities		
Task Segmentation		
Seasonal/Special Events		
Indoor/Outdoor		
Community Based Activities		
Cultural Activities		
Religious Activities		
Adaptations/Special Needs		
Activities For All Ages		
In-Room Activities		

Activity Program Review Form — Part 2

Questions to ask in reviewing the program (list examples for "yes" answers and ideas for the "no" answers):

                                                                                                            Yes/No

For individuals who do not attend group activities, do you provide individual projects? .... _____
Notes:

Do individuals give input to the design of the program? .... _____
Notes:

Is transportation assistance by nursing staff allowing all interested individuals to attend? ...... _____
Notes:

Are individuals informed of opportunities? .... _____
Notes:

Is the schedule of activities acceptable to the schedule of individual needs? .... _____
Notes:

Do individuals have a choice in regards to activities? .... _____
Notes:

Do you provide varied programming to meet the diversity of individual needs and abilities? .. _____
Notes:

Social Services Review Form

Tag F250 Social Services (OBRA Nursing Home Regulation)
"The facility must provide medically-related social services to attain or maintain the highest practicable physical, mental and psychosocial well-being of each resident."

Requirements	Interpretation	+ = Met - = Not Met
Identify the need of medically-related social services and pursue provision of these services	Maintaining or improving ability to personally manage everyday physical, mental and psychosocial needs.	
Adaptive equipment	Assuring provision of special devices and equipment to enhance functional and emotional independence.	
Restraint reduction	Providing alternatives to drug therapy or restraints by understanding and communicating to staff why individuals act as they do, what they are attempting to communicate and what needs the staff must meet.	
Clothing and personal needs	Assisting with identifying and purchasing needed supplies and items.	
Maintaining contact with the family about changes	Informing family about changes that occur in current goals, discharge plans and care plan meeting attendance.	
Referrals and outside services	Assisting with accessible transportation, talking books, absentee ballot forms.	
Financial and legal matters	Providing assistance with requests for attorney, pension information and updates, funeral arrangements.	
Health care decisions	Assisting individuals with information about current health status and decisions pertaining to treatment. Requesting others to be a part of this decision-making process.	
Discharge planning	Assisting with living situations, home health services, transfer agreements with other facilities.	
Counseling services	Opportunity for individuals to discuss concerns or assistance in obtaining outside counsel.	
Grief counseling	Meeting the needs of individuals who are grieving.	
Support individual needs and interests	Keeping staff informed of individual interests and preferences to enhance a sense of self and self-esteem.	
Building staff and resident relationships	Inservice training to continually assist understanding and support of individual needs.	
Self-determination and choices	Empowering the individual to make his/her own choices about lifestyle in the long term care facility.	
Promoting staff awareness of dignity and individuality	Role modeling, inservice training, family council, resident council.	

Social Services Program Review — Part 2

Questions to ask in reviewing the program (list examples for "yes" answers and ideas for the "no" answers):

Yes/No

Do facility staff implement social services interventions to assist the individual in meeting treatment goals? .... _____
Notes:

Do staff responsible for social work monitor the individual's progress in improving physical, mental and psychosocial function? .... _____
Notes:

Has goal attainment been evaluated and the care plan changed accordingly? .... _____
Notes:

Does the care plan link goals to psychosocial functioning and well-being? .... _____
Notes:

Have the staff responsible for social work established and maintained relationships with the individual's family or legal representative? .... _____
Notes:

Challenges and Techniques of Group Work

One of the most challenging and ever-changing roles that the professional plays is that of group leader. Many factors come into play in determining the overall composition and capacities of the group and, therefore, appropriate activities for that group. For example:

- When the majority of participants are frail and dealing with sensory and cognitive losses, the professional must radiate confidence and fine-tune activities to the capabilities of the group.
- When there is a high level of confusion or disorientation among group members, the leader will need to provide a high degree of structure and direction for the group.
- When the majority of the participants are cognitively aware and otherwise capable, the leader will need to be able to step back and allow the residents to assume natural leadership roles.

The following list presents some issues and needs that the professional should consider when leading a group. Each requires a constructive and compassionate response from the leader whether through action or attitude.

passivity	dependency	hyperactivity
lack of purpose	depression	feelings of uselessness
behavioral issues	anger	sensory losses
anxiety	loneliness	low self-esteem
apathy	wandering	cognitive losses
communication disorders	lack of response	embarrassment regarding
confusion	short attention span	condition

Here are some tools and techniques that have proven helpful in working with groups:

- When setting expectations and goals for the group, be sure to be realistic about what this group of individuals can successfully achieve.
- Structure each member's environment within the group to enhance his/her abilities and thereby increase involvement in socialization, improve attention span and provide a positive and successful experience.
- Always focus on the group member *today* and the abilities that s/he has *today*.
- Acknowledge the efforts and accomplishments of each group member individually.
- Offer time within each session for individuals to share past memories and experiences.
- Verbally acknowledge any information acquired through conversation regarding past occupations, accomplishments and interests of group members.
- Introduce the familiar themes of family, pets, foods, holidays and nature regardless of group members' cognitive levels.
- Remind the group of pleasurable experiences that are familiar to everyone.
- Allow opportunities to demonstrate what has been learned. Repetition and visual cues enhance learning.
- Remember that we all need to be needed. This can be a goal for a group — to be of help to others. Projects and gifts can be made for staff, visitors, entertainers and each other.
- Adults like to know that they are held accountable for their role in the group. Feedback from the leader is very important.
- Use touch to motivate and to help re-focus attention in the group. For individuals who do not have family visiting regularly, their only touch may be during therapy or activities. Never forget how strongly one is affected and nurtured by holding hands, hugging or just touching another in a loving and appropriate way.

Groups are important socially and are clinically used as a means of assessing one's social functioning. Social functioning tells us a great deal as it is always impacted by physical and mental changes. We can begin to see changes in how an individual responds to others. Some of these changes will be directly correlated to depression, medical change of condition, cognitive changes and/or sensory changes.

Because being with others enhances our ability to cope with changes in our lives, we are always in the business of encouraging an individual to spend time with others. The phrase, "friends can be good medicine" has been clinically researched. Friends do profoundly impact one's sense of well-being and the ability to cope and build resiliency.

Chapter 6
Activities

According to both federal and state regulations, and to meet the need of the people we serve, each setting is required to provide a meaningful and purposeful program of activities. This program should be for each and every individual regardless of ability or limitation. The intent is to assure that leisure and recreation needs are being met for people who no longer live at home or who have lost the ability to move about in the community. Therapeutic activities within a clinical setting are provided in order to meet specialized and individualized needs.

Activity Suggestions

This section of the chapter discusses the overall requirements for activities. If an activity program is going to be successful, it must provide all of these elements at the level appropriate for each individual:

1. Orientation and direction
2. Reassurance
3. Physical contact
4. Consistent routine
5. Choices that can be understood
6. Appropriate levels of stress
7. Verbal cues
8. Movement
9. Past identity
10. Socialization
11. Reminiscence

How do we accomplish this? Perhaps the best place to start is by modifying the environment. Decreased functioning can lead to situations in which the individual feels trapped in an environment that poses an apparently unsolvable problem and the person is unable to change or influence the situation.

1. Reduce noise and visual distractions
   a. Limit group size
   b. Limit number of people giving instructions
   c. Decrease background noises (TV, intercom, etc.)
   d. Show resident sound sources

2. Increase environmental clues
    a. Use color for identification (or shapes, animals, flowers, food, etc.)
    b. Reduce glare (carpet floors, move light sources, seat residents with their back to light source)
    c. Eliminate prints and patterns on floors, walls and furniture
    d. Choose strong contrasting colors for backgrounds
    e. Allow time to adjust from outdoor to indoor lighting

3. Re-direct wandering behaviors
    a. Camouflage doors with barriers or room dividers
    b. Increase staff awareness of their own entering and leaving
    c. Try to schedule activities at shift change as distraction
    d. Place two doorknobs on each door leading from the unit. Individuals with dementia usually cannot figure out how to open a door if they need to turn two doorknobs.

4. Maintain each person's normal schedule as much as possible (helps person's sense of control)
    a. Clothing/dressing
    b. Bathing/showering time
    c. Reading/buying newspaper
    d. Church services

Leisure, Leisure, Leisure

For most individuals the concept of leisure brings to mind *time* that is available to pursue hobbies and interests. The experience may be for relaxation or rejuvenation. It may be therapeutic or just recreational. Some individuals view leisure as a *state of mind*, having little to do with blocks of time. For these individuals, almost any activity, including work, can be viewed as a positive leisure experience. The way leisure is perceived is an important part of each person's personality.

The amount of free time available to individuals who are institutionalized is much greater than at any other time in their adult lives. In order to understand individuals, we need to understand their era and values. This is known as the "cohort factor." A cohort group is a group of people who share a common characteristic, life event or interest. Men who grew up in the United States during the depression, who fought together in World War II, then engaged in similar activities after the war (e.g., fraternal organizations) would be a cohort group. Many people, particularly those growing up in the early 1900's, give very little importance to this thing called leisure. Their work ethic usually made them value their work over the rest of their activities.

Often people view "leisure" as free time away from occupation or survival, but it can be so much more than that. Leisure is as much a state of mind as it is the availability of time. The people we serve tend to have a great deal of free time away from occupation (almost all will be retired) and may no longer be able to take care of themselves and others. Because of the functional losses they have experienced they may need our help to fill the day with leisure pursuits that increase their quality of life. The professional should keep in mind that:
- Leisure is a state of mind or an attitude.
- Leisure motivates us to recreate.
- Leisure is more the feeling experienced than the activity in which you are involved.

Some elements of leisure are
- antithesis of work
- pleasant expectations and recollections (reminiscing)
- minimal social role obligations
- psychological perception of freedom
- close relation to values of the culture (cohort factor)

Important factors of leisure for a recreation leader:
1. You need to be aware of your own definition and attitude regarding leisure and its significance to quality of life.
2. Before you can promote leisure involvement in others, you should look inside and determine your personal motivation.
3. Leisure experiences are energizing, relaxing, stress reducing, challenging, playful and freeing. They promote personal growth. They can be experienced both in a group and individually.
4. The desire to be involved in a leisure pursuit is innate. Leisure itself is learned. So if you are interested in quality of life in your older years, you need to nurture this aspect of your life when you are young. Start today.

Leisure Room[28]

While working as activity professionals, we realized there was a need to have resources more readily available and accessible to the people we serve and the people providing activities.

We felt that the answer was a room containing supplies and resources for a diverse population of individuals. The room would be available during the day and scheduled, with supervision. This leisure resource room would provide independence, access, creativity and learning opportunities both on a one-on-one and group basis.

The Leisure Resource Room provides a vast variety of tools for reality orientation, sensory stimulation, reminiscing, exercise and educational growth. There may be musical tapes, equipment and games. Pets can be brought in for visits and pet care.

The resources and supplies can constantly change as needs change. Newer equipment can be added and new ideas tried. Workstations can be developed and redeveloped. The people we serve and their families will add new ideas and be a good resource for future equipment needs.

In one area of the room, an individual with dementia may be engaged in a sensory stimulation activity, while another individual may be watching a movie with a headset on. People may come in to watch others or to see the promotions for the book of the week.

The table space can be used for small sensory awareness groups along with special events such as birthdays, showers and outside speakers.

This room is a wonderful space for those with busy therapy schedules during the day who would like to be involved in leisure events after dinner. The hours for this room would depend on individual needs and schedules.

How to Develop this Idea

The first step is a review of your budget. What is the monthly budget for activities? How is it spent? Divide the budget money so as to continue purchasing needed monthly items and begin to add new items and supplies for this new area. Each month you should be purchasing educational, musical and creative equipment that can be used for many reasons and with a variety of individuals.

If your budget does not allow for new capital expenditures, seek out donations, discounted merchandise and items found in garage sales.

---

[28] by Pat Hubbard, AC, SSD and Elizabeth Best Martini, MS, CTRS, ACC. Used with permission.

Finding a Room

Look around and reassess space usage in your facility. Do you have a large open area that the people you serve spend time in? Are there chairs, a table, a TV? Does it have potential for this type of resource room? If so, you could have cabinets made which can be locked when staff leave for the day.

Many older facilities have a large living area off of the front entrance. Perhaps there is potential in this area. People usually congregate in the front anyway and this would be bringing the activities to them.

These changes do not have to occur overnight. Begin by building onto what is already there. Add to this with activity supplies and equipment.

Use volunteers, family members and scheduled assistants to occupy the room throughout the day, facilitating small groups and assisting independent leisure pursuits.

Ask nursing assistants and other staff to bring individuals to the resource room. A few minutes of encouragement will make a difference.

This room could also be interdisciplinary in nature. The occupational therapist or speech therapist is always looking for a stimulating environment in which to work and the supplies are all accessible for ready use.

Who Uses the Room

All of the people we serve use the room. Now you have an area where all activity equipment is available for use. There will be no more running around to store and retrieve materials.

Think of the possibilities in helping to meet individual needs and provide a safe and structured environment for staff to bring all the people they serve. The possibilities are as endless as the imagination in developing activity goals and programs.

Of course you need to let the rest of the staff know about the room. At the end of the section is a suggested flyer to give to other members of the treatment team.

What to Purchase

Since the Resource Room is locked up when activity staff are off duty, you now can purchase valuable equipment that can be seen and kept for repeated use. Educational books and equipment are no longer kept in boxes or storage to be brought out on special occasions.

The equipment used in this room should meet the needs of the majority of the people you serve. Is there a larger population of individuals diagnosed with Alzheimer's or dementia-related disorders or are there alert individuals who are physically unable to be fully independent? The population dictates purchasing needs.

Create a wish list of supplies and keep a file of supply items and ideas for future reference. The next page has a list of ideas to start with.

Leisure Room Supplies

Supplies need to be safe, stimulating, purposeful, colorful, age appropriate, accessible and used as a resource by all staff.

Equipment and Supplies:

- VCR and tapes
- TV
- Slide projector
- Encyclopedias
- Typewriter
- Pens and paper
- Adult coloring books, art projects
- Poetry books, short stories, books on art, history, health
- Sensory supplies such as soft puzzles, stuffed animals
- Auditory discrimination games, sorting games, mirrors
- Adaptive devices for writing, hearing and seeing
- Trivia questions
- Etch-A-Sketch
- Mystery box to place hands in and guess object
- Exercise equipment and supplies of all sizes and shapes
- Rhythm sticks
- Tangle game
- Pictures sorted according to objects and themes
- Record player/CD player/tape deck with good speakers, head sets
- Records, tapes and CDs
- Guitar
- Video game player
- Aquarium
- Homemaking tasks — folding napkins, sorting silverware in a container, counting paper money
- Bird cage
- Large print books, fabric sample books, greeting card books, carpet samples
- Miscellaneous games and large puzzles
- Colorful posters
- Sorting games
- Collection of balls (large and small of various textures)
- Sensory boxes according to theme
- Magnetic letters and board
- Grooming kits (need to be individualized)
- Makeup mirror
- Familiar items such as kitchen utensils, hats, gloves, hankies, ties
- Large dominoes, cards, checkers
- Magazines and pictures to sort through and look at
- Large blocks and dice to move and stack
- Sensory apron
- Laundry baskets for storage
- Scarf collection
- Olfactory stimulation kit
- Woodworking ideas: hardware trays, sanding projects, key collections
- Velcro games
- Computer(s) with Internet connections

The Leisure Room Concept

The following is an example of a notice that could be posted on the bulletin board outside of the leisure room.

> The leisure room is designed to provide available leisure activities and supplies to the people we serve with varying levels of needs. The supplies and equipment are accessible for use by all staff to enhance interaction, socialization and a multi-dimensional sensory stimulation experience.
>
> Because this room is created to encourage active participation at all levels, the supplies are kept in this room and need to be supervised and protected by all staff members. This is a room designed to enhance quality of life for the people we serve. It belongs to all of us and needs to be watched over by all of us.

Supplies will be kept in clear bins, which are marked according to level of cognitive and functional abilities. If a CNA brings an individual into the room and provides him/her with one of these supply items, s/he must return to the room within a short time to reassess how the individual is doing.

The activity staff will schedule times when staff and volunteers will supervise the room. These hours will be posted. When there is no structured supervision, the responsibility lies with the CNA for both supervision and proper management of the materials (i.e. placing supplies within reach, introducing new activities and putting away supplies in appropriate places).

Any comments, recommendations and requests in regards to the room and supplies should be discussed with the activity staff.

Therapeutic Activities

The importance of therapeutic activities is that they focus on individual interests and personalities and that they focus on *abilities* as opposed to *limitations*. If we can assist an individual in focusing on the strengths s/he still has, his/her limitations seem somehow more manageable. If you are working with an individual who feels that life is over because s/he has lost the ability to write due to a stroke, you can support him/her in therapy goals, encourage trying something new or find another individual with a similar situation for mutual support. There are many options.

Many times, the importance of therapeutic activities is not measured by the activity itself, but rather in the value of the individual's involvement. Each activity has a purpose and a goal and within that activity each individual has a purpose and a goal.

For all people the daily pursuit for quality of life and meaning is of profound importance. Sometimes, the only way to characterize this pursuit is as a struggle. Nevertheless, it is a most worthy struggle and one that the professional carries on with dignity, courage, knowledge and professional expertise.

It is somewhat ironic that many professionals in charge of planning the activities of others do not look to their own lives and choices for insights into leisure options and motives. Ask yourself the following questions:
- What is it that you do in your leisure?
- Do you enjoy being alone or with others?
- Do your interests vary or do you always seek out the familiar?
- Do you value leisure time as an important component of your own quality of life?
- If you were living in an assisted living community or a long term care setting, could you still continue with your personal leisure interests? What help would you need from other people?
- Could these interests help you in dealing with new situations and problems?
- Could they bring meaning to your life? In what way?

Activity Supplies

Certain equipment is required for running activity programs. Even if you can't put together all of the supplies for a Leisure Room, we recommend that you have the following basic equipment somewhere in your facility which can be used for activities:

- Slide projector
- Large print books
- Cards
- Bingo games
- Newspaper
- Magazines
- TV & VCR
- Eraser boards
- Puzzles

- Stereo and tape deck(s) with 4 to 6 headsets, musical tapes and CDs
- Reality orientation boards

- Exercise balls
- Pens, paints, brushes
- Word games
- Bowling set
- Paper assortment
- Trivia

- Scrabble
- Crossword puzzles
- Pokeno
- Parachute
- Scissors

Keeping track of your supplies is an important part of running activities. The chart on the following page shows one format for keeping track of supplies used for sensory stimulation that are distributed throughout your facility. Whether you use the Leisure Room concept or not, you will still have some of your supplies in different parts of the facility. This form provides a way to keep track of where they are.

This is the kind of form that needs to be updated often if you are planning to use it to find out where something is. A white board that can be changed as supplies are moved or a computer program that is easy to use are ways to keep track of your supplies on an ongoing basis. This might be a good project for a volunteer.

If you really don't mind looking for supplies, then a form like this can be filled out every few months to be sure that you still have enough usable supplies where your volunteers, staff and/or the people you serve can get to them easily.

(Please note that the numbers of items in the activity supply list are not recommendations about the number of items you should have in your facility. That decision comes from your analysis of the needs of the people you serve.)

Activity Supply List

Date: _____

Supply Item	Leisure Room	Station One	Station Two	Station Three
Tangle	4	2		
Slinky	3	1		1
Magnetic letters	3 sets			
Frog Tac Toe	1			2
Sing-a-long radio	2	1	1	1
Stacking blocks	2 sets			
Tape recorder	2	1	1	1
Tapes	23	12	4	18
Ring toss	1			
Parachute	2			
Dominoes	2		1	
Large print cards	4	1	1	
Flash cards	3	2	2	1
Coaster sets for stacking	3			
Clothespins	1 box		1 box	
Grooming items		2	2	3
Writing materials	3	2	2	1
Trivia games	2			
Velcro catch game	2			
Pat mats		1	1	
Scissors and paper	1	1	2	1
Checkers	2			
Plastic puzzles	3			
Koosh balls	1	2	1	1
Eraser board	2			
Safety locks and bicycle chains	3			
Maps	6	2	2	1

Comments:

Activity Analysis

Therapeutic activities are designed and provided to enhance the individual treatment goals for each person that we serve. When you have determined what the activity treatment goals will be, the next step is to analyze each activity. You can do so by using the form on the next page.

The purpose of this process is to separate the components of the activity and to determine what skills are needed in order to successfully participate and complete the activity.

Analyzing an activity occurs separately from assessing the individual. These are two separate assessment processes. By breaking an activity down into separate components, the professional can recommend specific programs which will enhance interdisciplinary goals and can assist in adapting them to the needs and abilities of the individual.

The left side of the activity analysis form addresses the administrative components of an activity. Fill this in for each of the activities offered in your program. The right side of the activity analysis form focuses on the other components of the activity. Use this as a means of walking yourself through an activity experience to determine whom it would be most appropriate for and also to determine what adaptations may be needed in order to offer it to a wider range of individuals.

Each time that you design a new group activity, complete an activity analysis form. This documents your thoroughness and professionalism in designing a meaningful program.

In analyzing activities, you also want to recognize the type of social skills required to participate in the group. As the coordinator, you need to know what the purpose of the group is along with what type of interaction is expected of each individual. Will s/he be interacting with others, needing to work cooperatively, sitting with others but not required to socialize or share tools?

These are very important questions to ask. If you have an individual whom you have assessed as being in need of stimulation, but unable to tolerate other people too close to him/her, you need to closely evaluate and determine what type of setting would meet his/her needs. S/he could handle an independent project at one table alone while other residents are seated at another table in the same room.

If you are interested in outlining the activity without the additional analysis, there is an excellent form in *The Album of Activity Policy and Procedures Manual* written by Recreation Therapy Consultants, (858) 546-9003.

Activity Analysis Form

Activity _____

Type of Activity _____

Physical Aspects

Body Position Requirements:
sit _____ stand _____ walk _____
one handed _____ two handed _____
eye/hand coordination _____
gross motor _____ fine motor _____

Administrative Aspects

Goal: _____

_____

Equipment & Supplies: _____

_____

_____

Sense Requirements:
touch _____ taste _____ sight _____
hearing _____ smell _____

Skills/Limitations of Participants: _____

_____

_____

_____

Physical Requirements:
endurance _____ speed _____
strength _____
cardiovascular activity needed _____

Social Aspects

Procedures: _____

_____

_____

_____

_____

_____

_____

_____

_____

1:1 activity _____ small group _____
requires ongoing conversation _____
requires ability to share/cooperate _____
requires ability to listen _____
requires tolerance of close proximity _____
independent work within a group _____

Cognitive Aspects

attention span _____
memory: long term _____ short term _____
thinking: abstract _____ concrete _____
sequencing skills needed _____
problem-solving skills needed _____
time given for response:
    yes _____ no _____
object identification _____
directionality _____
amount of concentration needed _____
requires ability to follow _____ step
    directions

Length of Activity: _____

_____

_____

Precautions: _____

_____

Affective (Emotional) Aspects

use of past skills _____
use of past memories _____
highlights individuality _____
increases sense of self _____
promotes body awareness _____
fosters sense of belonging _____
experiences sense of success _____
anticipation, anxiety _____
requires use of new skills _____

_____

_____

Adaptations: _____

_____

_____

Coordinator: _____ Date: _____

Theme Activities

Before we look at the activities as they are divided into the different levels, we want to discuss theme activities. The basic idea behind a theme activity is to create an experience that is appropriate for residents with many different levels of functioning. Tying many activities in one theme area over a period of days or weeks helps facilitate memory as many activities reinforce one idea. Another benefit of using themes over a specific period of time is that it helps the people you serve measure the passing of time — helping create distinct units of time so that everything doesn't just blend together. An example of an activity based on a mountain theme is shown below.[29]

Mountain Theme[30]

Trigger Words: trees, streams, pine cones, log cabin, camping

Enhancing the Activity Environment:
- Gather bark, pine needles, pine cones, soil, rocks
- Paint trees on butcher paper
- Scent paper with wood musk perfume
- Burn incense of pine
- Play environmental tapes of the wind blowing, birds singing, thunder
- Hang Christmas lights on ceilings to simulate stars
- Use backpacks to hold supplies
- Have a parachute with a fan to simulate clouds and wind
- Wildflowers
- Potpourri sachet
- Pelts from furrier

Activities:
- Create nature trails indoors or out
- Make group mural using pine needles for forest floor, tissue paper for leaves or dried leaves. Apply with spray adhesive
- Make bird feeders with pinecones, peanut butter and sprinkle birdseed on the peanut butter. Hang it outside
- Paint a tree branch on fabric (drapery size) and hang. Use it for hanging valentines, shamrocks, etc.
- Create a campfire and sing songs
- Make toasted marshmallows or s'mores
- Invite SPCA to bring animals who live in the forest — rabbits, owls, birds
- Flashlight games/tracking
- Fishing game
- Storytelling

---

[29] An excellent resource addressing the issues of themes, special needs and programming for all levels is *Creative Forecasting*, PO Box 7789, Colorado Springs, CO 80933-7789. Phone: 719-633-3174, fax: 719-632-4721.
[30] From Ann Nathan and Elizabeth Best Martini, used with permission.

Theme Weeks

Here are four mini themes with ideas that can be used throughout a week. Expand and adapt these activities as desired and have fun.[31]

Humor

April Fools' Day Discussion
Origin of April Fools' Day: Source: Panti's Extraordinary Origins of Everyday Things.

There are many theories about the origin of this day, but the most accepted one seems to be that it originated in France in the 16th century due to a change in the Gregorian calendar. New Year's Day was observed on March 25, the advent of spring. The celebrations, which included exchanging gifts, ran for a week and ended with dinners and parties on April 1. King Charles announced that New Year's Day would be moved to January 1 in 1564. Many Frenchmen who didn't accept or hear about the change had parties and exchanged gifts on April 1 and were called "April Fools." People sent foolish gifts and invitations to nonexistent parties to those who celebrated on the old New Year's date. These individuals became known as a poisson d'Avril or "April fish" because at that time of year the sun was leaving the zodiac sign of Pisces, the fish. It took almost 200 years for the custom of the April Fool jokes to reach England and later, to America.

Pranks
Read the following pranks that others have done on April Fools' Day and ask the participants to discuss pranks they have done or heard about.
- Putting salt in the sugar bowl
- Putting pepper in fudge
- Substituting pickle juice for apple juice (in a glass at breakfast)
- Gluing a penny to the pavement
- Stuffing a biscuit with cotton
- Saying "You have a black mark on your face"
- Taping filing cabinets closed
- Taping down telephone hook so phone will continue to ring after being answered
- Stapling folders together

Funny Foods

Make the following recipes during a cooking activity.

April Fools' Candy
        1 cup milk
        1 envelope Knox gelatin
        6 oz (1 cup) chocolate chips

In the top of a double boiler pan, pour in milk, and stir in gelatin until dissolved. Place top pan over pan of water and turn heat to medium. Pour in chips and melt them in the milk and gelatin mixture, stirring constantly. Pour mixture into a greased, 9" square pan. Put pan in refrigerator, and the candy will be ready to eat in approximately 10 minutes. Yield: 25 pieces. Per Serving — 40 calories, 2 g fat, < 1 mg chol, 5 g carbo, <1 g protein, Exchanges — ½ starch.

---

[31] By Mary Anne Clagett, CTRS, ACC. Reprinted with permission from *Creative Forecasting*, A monthly publication for Activity and Recreation Professionals.

Ants on a Log

> celery, cheddar cheese spread, cream cheese, peanut butter, raisins

Wash and dry celery. Cut into 3"- 4" pieces. Stuff with cheddar cheese, cream cheese or peanut butter. Add raisins on top.

Funny Charades

Write each action listed on a slip of paper and put in a basket for participants to draw and act out. This would make an excellent intergenerational activity. The actions may need to be adapted depending on the ages of the children. For younger children, ask each child to imitate an animal for participants to guess.

- Pose like the Statue of Liberty
- Sing a lullaby to a baby
- Pantomime shaving
- Play a harp
- East very spicy food
- Imitate a girl scared by a mouse
- Eat spaghetti
- Roll out cookie dough
- Put on makeup
- Drive a car on a bumpy road
- Paint a portrait
- Fly a glider
- Polish shoes
- Catch and reel in a fish
- Hang a picture on wall
- Play marbles
- Fly a kite

Sensory Stimulation

Here are some items to use with your participants who are low functioning. Encourage them to touch, hold and identify: pictures of clown (or a visiting clown), unusual hats, comic books and Sunday comics.

Broadway

Discussion Topics

History (Source: *Broadway* by Brooks Atkinson)

New York City's world-famous Broadway area is the center of professional theater in the United States. Broadway is the theater district in midtown Manhattan. In 1900, it was 1 ½ miles long; it was less than half that length in 1950 and was six blocks in 1970. In 1900, sixteen of the Broadway theaters were located on Broadway; in 1950, only three were located there; in 1970, two. Most of the houses for legitimate theater are on side streets but are known as Broadway Houses.

From 1900 to World War I, Broadway attracted large audiences of middle class people who were in search of amusement, excitement and romance. The shows did not seem to depict any relation to art or life. Between the two World Wars, Broadway was bursting with energy and enterprise; the new dramatists and people of the theater were full of hope and fresh ideas and were enthusiastic about new styles of craftsmanship. During those dynamic years, Broadway greatly influenced the theater of the world. During World War II, and even a few years before the war, Broadway began to lose originality and drive. There were fewer dramatists, and there was competition from television and motion pictures.

Reminisce about the Following Topics
- Ask participants to tell about the Broadway and off-Broadway productions they have seen.
- Ask each participant to tell about the best theater show/play s/he has seen (not necessarily on Broadway).

- Encourage individuals to share experiences of acting on stage at any level (i.e., school, church, professional).

Guess the Musical Word Game

Ask your participants to complete the names of the popular musicals that appeared on Broadway.

- Annie Get Your _____ GUN
- Bye Bye _____ BIRDIE
- Damn _____ YANKEES
- Fiddler on the _____ ROOF
- Finian's _____ RAINBOW
- Funny _____ GIRL
- Gentlemen Prefer _____ BLONDES
- Guys and _____ DOLLS
- Hello, _____ DOLLY!
- Jesus Christ, _____ SUPERSTAR
- The King and _____ I
- Kiss Me, _____ KATE
- Li'l _____ ABNER

- The Music _____ MAN
- My Fair _____ LADY
- Paint Your _____ WAGON
- Peter _____ PAN
- The Pirates of _____ PENZANCE
- Show _____ BOAT
- The Sound of _____ MUSIC
- South _____ PACIFIC
- A Tree Grows in _____ BROOKLYN
- The Unsinkable _____ _____ MOLLY BROWN
- West Side _____ STORY

One-word musical titles (that could not be included in the word game) include *Brigadoon*, *Cabaret*, *Camelot*, *Carousel*, *Cats*, *Gypsy*, *Hair*, *Kismet*, *Oklahoma*, and *Oliver*.

Lights, Cameras, Action

Form a Drama Club. If some of the participants want to act out a scene from a Broadway play or learn some songs from a musical, this would be an excellent opportunity. Many public, college and university libraries have scripts that can be checked out. Participants can perform for the club or, on a larger scale, before an audience. Invite a Drama Club from a high school to visit and perform an act of the play they are working on and/or take an outing to see the school's production.

Sensory Stimulation

Here are some items to use with low functioning participants. Encourage them to touch, hold, and identify; top hat, cane, songs from poplar musicals (use list in word game) to listen to, and camcorder.

Ask participants to do some simple pantomimes. These movements are meant to stimulate long term memories. Suggestions include: play a piano, knead bread dough, stir cookie dough, open a book, type on typewriter, catch and reel in a fish, play a violin, hang clothes on the line, shake wrinkles out of a scarf, nod head yes, shake head no, shrug shoulders.

Rain Showers

History of Umbrellas Discussion Topics

The umbrella is one of the oldest artifacts in man's history and was a familiar item in many cultures by the time man began to write. The umbrella originated in Mesopotamia (an ancient region of southwest Asia in modern-day Iraq) in 1400 B.C. It was an extension of the fan, protecting people from the harsh sun. The word "umbrella" is derived from the Latin umbra, meaning shade. This use of the umbrella continued for centuries. Greek and Roman women used umbrellas or parasols, as they were also called, as sunshields, but the cultures regarded them as effeminate. Roman women began the practice of oiling paper sunshields, to waterproof them. Sun parasols and rain umbrellas were used by women well into the 18th century in Europe and later in America. Men continued to wear hats in the rain and got soaked. It took a British gentleman, Jonas Hanway, more than 30 years to convince other British men that umbrellas were more practical and cheaper than hailing a coach every time it rained. By the mid-1780's, British gentlemen were using umbrellas, also called "Hanways."

"April Showers Bring May Flowers"

Ask the participants to share old wives' tales about how to predict rain. Here are some common weather superstitions to stimulate conversation.
- Rain will come when the north wind shifts to the west and then to the south.
- It will rain when the sky is dark to the west.
- It will rain when there is a ring around the moon.
- If dogs eat grass, there will be rain, maybe a storm.
- If a pig carries straw in its mouth, a storm is on the way.
- When cricket chirps grow long or strong, a storm is coming.

Rainbows

When sunlight passes through raindrops (or fog or mist), the water bends the light rays and forms bands of color. The most brightly colored rainbows occur when the raindrops are large. A person can only see a rainbow when his back is to the sun.

The colors of a rainbow always appear in the same order: red, orange, yellow, green, blue and violet. Red is the brightest band of color, running along the top of the bow. Then come the other colors, each paler than the last. Violet is the hardest to see.

Rainbow Party

Decorate the area with rainbow colors. Place a pot of gold (gold-foil covered chocolate coins or other treats) at the end of a rainbow on the refreshment table. For an activity, play the word game below.

"Bow" Guessing Game

All answers begin with "bou" or "bow."
- Clear, thin broth BOUILLON
- Something that indicates a border or limit BOUNDARY
- Container used for holding food or liquid BOWL
- Cluster of flowers BOUQUET
- Small, retail shop that specializes in goods BOUTIQUE
- Another name for a derby hat BOWLER
- One who pursues a criminal or fugitive for whom a reward is offered BOUNTY HUNTER
- Marked by abundance BOUNTIFUL
- Game played by rolling a ball in an attempt to knock over pins BOWLING
- Knot with large, decorative knots BOW KNOT
- Knot that forms a loop that does not slip BOWLINE
- Type of whiskey BOURBON
- Rubber ball does this when thrown on the ground BOUNCE
- Broad city street, often tree-lined and landscaped BOULEVARD
- Cord attached to both ends of an archer's bow BOW STRING
- Another word for a match BOUT
- Former name of Hoover Dam BOULDER DAM
- Short necktie BOW TIE
- Held at the end of the college football season BOWL GAMES
- Flower or small bunch of flowers worn in a buttonhole BOUTONNIERE
- Bark of a dog BOW-WOW

Ask a staff or family member to sing "Somewhere Over the Rainbow" from the movie, *The Wizard of Oz*, to close the party. (Arrange this before the party.)

Sensory Stimulation

Here are items to use with low functioning participants. Encourage participants to touch, hold, and identify: different types of watering cans, umbrellas raincoat, rain gauge, items with rainbows on them and prisms shining in sunlight (so participants can see their reflections).

World of Disney

Walt Disney's Life Discussion Topics

SOURCE: *The Story of Walt Disney* by Bernice Seldon
- 1901 Walter Elias Disney is born on December 5.
- 1918 Walt goes to France to work for the Red Cross Ambulance Corps.
- 1919 Walt gets his first job as an artist and later starts the Laugh-O-Gram Company.
- 1923 Walt creates the Alice in Cartoonland series. He moves to Hollywood and forms the Walt Disney Studio.
- 1928 Mickey Mouse is born. Steamboat Willie (the cartoon Mickey stars in) opens in New York City.
- 1933 Walt creates The Three Little Pigs.
- 1934 Donald Duck makes his debut.
- 1937 Walt creates Snow White and the Seven Dwarfs.
- 1940 Walt creates Pinocchio. The Disney Studio moves to Burbank.
- 1941 Walt creates Dumbo.
- 1942 Walt creates Bambi (Disney's favorite film).
- 1948 Walt produces his first nature film, Seal Island.
- 1955 Disneyland opens in Anaheim, CA. The Mickey Mouse Club TV show begins.
- 1964 Walt produces Mary Poppins.
- 1966 Walt Disney dies on December 15.
- 1971 Walt Disney World opens in Orlando, FL.
- 1983 Tokyo Disneyland opens in Japan.
- 1986 Walt Disney Productions changes its name to Walt Disney Company.
- 1989 The Disney MGM Studios Theme Park opens at Walt Disney World in Florida.
- 1992 Euro-Disneyland opens near Paris, France.

Use the Following Topics to Stimulate Conversation:
- First Disney film you saw
- Favorite Disney film
- Favorite Disney character
- Disney's approach to song as story
- This quote was made in 1937 during the production of his first animated feature, Snow White and the Seven Dwarfs. "It can still be good music and not follow the same pattern everybody in the country has followed. Really, we should set a pattern — a new way to use music — weave it into the story so somebody doesn't just burst into song."

Disney Movies' Music

Ask participants to tell the name of the movie that each song is from.
- Whistle While You Work SNOW WHITE AND THE SEVEN DWARFS
- Chim Chim Cher-ee MARY POPPINS
- Once Upon a Dream SLEEPING BEAUTY
- Zip-A-Dee-Doo-Dah SONG OF THE SOUTH
- You Can Fly! You Can Fly! You Can Fly PETER PAN
- Who's Afraid of the Big Bad Wolf? THREE LITTLE PIGS

- I've Got No Strings PINOCCHIO
- Cruella De Vil 101 DALMATIANS
- The Siamese Cat Song LADY AND THE TRAMP
- When You Wish Upon a Star PINOCCHIO
- Heigh-Ho SNOW WHITE AND THE SEVEN DWARFS
- Supercalifragilisticexpialidocious MARY POPPINS
- A Whole New World ALADDIN
- Under the Sea THE LITTLE MERMAID
- I'm Late ALICE IN WONDERLAND
- The Bare Necessities THE JUNGLE BOOK
- Bibbidi-Bobbidi-Boo CINDERELLA
- Be Our Guest BEAUTY AND THE BEAST
- Hakuna Matata THE LION KING
- Colors of the Wind POCAHONTAS

Intergenerational Disney Character Party

Involve participants in choosing the theme and planning the party. Choosing a theme will help plan the decorations, activities and food. Invite a group of children to the party. Activities could include the showing of the movie (used for the theme), Disney Fashion Show (individuals showing off their Disney clothes) and songs from Disney movies sung by volunteers (this will need to be planned beforehand so singers can prepare). Ask participants and the children to wear their favorite Disney clothing. If some individuals don't have clothing with Disney characters, give them mouse ears made out of construction paper.

Sensory Stimulation

Here are some items to use with low functioning participants. Encourage them to touch, hold, and identify a variety of Disney characters ranging from stuffed animals, pictures, and memorabilia; music and song from early Disney films; videos from early Disney films (i.e. Snow White and the Seven Dwarfs, Pinocchio, Bambi). Show first 10 minutes of the videos as participants may recall some of the characters.

Intergenerational Programs[32]

"People of all ages can be friends," Daisy answered when I asked her why she, an eight-year-old girl, enjoyed participating in an intergenerational program.

"My own children, even my grandchildren, are grown-ups now. An adult is not nearly as interesting as a bright, young child. I enjoy sharing ideas with them and hearing about their lives," explained Ted, a former college professor, when asked the same question.

These simple statements contain the components for a successful intergenerational program. These components are 1. acceptance and enjoyment of each other's differences, 2. sharing ideas and 3. caring. The task is to provide an atmosphere that will allow these characteristics to flourish.

In 1989 we wanted to start a program that would provide a framework for children's and senior's natural affinity to blossom. There wasn't a lot of information available on the sort of program that we envisioned, so the learning process has been through trial and error. We have had a few disasters and many high points. As our awareness of our strengths and limitations has grown, along with our ability to trust the process, our program has become a happy event for all of us.

---

[32] *Intergenerational Program* is from Marcia Weldon. Used with permission.

Know Your Participants

However, don't assume that all seniors will enjoy children and that all children will enjoy seniors.

A new woman in our group was a retired schoolteacher. Because of this we assumed she would be ideal for our intergenerational program. It soon became apparent she felt that children were just one step above slime on the evolutionary ladder. Fortunately, we discovered this before she joined the program or her presence would have caused a few tears and nasty comments.

Another woman, Esther, was also a retired schoolteacher. On our visits with the children there were always at least four little girls hovering around her. She was able to hold an audience of 20 seniors and 30 children listening in rapt attention to her stories. (She must have been a fabulous teacher). The rule we learned from this is to know the seniors in the program and not to push anyone. Don't assume that because a person was a schoolteacher s/he loves children. Conversely, don't assume that a well-worn Merchant Marine won't melt when s/he is around the kids. Children bring out qualities in seniors that will surprise you!

How to Get a Program Started

The ideal situation is if you have a school-aged family member or a friend who can introduce you to a teacher. Most teachers are open to having an intergenerational program. If you don't know someone who is a teacher, make an appointment with the principal of the grade school closest to your facility. Discuss your program idea. They will tell you which teacher would likely be interested. (Usually it is a teacher with an interest in history.)

Set up an appointment with this teacher. Ask him/her the level of the children's writing and reading abilities. We've done this program with preschool, second, third and fourth graders. Our personal preference is the fourth grade. Nine and ten year-olds are young enough to be openly creative and harbor fewer preconceived notions than adults while possessing good verbal and writing skills.

Our favorite teacher has the qualities that work best for our program. She is flexible and organized. You may have very different needs. What is important is to determine your needs and find someone who will fulfill them.

The Seniors Who Are Involved

Having tried this with both the frail elderly and with those who attend adult day health centers, our preference is for the latter. However, if you have a stable population of high-functioning adults in your assisted living or long term care facility, this activity could be perfect for them.

If your seniors will forget the children's visits or if you have a largely fluctuating population due to death, your program will be of a different sort than the one described here. The seniors and children will still enjoy each other's company, but they might not experience connections that are as deep or lasting.

The Time Involved

1.   1 – 1½ hours of group work each week, reading and responding to children's correspondence.
2.   One visit every 1½ – 2 months, alternating between the school and your facility.

Your Facility

Please don't invite children to your facility if you have a lot of people sitting in the halls, people screaming or strong odors. One of the positive aspects of this program is to familiarize children with the elderly and to those people with physical disabilities. Ideally, they will take this comfort into their adulthood. Scaring them will have the opposite effect. If your facility sounds like the one above, meet the children in a park or only go to their school.

Introduction — A Beginning

After finding a teacher and a classroom, you can begin your program a few weeks after school begins. We start the program by taking photographs of our participating seniors. We mount them on a poster board. When that is completed, we spend an hour asking the seniors in our group to dictate an introductory letter for us to take to the children's classroom. (They might include anecdotes, jokes, their philosophy of life, etc. How they describe themselves as a group is enlightening.) We take the letter to the children's classroom and read it to them.

We leave the poster with our pictures in their classroom and take pictures of the children to hang on the wall of our facility. We use the pictures as a stimulus for the seniors to discuss the activities they'd like to participate in with the children. We make lists.

Remember: You build the frame; let the seniors and children paint the picture. This is their project!

First Visit

Before the first visit we have exchanged several letters and/or drawings. (As group leader it usually works best to let the seniors dictate what they want to say. You write it down in one joint letter.) This creates a discussion group and the seniors get to learn things about each other they never knew before. Also, it allows participation for everyone, regardless of dexterity with a pen.

The children enjoy sending separate letters and drawings. Resist the temptation to tie specific children and seniors together in a pen pal, one-on-one situation. If someone is sick during a visit or drops out of the program, their pen pal will be very disappointed. It's best to let friendships develop naturally.

Halloween is the perfect time for a first visit. If the children come to your facility, ask the teacher if they can wear their Halloween costumes. The seniors can also wear costumes, hats and/or makeup applied at the facility or at home. Get your staff involved. We have made trick-or-treats and created a spook house in a bathroom.

Throughout the school year, every month and holiday will suggest a project. Here are a few ideas we have enjoyed sharing with each other. These are a sampling of the activities our children and seniors have participated in together. You are limited only by your imagination and the excitement of your participants.

1. Letters on construction paper leaves: "What I'm Thankful For."
2. Letters at Christmas, i.e. "My Favorite Christmas."
3. Making and exchanging Christmas gifts.
4. Hopes, fears and wishes for the New Year
5. "The First President I Remember." (Some seniors remember hearing a president speak in their hometowns when they were children, etc.)
6. Making Valentines.
7. Making a huge paper quilt (1–2 children and 1 senior per square), collage forms.
8. Seniors begin story/poem; child finishes it.
9. Child or senior tells dream; child or senior illustrates it.
10. Trading riddles and jokes.
11. EAT LUNCH TOGETHER!!!
12. Overlaid and printed hand prints.
13. Sock hop.
14. Compile a book of all the stories, poems, etc., you've created. Give a copy to all involved and present one to the school library during a visit to the school.
15. Time capsule.

Final Visit

Two weeks before school ends, make your final visit to the school. Eat together. With the teacher, plan a closing ritual. **This is the best day of the year!!!** Some kids cry, some seniors cry and even some activity staff members get teary-eyed. Take your camera or, better yet, bring a friend to film for you. You'll want to have pictures for your bulletin board and scrapbook. A videotape is nice for starting off your next year.

Everyone Wins

Seniors and children have a natural bond. Both groups of people get tired of being bossed around by middle-aged members of society. Both groups are willing to have fun, relax and enjoy simple pleasures.

The benefits of an intergenerational program for seniors are numerous. Children are not only willing to listen to their stories, they listen with enthusiasm. The children's attentiveness and genuine respect raises the senior's self-esteem. Sometimes the children bring books and read to seniors on a one-on-one basis. In this activity the seniors are able to provide a real and valuable service to the children. We have seen children read to seniors who were unable to read aloud in the classroom.

"The children are so well-mannered, polite and considerate." We cannot tell you how often we have heard this after our first visit. The program provides the seniors a sense of peace, safety and satisfaction by letting them know there are good children in the world despite what they hear and read in the media.

Seniors also benefit from an intergenerational program, because when they are with the children they absorb their energy like a sponge. We have seen elders who shuffle around the facility swinging on swings, playing tetherball and doing the hokey-pokey. **Proximity to youth is a powerful medicine.**

The children derive a sense of history and continuity from the seniors. The seniors let the children fuss over them and worry about them. This sort of nurturing empowers the children and gives them a positive role model to carry into their adulthood. They lovingly push the elderly who are in wheelchairs. They walk slowly with those who are able to walk, taking their arm. We have seen several classroom "bad boys" surprise their teacher with their tenderness and compassion.

The old adage, "You get as much out of something as you put into it" aptly describes an intergenerational program. It takes work and planning, but the rewards are enormous.

Everyone wins. The children gain a feeling of stability; the seniors are given the gifts of energy, meaning and purposefulness. Both gain a sense of community and fun. During your final visit when the children and seniors are hugging each other, when people are smiling and crying simultaneously and you have witnessed small miracles of health and communication — you may feel the biggest winner is the group leader. You created a garden where love and understanding could grow. It doesn't get any better than that!

Levels of Participation

Just because a participant attends your activity does not mean that s/he is benefiting from the activity. David Dehn[33] has developed a model to be used by both the participant and the professional to measure more than just attendance. To help the participants understand the difference in the five levels of participation, the professional may want to start with a collage of pictures and words. Have the participants find words and pictures in magazines and newspapers that show one of the five levels of participation. After tearing out the word or picture it is glued onto the participation collage. The rule is that at least two participants have to agree on which level the word or picture should be placed.

Supplies needed for activity:
- Large piece of paper (at least three feet by four feet).
- Magazines and newspapers
- Glue sticks

Level +2	The participant is very involved in the activity and is receiving beneficial consequences as a result.
Level +1	The participant is moderately involved in the activity. Involvement may be only mentally involved *or* physically involved *or* socially involved but not to the extent normally required to fully participate in the activity.
Level 0 (Zero)	The participant is attending the activity but receiving no benefit and receiving no harm.
Level -1	The participant's behavior is distracting or harming him/her.
Level -2	The participant's behavior is distracting or harming both himself/herself and other participants.

After the collage is done, hang it up on the wall and talk to the participants about their collage. After each activity, ask each participant what s/he feels his/her level of participation was during the activity. Asking the participant what s/he thought his/her participation level was after each activity helps the participant understand that his/her actions make a difference.

---

[33] Dehn, David (1995). *Leisure Step Up*. Ravensdale, WA: Idyll Arbor, Inc.

Chapter 7
Programming for Low Function

The types of activities included in this chapter are activities that are appropriate for individuals with severe cognitive impairment. We discuss two different levels of programming for individuals who have little to no ability to take care of their most basic needs: Level One, Sensory Integration and Level Two, Sensory Awareness/Sensory Stimulation. The primary goal of Level One, Sensory Integration, is for the professional to provide basic stimulation of the individual's senses: eyes (seeing), ears (hearing), proprioceptors (awareness of the position of the body), vestibular system (balance), tactile systems (touch, feel) and olfaction (smell). Individuals who are functioning at this level will not respond to this stimulation with any clear and meaningful responses. Individuals in a deep coma, in the later stages of Alzheimer's and other dementias and individuals with profound mental retardation would fall into this category.

The primary goal of Level Two, Sensory Awareness/Sensory Stimulation, is to provide various types of stimulation with the express purpose of eliciting a response from the individual. The responses given by the individuals may or may not be a logical response to the type of stimulation provided but the individual's response appears to be related to or because of the stimulation.

Programming for Individuals with Cognitive Impairments

If you have individuals with significant cognitive impairments, you need to be especially careful to provide activity programs for them. If you work in a nursing home, OBRA requires that you develop programs that meet their leisure needs, too.

The basic goal of activity programming for individuals who are cognitively impaired, as it is for any activities program, is to stimulate a person's response and to promote the highest level of functioning of which s/he is capable. Specifically, the goal is to continually simplify tasks so they remain within the individual's diminished abilities, thus allowing her/him to retain as much control over her/his life as possible and to maintain a sense of personal dignity.

Although these individuals may have lost the ability to amuse themselves, because that requires memory capacity they no longer possess, they have not lost the ability to be amused or to feel good. Total inactivity is frustrating for anyone. Meaningless activity in which there is no sense of usefulness or challenge is deadly, even for the person who has memory loss.

In addition to memory loss, we are talking about programming for people who may also be experiencing increasing losses in judgment and initiative, the abilities to problem solve, attach meaning to sensory impressions, recognize familiar objects and express themselves. They may also exhibit aimless wandering; carelessness in their appearance; disorientation to person, time and place; irritability; personality and mood changes; and compulsive repetition. Physical changes may include muscular weakness, gait changes, loss of balance and difficulties in performing Activities of Daily Living (ADLs). Cognitive deficits are often characterized by the decreasing ability to use past experience to solve current problems.

General Activity Goals

1. To prevent or reverse the tendency to withdraw or deteriorate.
2. To retain or retrain recognition of articles once familiar.
3. To utilize physical and mental capabilities.
4. To accept the present surroundings.
5. To maintain or stimulate interests and social contacts.
6. To focus attention on one's human worth or self-value.
7. To focus concentration away from physical condition.
8. To alleviate worry and distress.
9. To provide an outlet for irritation and resentment.
10. To promote speech.
11. To promote controlled fatigue and prevent excessive sleeping during the day.

Level 1: Sensory Integration Activities

Each individual is born with the potential to organize input from their sensory system: proprioception, touch, hearing, taste, smell and vision. The sensory input needs to be "integrated," otherwise we experience a profound sensory overload on one extreme or deprivation on the other.

If everything that we felt, saw, heard and tasted at one time were processed in the upper brain simultaneously, we would be bombarded. Sensory integration is "the ability to organize all of the information that we process so as to better manage ourselves within our environment."[34]

As an infant, we make motor responses to the world around us. These responses are global as the entire body learns to move towards the stimuli. With integration of the senses, the motor responses become more coordinated and purposeful. Each component of the sensory system operates separately and also as a part of the whole system.

An experience incorporating all of the senses leaves an indelible mark, much greater than with only one sensory input. It is as though the inner eye captures the experience so that all five senses can bring up the memory. How often do you smell a scent that reminds you of a past experience? The smell stimulated the memory but was not itself the focal point of the real experience.

When the developmental process has been altered in any way, individuals may not have the sensory motor capacity to respond to their environment. They also may not have attained a normal cognitive level due to the sensory motor deficits.

Individuals experiencing sensory losses or cognitive losses can use the rest of the sensory system to respond to their environment and also to rekindle past memories and learned responses. "A

---

[34] Ayres, A. Jean, 1971, *Sensory Integration and Learning Disorders*, Western Psychological Services, Pages 1-2.

sensory integrative approach differs in that it does not *teach* specific skills — rather the goal is to enhance the brain's ability to learn to do these things."[35]

Deficits in Sensory Integration

Any alteration in the developmental pattern of one's growth will impact the integration process and present one or more of the characteristics listed below:
1. Poor body posture, balance
2. Reduced visual discrimination
3. Short attention span
4. Irritability
5. Physical rigidity
6. Tactile defensiveness (lack of integration of the somatic sensory system)
7. Poor judgment skills
8. Limited cognitive function
9. Diminished tactile discrimination
10. Distractibility

Many of the people you serve will exhibit seven out of the ten deficits listed above. Any individual who exhibits even a few of these will benefit from sensory integration activities because body and self-awareness are central components for participating in activity and social services groups.

Goals of a Sensory Integration Focus

1. Use recreation and leisure to improve, habilitate or rehabilitate the physical, social, emotional and cognitive functional abilities of the individual.
2. Educate toward quality leisure functioning regardless of level of functioning.
3. Increase attention span.
4. Build tolerance to physical prompts.
5. Practice fine motor and large motor skills.
6. Increase capacity for interactions.
7. Increase tolerance to task levels of social and physical interaction.

Basic Introduction to Sensory Integration

As an introduction to sensory integration, we will look at some of the systems involved in an everyday activity. The components that are involved include:
- Eyes (see)
- Ears (hear)
- Proprioceptors (awareness of the position of the body)
- Vestibular System (balance)
- Tactile Systems (touch, feel)
- Olfaction (smell)

These sensory nerve impulses are received and coordinated by the "brainstem" which in turn sends nerve impulses to our eye muscles so we can see; body muscles so we can sit, stand, walk, turn cartwheels and still maintain a sense of balance. It takes all of the parts of our body working together to successfully interact with things around us.

---

[35] Ayres, A. Jean, 1971, *Sensory Integration and Learning Disorders*, Western Psychological Services, Page 2.

A Stroll on the Beach

Imagine that you are walking on the beach barefoot. Your feet are being stimulated by their movement through the sand, your auditory system is processing the sounds of the ocean, you can taste the ocean on your lips and your eyes are guiding the way (along with enjoying the experience). Looking closer, you might ask, "How do my legs know how to maneuver in sand?" The sensory nerve impulses are responding to stimuli sent to the brainstem to be processed and sent back to the eyes to see, the spine to hold the body upright and the legs to move in symmetry with the arms for movement. Within each ear you have both your hearing mechanism (cochlea) and your balance center (the vestibular system).

The vestibular system enables the organism to detect motion, especially acceleration and deceleration and the earth's gravitational pull. The system helps the organism to know whether any given sensory input — visual, tactile or proprioceptive — is associated with movement of the body or is a function of the external environment. For example, it tells the person whether s/he is moving within the room or the room is moving about him/her.[36]

The vestibular system is your organ of adaptability. This process carries over to cognitive functions. Sensory impulses bring about biochemical changes in the brain that are critical to the learning process.

The muscles, joints, ligaments and receptors associated with bones provide information to the brain stem about your relationship to the world around you. This is the proprioceptive system.

The relationship among the proprioceptive, vestibular and tactile systems gives you the ability to carry out the seemingly easy task of enjoying a stroll on the beach.

The vestibular system provides information about changes in your head position with respect to gravity. The objects you see around you and the surfaces you touch or stand on may be changing continually. When your head moves, a biochemical reaction occurs in your inner ear. This biochemical reaction enables learning, increases attention span and increases memory.

Tactile stimulation refers to the use of the nerves directly under the skin, "touching." Through experience you learn to identify textures, temperatures and hardness. Just like the muscles, all nerves need to be exercised. Because disability or living situation tends to decrease opportunities to touch and be touched, purposeful tactile stimulation should be planned.

The vestibular/ocular (ear-eye) nerve literally "holds" the image of what was last seen. For maximum learning, an individual needs sensory stimulation and input into all sensory systems (vestibular, tactile, proprioceptive, hearing, visual and olfactory).

Therapeutic Program Ideas

1. Encourage movement of the head in groups and individual interaction with an individual.
2. Create activities that encourage use of fingers and hands. (This movement allows brain to open up to new information.)[37]

   - clapping and rubbing hands
   - string games
   - painting
   - hand holding
   - Velcro
   - hand puppets
   - taffy pulls
   - window wiping
   - hand massages

---

[36] Ayres, A. Jean, 1971, *Sensory Integration And Learning Disorders,* Western Psychological Services, Pages 5-6.
[37] Adapted from Marsha Allen Workshop on Sensory Integration.

3. Provide tactile discrimination activities (sandpaper, soft, hard, cold, warm).
4. Always add scents to activity (scented objects, room sprays, scented pens). Try to avoid scents that are alcohol based. They actually stimulate a different set of olfactory nerves than a pure scent would. You reach more nerves if you use pure scents or oil-based scents instead of alcohol-based ones.
5. Create activities which provide body awareness experiences:
   - facial brushes
   - marbles and sand in a shoe box for foot and hand massage
   - parachute games
   - vibrators
   - rhythm balls rolled over joints of the body
6. Use art experiences with paint rollers. This activity moves the left arm across to the right and vice versa, which crosses the midline of brain hemispheres. By crossing midline you are helping to strengthen both hemispheres so the individual has a greater repertoire for responsiveness.
7. Create activities that encourage and promote body movements (leaning forward or with head leaning back).

Suggested Group Ideas[38]

Relaxation and Therapeutic Touch Group

Ocean sounds can be the musical background for the activity. Each individual would receive a hand massage, a shoulder rub and the vibrator used after s/he is relaxed enough to accept the stimulation.

Body Awareness Musical Group

Choose music such as Simon Says or songs that refer to noses, faces, hands, etc. The leader may touch the individuals' hands for body identification.

Animal Assisted Therapy Group

Provide the combined sensory experience of holding an animal up to the individuals, on their lap or in their hands.

Fur Touch

Leader places individuals' hand or hands into a piece of soft furry fabric. This piece of fur could be of value with individuals who are highly sensitive to touch.

Exercise Group

Any exercise group or one-on-one experience can help an individual to be aware of a body part or to move that part.

The Breath Experience

Incorporate breathing exercises into many of your activities. Our breath not only enhances circulation and focuses attention, but also encourages relaxation and a multi-sensory experience of self.

---

[38] A good book with 86 additional activities for residents with significant cognitive impairment is Parker and Will, 1993, *Activities for the Elderly, Volume 2, A Guide to Working with Residents with Significant Physical and Cognitive Disabilities,* Idyll Arbor, Ravensdale, WA.

Begin many of your activities with an awareness of body and breath in whatever way is possible.

Activity Ideas
1. (A E I O U) vowel repetition by all participants.
2. Blow a feather or Ping-Pong ball across the table.
3. Party blowers, whistles, kazoos or pinwheels provide visual and/or auditory stimulation; then incorporate or reinforce the activity with use of one's breath.
4. Blow bubbles. Client touches falling bubbles and blows bubbles as they fall close to him/her.
5. Play a familiar (or just active) song and encourage humming along with movement to the music.
6. Play an environmental tape of the ocean and assist individuals in stretching arms up and breathing.
7. As in all groups, let the participants know that the group has ended (closure) with a special song, handshake, hug, clapping, etc.

Level 2: Sensory Awareness/Sensory Stimulation Activities

One of the professional's most important goals is to provide each individual with a good quality of life. Obviously, this presents many challenges. One of the most critical and inclusive is that of providing adequate stimulation to each individual. The importance of stimulation must not be minimized. If an individual fails to receive stimulation to his/her senses, the natural developmental process is thrown off track. In infants and very young children, for example, the lack of a loving human touch may produce a condition called "failure to thrive" which can threaten the very survival of the baby. This failure to thrive is also a critical risk to the very old if they no longer receive the most basic level of sensory stimulation that life requires.

Stimulation can be sensory, emotional, social and cognitive. When an individual at any stage in life is unable to reach out for stimulation, it must be provided through activity, environment and one-on-one interactions. Meeting these stimulation needs is one of the most crucial components that must be addressed when planning an individual's program.

This need should be addressed throughout the comprehensive assessment process. The professional's goal of providing each individual a high quality of life can be furthered when an interdisciplinary approach is used. Notions that may seem abstract such as culture, individuality, autonomy and environment become real and down to earth when seen as opportunities for individual stimulation and growth.

Because people need a variety of sensory input and involvement to maintain their contact with reality, sensory stimulation is often an important aspect of an activity program. Individuals who have not been responding for an extended period will often respond to changes in the sensory environment. All of the feeling, hearing, seeing, smelling, tasting and moving that an individual does during his/her waking hours makes up his/her sensory input; if this is limited, s/he will lose contact with reality.

Stimulation occurs when an individual interacts with the world and people around him/her. Stimulation helps one stay able to identify, process and then respond to stimuli and events. It is how we understand and interpret the experience of being alive. The charts on the next page show the types of stimulation and sources of stimulation that are important for the people we serve.

Categories of Stimulation

	sensory	emotional	social	cognitive
level of involvement	basic neurological stimulation — body responds at the basic nerve level	more complex reaction to stimulation— the interpretation and recognition of stimulation from the sensory level which is then interpreted by past memories		
types of stimulation	touch proprioceptive smell sight vestibular taste hearing	anger insecurity pleasure desire	feed me, I'm empty desire for others need for friendship	memory (long and short term) problem solving sequencing

Sources of Stimulation

Environment	People	Internal
Natural (uncontrolled) or controlled stimulation in the individual's environment which stimulates the basic senses as well as the higher senses of emotions and cognition	This is separated from environment only because we are so purposeful in the way we try to use ourselves (and tools) to make up for a lack of stimulation in the individual's environment	Stimulation originating within the individual him/herself. Includes proprioceptors and things like pain (e.g., from gas) or hearing voices.

The goals of sensory awareness and sensory stimulation activities are to:
- elicit response or increase level of arousal
- prevent sensory deprivation
- encourage the individual to use the senses to respond to stimuli

The type of individuals who need these activities include those who show problems with:
- severe disorientation
- cognitive and sensory deficits
- lack of ability to respond without sensory inputs
- self-stimulation
- deficits in sensory/perceptual integration
- rigid body and posture
- avoiding eye contact
- constant movement whether in wheelchair or not

The way you need to lead these activities includes:
- using touch
- being consistent
- being respectful
- expecting a response (self-fulfilling prophesy)
- speaking to the individual in an adult manner regardless of the lack of response
- using direct eye contact
- repeating, repeating, repeating
- letting them know you enjoy being with them
- being yourself
- using visual and verbal cues
- analyzing the stimulation level to avoid over-stimulation

Staff Involvement in Sensory Stimulation

In order for a sensory stimulation program to be successful, all staff members need to understand not only its therapeutic value, but also how they can use this type of stimulation in their work with the people we serve. The professional should provide inservice training and various tools and forms for staff use. Examples of the forms are shown on the following pages.

Sensory Stimulation Supply List and Assessment Form

This form identifies supplies to be used in this program. Each item should be assessed for *all* possible types of sensory stimulation. As an example, "magnetic letters" would be assessed as a supply item that could be used for tactile and visual stimulation. It could also be a kinesthetic (body in motion) stimulation. If the staff person was requesting that the individual move the letters around and spell a name, this could be a cognitive stimulation tool also. The intent of the form is to be sure that all of the supply items have been assessed as to types of stimulation, safety issues and appropriate use. The comment section should be used to address safety and specific uses of the supply item.

We recommend that you have the following items available for a sensory stimulation program:

- Tangles
- Slinky (plastic)
- Magnetic letters
- Ring toss
- Parachute
- Dominoes
- Large print cards
- Flash cards
- Coasters to stack
- Hankies to fold
- Clothespins
- Maps
- Grooming items

- Velcro catch game
- Velcro strips
- Koosh balls
- Writing materials
- Eraser board
- Water puzzles
- Texture books
- Scratch & sniff
- Scents
- Pictures to sort
- Photos to look at
- Stuffed animals
- Name cards

- Cooking items
- Busy boards
- Busy aprons
- Gardening items
- Mystery box
- Fabrics & textures
- Musical instruments
- Etch-a-Sketch
- Hardware trays
- Wood working games
- Pat Mat (plastic pillow filled with water and a sponge)

We also recommend that each facility have at least one "Spinoza Bear" for use with individuals. The Spinoza Bear is not only a soft, cuddly teddy bear. It is also a carefully designed, dynamically effective therapeutic tool that provides sensory stimulation. It comes with a library of tapes. You can order a Spinoza bear from Spinoza, 245 E. 6th Street, St. Paul, Minnesota 55101-1940. Phone: 1-800-CUB-BEAR.

Sensory Supply Card

Each sensory supply item should have a separate card filled out on its use and goals. These should be available on a ring or in a binder attached to the supply box. We can never assume that everyone understands how to use a specific supply item. A photo of each supply item could be attached to the card describing it. It is a good idea to laminate the card.

Individual Activity Cards

Each individual who has been assessed as in need of sensory stimulation should have a card filled out with specific and individualized information about his/her interests, responses and types of supplies that s/he has responded well to. Also include any activity that seems to decrease anxiety and elicit interest and focus away from an undesired behavior.

Sensory Supply List

Supply Item	Tactile	Auditory	Olfactory	Type of Sensory Stimulation Provided Gustatory	Visual	Kinesthetic	Cognitive	COMMENTS

Sensory Supply Cards

Name of Supply Item: _____

How to Use It: _____

_____

_____

Goals: _____

_____

_____

Comments and Precautions: _____

_____

_____

_____

Date Written: _____

Author: _____

Activity Card

Name Of Individual: _____

Identified Leisure Interests: _____

_____

_____

What does this individual respond well to? Explain:

_____

_____

_____

What specific sensory supply items work best with this individual?

_____

_____

_____

_____

Safety Precautions and Interventions:

_____

_____

_____

_____

Additional Comments: _____

_____

_____

_____

Date Written: _____

Author: _____

Sensory Awareness Ideas[39]

Flashlight games to increase visual tracking. One game might be flashlight movement to music. Cover the light with colored cellophane to increase interest.

Glow in the dark balls and other materials can be used for games of toss and catch or hide and seek.

Straws to blow Ping-Pong balls or paint across paper (group or individual) or cotton balls or whatever a straw can blow. Good for increasing lung power and speech skills.

Tearing newspaper or colored paper and playing freely as if they were Fall leaves. Then recycle into papier-mâché or stuff paper sacks of various sizes and play games of toss and catch or make a collage or seasonal decorations.

Use paper punches for activity similar to the one above. Increases hand strength and eye-hand coordination.

Matching a pile of shoes or socks or shirts. Teaches sorting and categories.

String painting with paint applied between two pieces of paper.

Milk cartons for bowling and building. They are inexpensive and lightweight.

Shadow Design

Equipment:	Slide projector or some similar light source.
Activity:	Aim projector light at wall or sheet or large piece of paper.
For:	Gross motor development and body awareness. To learn concepts; i.e., large and small, right and left. For increasing imagination/creativity. To have fun.
Examples:	Make yourself tall/small, move right or left, up or down pretend to be a bird, giant rock, move only your arms, for dancing and movement to music.

Hair Dryer Bubble Blow

Equipment:	Old 1960's hair dryer or a fan and bubble soap.
Activity:	Empty room of objects and start making lots of bubbles by holding bubble wand in front of blower. Touch the bubbles in free form movement.
For:	Increasing visual tracking skills as measured by following the movement of the bubbles, eye-hand coordination, enhancing imagination, for fun.
Cautions:	Bubbles make floors slippery. Use carpeted areas.

---

[39] The ideas through **Tactile Finger Walk** are from Lois Herman Friedlander, RMT, MFCC.

Free Form Ball Toss

Equipment: A dozen or more balls of soft texture in varying sizes.

Activity: Empty the room of obstacles and throw balls at each other, kick balls to each other, roll them, kick backwards, etc.

For: Increase body awareness through hand, eye and foot movements. Increase balance.

Free Form Pillow Toss

Activity: Variation on above ball activity but pillows have the advantage of being easier to manipulate for catching and throwing or kicking with feet.

Powder and Facial Scrubber Time

Equipment: As many Clairol Facial Scrubbers as necessary for your group.

Activity: Put hypoallergenic powder on arms and "erase" it with the scrubber.

For: Utilizing visual tracking skills, eye-hand coordination, enhancing imagination, for fun.

Tactile Finger Walk

Equipment: Peach packing materials from the local grocery or newspapers or Mylar.

Activity: Place materials on table. Have participants manipulate material.

For: Utilize tactile awareness and discrimination, increase gross motor movement.

Humor

1. Humor has been defined as "A sense of joy in being alive." Humor should be incorporated in all activities. It creates a sense of playfulness and should be provided on an age-appropriate basis.

2. Individuals in stress and confusion oftentimes revert back to a happier time. We see this often in individuals who are no longer in touch with reality.

3. If we can offer a setting that is safe and playful, we may be providing a wonderful gift of not only reality but also reminiscence to a happier time.

Potpourri Sachet

Purpose:	Olfactory Stimulation
Skills Necessary:	Verbal, fine motor coordination, ability to follow directions, moderate cognitive ability
Goals:	Utilize motor coordination (gross and fine) Stimulate sense of smell Complete a short-term task Increase self-esteem by successfully completing the project
Objectives:	Each participant will make one potpourri sachet. Each participant will participate in the use of a sachet.
Materials:	Cloth (to be cut into 4" to 5" square pieces) Yarn or thin cloth ribbon Fragrant dried flower petals (rose, lilac, gardenia or cedar chips) Small bottle of fragrance oil
Process:	(Prior to activity pick and dry flower petals and treat with a few drops of fragrance oil — gardenia, rose, floral, etc.)

1. Seat participants around table.
2. Have prepared:
   - cloth cut into 4" to 5" squares
   - yarn or thin cloth ribbon in 4" to 6" lengths
   - rubber bands
   - mixed dried petals, enough for each participant.
3. Have each participant smell potpourri.
4. Have each group member:
   - lay piece of cloth flat
   - place dried petals in the center of the cloth
   - fold edges up around the potpourri
   - secure at top with a rubber band (may need assistance)
   - tie ribbon in a bow around the rubber band.

Optional — add string, yarn or thin cloth ribbon for hanging in room or bathroom or leave plain to freshen up drawers.

Provide closure for group. Thank each participant for attending.

Spice Kitchen

Purpose: Olfactory Stimulation

Skills Necessary: Verbal, moderate cognitive functioning

Goals: Promote/utilize stimulation skills
Practice interpersonal skills
Utilize discrimination skills
Access long term memory
Promote/utilize expression

Objectives: Each participant will smell and identify at least one spice.

Materials: Herbs and spices (cinnamon, anise, pepper, sage, cloves, lemon peel, orange peel, onion, chives, garlic, mint, oregano, horse radish, etc.)

Process:
1. Gather participants around a table.
2. Give each participant an herb or spice (may have to distribute scents individually throughout activity to preserve group structure).
3. Choose starting participant.
4. Allow each group member to smell and identify his/her herb or spice.
5. Repeat process until all participants have had a turn.
6. Summarize participants' reactions related to herbs and spices.
7. Thank each participant for attending.

Potential Problems and Solutions:
1. If participant is nonverbal, s/he can identify scent through gestures and facial expressions or by group leader using questions in which responses are yes/no.
2. It is important to allow time for reminiscing between smelling of scents to allow "smell" sensors to become neutral.

Adaptation: Activity can be done on a one-on-one level and have participant identify several "kitchen" scents.

Sensory Stimulation Activities[40]

Sight/Vision

Contrasting colors are most important to enhance visual stimulation. Colors such as red and orange are the easiest to see. Large cards and pictures of bright colors work well with individuals who have poor vision. Other ways of using visual stimulation include showing slide pictures or using playing cards with pictures.

Play a game that increases visual experiences by placing a number of objects on a tray and having the participants name the objects. After the participants observe the tray for 3 minutes remove it and have the participants try to name all the objects on the tray. A variation would be to remove one or two of the objects and have the participants try to remember what was removed. Start with 6–8 objects and increase or decrease appropriately. Some other activities and objects to use for visual stimulation include:

• hiding activities	• electronic games	• posters
• colorful objects	• maps	• TV
• slides	• mirroring/mirrors	• photos
• tracking activities	• different colored glasses	• flash lights

Other ways to stimulate the sense of sight include:

1. Using a flashlight, move the light slowly in different directions for the individual to focus on and track.
2. Turn the light off and on slowly, and then move quickly.
3. Shine light on different parts of individual's body.
4. Shine light on different people. If they are able to, ask the individuals to identify or acknowledge those people in some way.

Touch/Tactile

The fingers are filled with receptors that are stimulated by shapes and textures. The lips are also very sensitive to touch. The skin is the largest sensory organ of the body and touch is perceived differently in various areas of the skin. The entire surface of the body is capable of receiving sensory stimuli from the environment. Besides touch, the tactile senses also include pressure, temperature and pain.

Three of the most pleasurable tactile experiences include:
1. to be lovingly touched by another person i.e. hug, massage.
2. to feel the warmth of the sun on one's skin.
3. to hold an animal, i.e. pet therapy visits or adopt an animal at the agency.

Remember:
1. Use tactile stimulation to arouse as well as to quiet.
2. Verbally describe activity or object, feel it, taste it. Ask about sensation received from an individual who is verbal; describe it for an individual who is nonverbal. Ask about preference and feelings. Describe the properties — soft, hard, rough, firm, warm, cold.
3. Introduce gradually. No more than three things at a time. Use each object at least four consecutive sessions before introducing new things. Return when nine have been presented. Repeat set of nine three times before introducing new textures and sensations.

---

[40] This section (through the Paint Bags Activity) was written by Ann Nathan, MS, CTRS and Elizabeth Best Martini, MS, CTRS, used with permission.

To stimulate an individual's tactile sense, objects may be placed in old socks, passed behind backs or under the table. Participants may try to determine what the objects are. A variation is to label paper bags with each letter of the alphabet, fill them with one or more items beginning with that letter and have the participants guess the object. Keep in mind that putting more than one item in a bag may be confusing to some individuals. Be careful with small items that could be put into the individual's mouth and cause choking. Rubber balloons are especially dangerous in this regard.

Some items that might be included are

• apple	• hair brush	• oyster shell	• sticky tape
• balloon	• harmonica	• pipe	• thimble
• clothespin	• ice tray	• pliers	• under shirt
• cotton ball	• jelly beans	• quill	• vegetable
• cuff links	• key	• raisin	• Velcro
• dice	• lemon	• rubber ball	• wishbone
• eraser	• marshmallow	• softball	• letter X
• fork	• nut	• spool	• yarn
• golf ball	• orange	• spoon	• zipper

Another touching exercise is to give the participants a variety of objects to feel one at a time. If they are able to, the participants may be asked to describe one element of what they feel or they may guess the object. Some possible objects include:

• cork	• candle	• thimble	• peeled hard boiled
• sandpaper	• make-up	• lotions	egg
• shaving cream	brushes	• velvet	• ice
• rope	• leaf	• wet sponge	• flower
• bird feather	• Styrofoam	• raw potato, half	• rubber glove filled
• powder puff	• emery board	peeled	with sand
• corn silk	• moss		

The rubber puzzles that are manufactured commercially provide good tactile stimulation also. One can make his/her own game by selecting a shape such as a heart, circle or other geometric shape and cutting the pattern from materials with a variety of textures i.e. velvet, cork, card board, burlap, satin, plastic. Each shape is then cut into several pieces and all are put together in a box. Participants pick out the pieces and match them by their texture. When all pieces have been separated, the puzzles can be put together.

Sensory integration utilizes many of the same modalities. Refer to the previous level, Sensory Integration, for proprioception and vestibular stimulation activities.

Taste

The sense of taste depends on receptors located on the taste buds, which are on the tongue. There are four taste sensations: sweet and salt on the tip, sour along the sides and bitter along the back. After the age of fifty, there is an increase in the threshold of sensation for all four taste qualities. Because of these changes, those who are older need an increased amount of stimulation in order to get an adequate taste sensation.

Any experience with eyes closed increases taste awareness. It is interesting to see how many tastes people can identify with their eyes closed. Some tastes that they might identify:

• allspice	• pickles	• lemon	• peppermint
• licorice	• syrup	• honey	• root beer float
• mocha	• orange	• wintergreen	
• berries	• vanilla	• peanut butter	
• chocolate	• nutmeg	• cinnamon	

Smell/Olfactory

A sense of smell seems to have an effect on emotions (i.e. pleasant, unpleasant, harmful etc.). Care should be taken to prevent the individual from tasting some of these items. Use sharp, distinct smelling substances (i.e. perfumes, colognes, soaps, flowers, herbs, food products, etc.). What smells are common to your environment? Refer to other segments of this chapter. A small amount of different substances may be put into jars and participants may guess the contents. Some suggestions include:

• vinegar	• nutmeg	• apple	• banana
• vanilla	• cloves	• rose	• almond
• bay rum	• coffee	• sherry	• tea
• lavender	• lemon	• lilac	• fresh cut grass

Hearing/Auditory

To stimulate the sense of hearing, a leader or participant may make a series of sounds and may ask for identification and/or direction. The following are some suggestions:

• pouring water	• rubbing wood against wood
• striking wooden matches	• shaking a wind chime
• balling up a piece of paper	• clinking ice in a glass
• own voice on tape	• jingling coins together
• slamming a door	• balling up dry leaves
• rubbing two pieces of sandpaper together	• banging an aluminum pie plate
• ripping a newspaper, tearing paper	• thumbing through a book
• hitting a spoon against bottles with different amounts of water in them	• common sounds in your particular environment

Another suggestion to stimulate hearing is to drop different items and let the participants guess what was dropped, i.e.:

• rubber ball	• marbles	• keys
• book	• coins	• golf ball
• plastic dish	• soft drink can	• basketball
• tennis ball	• Ping-Pong ball	• aluminum pie plate

Participants may produce their own variety of sounds by utilizing their voices and bodies. Many people can make sounds by clapping hands, snapping fingers, stamping feet and rubbing palms together. Vocally, sounds may include: clucking, whistling, blowing air through loosely closed lips, coughing, crying, laughing, humming and using a variety of pitches and degrees of loudness.

Listening and identifying nature sounds and the everyday environmental sounds are also good listening experiences. Other ideas:

• indoor recirculating fountains	• chanting
• large bird cage	• roving reporter exercise
• symphony of emotions exercise	• conversation
• tapes — personal ones made by family, friend, therapist	• radio/TV
	• singing

See the activity description on the next page for one way to run this activity.

Auditory Discrimination/Sequencing

Skills Necessary: Verbal/nonverbal, functional attention span, moderate auditory functioning, moderate cognitive functioning

Goals: To promote/enhance auditory awareness
To promote/enhance memory recall
To promote/enhance socialization
To maintain/increase sequencing skill
To maintain/increase attention span
To maintain/increase discrimination ability

Objectives:
1.   Each participant will differentiate between at least two different sounds played by group leader.
2.   At least 50% of group participants will appropriately sequence more than two sounds (i.e. sticks, bell, drum, snap, clap, hand swish).
3.   Each participant will verbally identify (or point to flash cards for) two sound producers.

Materials: Variety of sound producing instruments or objects (not exceeding more than five per activity).
Hide sound producers in a box, under the table, behind chalkboard, etc.

Process:

1.   Seat participants around a table.
2.   Explain to participants that various sounds (hidden to them visually) will be produced for them to listen to and identify.
3.   Begin by having the group identify the individual sounds that you have selected.
4.   Choose a starting participant.
   a.   Produce a sound and have the participant identify it, turn toward the sound or respond in any way possible.
   b.   Produce a second sound and have participant identify it.
5.   Repeat process with each participant.
6.   Select a participant.
   a.   Produce three successive but different sounds.
   b.   Ask participant to identify them in the order that they were produced.

Problems and Solutions:

1.   Try to use sounds that are distinctly different. Some sounds may be too similar for participants to differentiate.
2.   If a sequence of three sounds is too difficult, encourage the group to help or cut back to two.
3.   If three sounds are too easy, add more sounds.
4.   Flash cards of each sound can be made to assist those with verbal limitations.

Adaptation:

Sounds could be categorized by certain themes (i.e., air sounds, animal sounds or sounds in the facility).

Sand Hide 'N' Seek

Skills Necessary:	Verbal/nonverbal, minimal fine motor skills, low to moderate cognitive skills
Goals:	To promote/enhance memory recall To promote/enhance visual and tactile stimulation To maintain/increase fine-motor coordination
Objectives:	Each participant will attempt to find an object in the sand at least once.
Materials:	Plastic tub, bucket or box filled with sand and/or cornmeal Ten small objects of various sizes and shapes (i.e. comb, ball, blocks)

Process:

1. Arrange group around table (if group is large, use two tables and two tubs).
2. Group leader will identify objects being placed in the sand.
3. Place tub next to starting individual.
4. Place five objects in tub and bury in sand.
5. Request participant to put hands or foot in sand to become accustomed to its texture.
6. Request participant to find one object with hand and remove it from the sand.
7. Replace the chosen object with one not yet used, always keeping the same number of objects in the tub. When all ten have been used, repeat process.
8. Thank each participant for attending.

Potential Problems and Solutions:

1. Participants who are low functioning may attempt to eat sand. Cornmeal may be used as a substitute.
2. For participants who are nonverbal, promote the use of physical gestures (such as head nods, simulation of object use) as responses to questions asked by the group leader.
3. If participants are unable to follow directions, use hand-over-hand method.

Adaptations:

1. Use shapes and colors rather than actual objects.
2. Use large puzzle pieces. Each member pulls one piece from sand and, when all the pieces have been removed, the group attempts to put the puzzle together.
3. Place marbles in sand and move hand or foot over them.

Scented Group Mural

Skills Necessary:	Verbal/nonverbal, minimal fine motor ability, minimal cognitive functioning
Goals:	To promote/enhance olfactory stimulation To promote/enhance visual and tactile stimulation To maintain/increase fine motor skills To encourage cooperation within a group
Objectives:	Each member of the group will contribute 1–2 pieces of yarn to the picture. Any group members who are verbal will contribute at least one statement each concerning the scent of the yarn and its relation to the picture.
Materials:	Large cardboard sheet Various colored yarn (cut in 1" strips) Scissors Glue Oils or perfumes to pre-scent yarn according to the theme (Could also use fresh fruit juices)

Preparation:

1. Group leader adds scent to the yarn the night before by dabbing yarn with various oils or perfumes of flowers, fruits, etc., according to chosen theme. Allow the yarn to dry.
2. Group leader draws items from theme on cardboard, for example: fruit (apples, watermelon, grapes, etc.).

Process:

1. Gather group participants around table.
2. Group leader explains theme and the project, displaying the cardboard drawing.
3. Give each participant yarn strips.
4. Have group participants choose a strip.
5. Put glue on small area of cardboard and demonstrate putting yarn on the board.
6. Have first participant choose strip of her/his choice; glue the chosen area and place yarn on area.
7. Repeat procedure for each participant.
8. Discuss finished picture.
9. Thank each participant for attending.

Texture Collage

Skills Necessary: Verbal/nonverbal, minimal fine-motor skills,
                          Low to moderate cognitive functioning

Goals: To promote/enhance tactile and mental stimulation
                          To promote/enhance socialization and awareness of others
                          To promote/enhance group cooperation
                          To promote/enhance self-expression
                          To increase eye-hand coordination

Objectives: Each participant will place 2–3 objects on the collage.

Materials: Large paper or cardboard piece
                          Textured items preferably centered on a theme
                          Glue

Process:

1.   Place participants around table.
2.   Discuss already chosen theme (i.e. nature, spring, flowers, sports, games).
3.   Spread out items that the group leader brought in related to theme. Have each participant choose at least 2–3 items that s/he will place on collage.
4.   Place large cardboard in front of starting individual.
5.   Have participant point or express where s/he would like to place his/her item.
6.   Assist participant to put glue there.
7.   Ask/assist participant to place item on glued area.
8.   If able, participant pushes cardboard to next individual.
9.   Repeat steps 5-8 until all participants have placed their items on the collage.
10.   Discuss finished collage.
11.   Thank each participant for attending.

Potential Problems and Solutions:

Some participants may try to eat the items. Hold back stimulation item until time to be used or implement close supervision.

Surprise Bag

Skills Necessary:	Verbal/nonverbal, finger sensation to feel objects, moderate cognitive function
Goals:	To promote/enhance tactile stimulation To promote/enhance mental stimulation To promote/enhance memory recall To maintain/increase fine motor skills
Objectives:	Each participant will touch and may identify (if able) at least one object in the grab bag.
Materials:	Bag(s) (preferably cloth) Ten small objects of various shapes and sizes

Process:

1. Seat participants in a circle.
2. Explain to participants that there is a bag of objects and they are to:
   a. Reach in the bag.
   b. Feel for an object that they can identify (if able).
3. Remove the object from the bag to confirm the identification.
4. Choose a starting participant.
5. Repeat process #2 and #3 with each participant.
6. Optional: Reminisce about objects.
7. Thank each participant for attending.

Potential Problems and Solutions:

1. The group leader may need to give verbal clues to assist in identification.
2. Flash cards of each object could be made in advance for participants who are nonverbal or for easier identification.

Adaptations:

1. Objects can be based thematically such as kitchen items, babies, environmental themes, holidays, seasons, vocations, etc.
2. Objects can be based on various shapes or colors.

Paint Bags

Skills Necessary: Verbal/nonverbal, minimal fine motor skills, low cognitive skills

Goals: To maintain/increase fine motor dexterity
                                   To maintain/increase direction following
                                   To promote/enhance creativity and self-expression

Objectives   Each participant will move finger, hand, foot, etc. along bag creating a design.

Materials: Zip-lock bags
                                   Various colors of tempera paint

Process:

1. Group leader makes bags taking each zip lock bag and filling it with one color of paint (medium consistency). Use just enough paint so that bag is fully covered but can still lie flat.
2. Gather participants around one table, if possible, or two pushed close together.
3. Place a paint bag in front of each and explain (while demonstrating) that it is to be used like a writing tablet.
4. Suggest simple designs, letters or numbers to be drawn on the paint bag with finger. Allow time for participants to comply, repeating and assisting when needed.
5. Explain and assist participants in smoothing design off bag front.
6. Repeat process 4 and 5 using various suggestions according to group skills.
7. End the activity by having participants sign their names or make a handprint in the paint bag.
8. Thank each participant for attending.

Problems and Solutions:

1. Participants who are lower functioning may not be able to independently move fingers or to follow directions. Provide assistance while allowing participant to utilize maximum capabilities.
2. Suggest more complex designs for participants who are higher functioning or allow them to create pictures of their own choosing.

Adaptations:

1. Various liquid mediums could be used (i.e., colored vegetable oil, colored sand, etc.) to provide a variety of tactile stimulation.
2. More than one primary color can be used for some participants.

Therapeutic Use of the Vibrator[41]

Always request physician approval for vibrator stimulation.
A vibrator is an excellent tool to be used in conjunction with other sensory awareness experiences.

Values of this tactile experience:
• To assist the participant in body awareness and specific body parts.
• To stimulate sensory receptors and the kinesthetic/proprioceptive sense of self.
• To experience the sense of touch in a safe and relaxed setting; this is especially helpful in work with tactile defensive individuals.
• To encourage a sense of exploration and curiosity of the world around them.
• To facilitate the experience of "feeling rooted" in one's body — even if only for a short time.

Techniques for the use of the vibrator:
• Always tell the participant what you will be doing and what s/he will be experiencing. If possible, let the individual touch and feel the vibrator both on and off.
• Approach slowly to determine tolerance to touch and to the vibrator.
• Stop use of the vibrator if you sense the individual is experiencing any pain or discomfort — you want the experience to be pleasurable.
• Begin to touch individual on shoulders, arms or hands; avoid extremities if you are unfamiliar with the individual's medical condition.
• Vibrator use is most beneficial and successful with drug free participants; some medications will decrease one's sense of touch and awareness.
• The average amount of time to use a vibrator is 2–3 minutes per participant.
• Literature indicates that 10 seconds on and then 5–10 seconds off may be the most effective way of building sensory receptivity.

---

[41] Ross, Mildred, OTR and Dona Burdick, CTRS. *Sensory Integration*, p. 72, 1981, Slack, Inc., Thorofare, NJ.

The Sensory Box

The sensory box is a concept created to stimulate the professional's imagination in working with individuals who are limited in sensory and cognitive abilities. This can either be a box, a tray, an apron or any other idea that you create to reach out to those most in need.

This box or tray will be designed, used and adapted as you work with it. Design new changes or additions to meet individual needs. When designing it, design it so that it is easy to clean between sessions with different individuals.

Description

When working with individuals who have regressed, a leisure goal could be to elicit focus, curiosity, response and involvement in a sensory experience — if possible. This would be through a multi-sensory experience. The response may be movement of the eyes or tracking of an object (visual), reaching to touch a bright object (proprioceptive, tactile), moving to music (auditory), tasting a piece of fruit (gustatory), recognizing or responding to a familiar scent (olfactory).

Curiosity = Exploration = Learning = Recreating

Creating the Sensory Box

The sensory box or tray can be created with almost any safe, non-toxic, non-edible objects. Use a variety of objects to elicit responses to as many of the senses as possible. Determine if the box or tray is for:

An initial sensory curiosity experience where the individual is not directly touching the objects, but receiving auditory and visual stimulation

OR

A hands-on sensory experience.

Create a box or tray that can be used as part of your inventory of supplies for special needs. Be sure to include a written picture and description of your creation.

Some Sensory Box Ideas:

A gift box with scarves to fold and tie together. Scarves can also be attached to Velcro to attach and remove.

Musical instruments in a box. Some of the smaller items can be Velcroed onto the box sides. An individual can touch them or pull one out and use it.

A box of familiar items to rekindle memories. It could be a box of ties, socks, chains, a wallet, a pocket watch or photos.

A television tray with magnetic letters and magnets attached, which can be used as a communication board, color sorting or letter identification experience. (Remember, never place your magnetic letters near a computer or computer disks.)

A basket of balls of all colors, sizes and shapes.

A bed rail cover with Velcroed objects to stimulate an individual on bed rest during a one-on-one visit.

A plastic shoe bag with twelve pockets. Add gloves of different types and fabrics. They could be gardener gloves, evening gloves, plastic gloves, bicycle gloves, etc. This could be a visual experience or a tactile and sorting experience.

Different scents and oils on cotton balls. Each cotton ball can be placed in a zip lock bag with pinholes in it or in a nylon stocking kept in a plastic container.

Musical gloves. These are commercially purchased in a toy store. They are battery operated and make music when touched on the fingertips. They are also great for teamwork.

Closing a Sensory Stimulation Session

In order to close the Sensory Stimulation Session, any of the following may be used:
1. a song,
2. a poem,
3. a story with a theme,
4. a story book with moveable parts for group members to try, or
5. a review of the time spent together in the group sessions.

Always reassure members that it was good to have shared the time together. Offer a handshake or a hug. Holding hands increases attention span. The day and date should be reviewed. A reminder statement should be given regarding the next group meeting time.

Activities for Individuals with Cognitive Impairments[42]

These pages show a set of activities that are appropriate for individuals with cognitive impairments and the goals of the activities. These activities may be done in groups or during one-on-one time with staff or volunteers.[43]

Type	Activity	Goal
Reality Activities	• Review of day's activities • Sensory stimulation	identity, socialization, improve/maintain memory, recognition, communication
Art Activities	• Filling in silhouettes • Copying figures • Collage • Assembling pre-cut shapes • Group murals • Paint bag art • Edible art	eye/hand coordination, recognition, sensory stimulation, creativity, accomplishment, follow directions, fine motor movement

---

[42] ©1991 E. Best Martini, MS, CTRS and R. N. Cunninghis, MEd, OTR, used with permission.

[43] Two resources to find out more about working with people with dementia are *Wiser Now* (a monthly publication from Better Directions, PO Box 3064, Waquoit, MA 02536-3064) and Cunninghis, Richelle, 1995, *Reality Activities: A How To Manual for Increasing Orientation, Second Edition*, Idyll Arbor, Inc., Ravensdale, WA.

Type	Activity	Goal
Activities of Daily Living	• Tying shoes/fastening buttons • Preparing vegetables • Gardening • Cooking • Grooming	retain skills, sense of accomplishment, eye-hand coordination, object identification, memory, following directions, multi-step tasks
Physical Activities	• Fitness exercises (purposeful) • Supervised walks • Movement therapy • Kick ball • Bean bag toss • Dice games	use excess energy, retain knowledge of body parts, competition, stimulation, socialization, maintain or increase range of motion, maintain or increase muscle tone, alertness, cardiovascular conditioning
Drama Activities	• Musical plays • Act out themes • "Share a Face" • Improvise with props • Story telling • Pantomime/charades	immediate enjoyment, socialization, cognition, communication skills, release of frustration, creative expression, problem solving
Music Activities	• Rhythm band • Sing along • Movement & music • Follow the leader • Old time dance steps	sensory stimulation, fun, exercise, reminiscence, coordination, following direction, socialization
Word and Quiz Games	• Unscramble 3 or 4 letter word • Hangman • Categories • Matching pictures • Homonyms, synonyms, antonyms • Old sayings, proverbs • Discussion questions • Trivia • Spelling bees • What's in a Name	improve cognition, sense of accomplishment, pride, socialization, increase memory, communication skills, competition, mental stimulation, problem-solving ability, attention span, increase self-esteem, reading skills, matching skills
Group Activities	• Discussion groups • Reminiscence groups • Simple card games • Food & culture	decrease anxiety, encourage use of memory, socialization, past knowledge, creative expression, listening skills
Individual Activities	• Looking at photos • Large puzzles • Memory Box	past memories, manual dexterity, accomplishment
Special Areas/ Undirected Activities	• Opening/closing containers • Opening/closing drawers • Leafing through magazines • Articles of clothing activity • Art projects • Tub of water with boats • Fabric fold	exercise creativity, use past skills, coordination, use excess energy, meaningful activity, identifying use/purposes of common objects, fine motor skills

Type	Activity	Goal
Body Imagery	• Sensory boxes • Tactile experiences (e.g. hugging, touching) • Movement exploration • Drawing hands & feet • Portraits of each other • Writing name in the air	sensory stimulation, identification of body parts, cognitive awareness, socialization, increased awareness of tactile stimulation, range of motion, eye-hand coordination, spatial awareness
Sensory Activities	• Touching/feeling • Taste • Smelling • Seeing • Hearing • Proprioception	sensory stimulation, environmental awareness, reminiscence, body imagery, tactile awareness

Touch for Individuals with Alzheimer's Disease and Other Types of Dementia

By Lorraine J. Brown, MS, CTRS

Webster's Dictionary describes touch as "to put the hand, finger, or some other part of the body on, so as to feel: perceive by the sense of feeling." There are many types of touching including hugging, patting, stroking, hand-holding, handshaking and massaging. Being touched in a manner that is comfortable is essential for everyone.

Touching is more than the act of two people experiencing their bodies physically connecting. Touch is a psychological, social, emotional and physical experience. And welcomed touch keeps on producing benefits after the touch is released. Some of the benefits of being touched are

- **Psychological:** increases a sense of well-being and self-esteem; reduces stress; focuses attention; increases patients' will to live; empowers the individual; overcomes fears; provides security, support, and feelings of being needed.

- **Social:** facilitates social interaction, increases communication, conveys unspoken messages and dispels loneliness.

- **Emotional:** provides cheer, relieves depression and anxiety, imparts feelings of belonging and enhances spiritual feelings.

- **Physical:** increases the feeling of being connected with surroundings, promotes feelings of well-being, aids in healing, relieves pain, improves body image, produces measurable physiological changes in both the person who is touching and the person being touched and contributes to health and healing.

Purpose of Study

Because touching is such an important part of everyday life, Lorraine Brown, MS, CTRS conducted a study on touch in nursing homes. The purpose of this study was to determine the differences in touching behaviors of caregivers of individuals in a nursing home setting with Stages 1, 2, and 3 of Alzheimer's disease, as well as those with other types of dementia. With the estimated four million Americans diagnosed with Alzheimer's disease, every effective intervention should be utilized to reach these individuals. Since touch has been identified as such a big part of our lives, its use should be considered as an integral component to help maintain or reconnect cognition and promote communication with individuals diagnosed with Alzheimer's disease or other types of dementia.

Findings

1. Female nurses' aides had the highest number of touch behaviors of all caregivers observed (nurses, nurses'-aides, non-nursing staff, family, visitors and other residents).

2. Residents were more likely to be touched during or after the noon hour.

3. Residents had an increased likelihood of receiving touch behaviors when in close proximity to the nurses' station.

4. Residents diagnosed with Stage 2 or 3 of Alzheimer's disease or other types of dementia received the most touch behaviors related to medical, personal and familiar needs by caregivers.

5. Overall, female caregivers engaged in familiar touch behaviors more often than male caregivers. A true understanding of cross-gender touch behaviors cannot be arrived at because no male residents participated in this study.

6. Residents in Stage 2 of Alzheimer's disease responded positively to touch, while residents diagnosed with other types of dementia responded negatively to touch. Residents in Stage 3 of Alzheimer's disease reacted inconsistently with the context of the touch behaviors.

Lack of Touch

This study, while limited in scope, did show that residents were touched by others far less often than they could have been. Moreover, it is the opinion of the researcher that even though this group of individuals received a very limited amount of touch and much of the touching was associated with receiving medication, clothing changes and cleaning, feedings, and being moved from place to place. This study revealed that residents diagnosed with Stage 1 of Alzheimer's disease and other types of dementia did not provide conclusive reactions to touch because of the limited amount of touch behaviors received by these groups. None of the residents observed in this study received the minimum of touch behaviors they could have received.

Suggestions for Touch and Frequency

Touch may be part of a greeting, gaining attention, communication, friendliness, warmth, comfort, acknowledgment of being, direction, emotional and/or physical support, a cautious gentle refrain, being included and an expression of farewell. There is no specific amount of touch recommended because each person's need for touch varies. The amount of touch each individual needs is contingent upon several factors including: beliefs, attitudes, culture, experience, fears, likes and dislikes, gender, age, physical, mental, and medical conditions, and socio-economic background. While, there are no specific recommendations for frequency of touching, each individual may give an indication of wanting or avoiding touch. An individual needs to be acknowledged by touch several times a day (for example, a handshake or a pat on the shoulder). Caregivers should take their cues from an individual's reactions (positive/negative) towards touch behaviors, to be able to gauge the need for more or less touch.

Suggestions for Reading about the importance of touch:

Davis, P. K. (1991). *The Power of Touch*. Carson, CA: Hay House, Inc.
Montagu, A. (1986). *Touching: The Human Significance of the Skin (3ʳᵈ Ed.)*. New York: Harper & Row.
Schweitzer, J. (1994). "The power of touch: Finding the courage to care." *Nursing*, 24 (10), 112.

Chapter 8
Programming for Moderately Impaired Function

Many of the people we serve will have impairments and disabilities that are significant enough to lower their awareness of themselves and/or of others. They lose some of the past that helped define who they are. Activities that reinforce their past benefit their social skills and improve their general interactions with others. The previous chapter addressed individuals who were very impaired — at Level 1: Sensory Integration and Level 2: Sensory Awareness/Sensory Stimulation. This chapter offers you information about, and activities for, individuals who function at three levels in the moderately impaired range.

Building on the levels in the previous chapter, this chapter covers Level 3: Validating Activities, Level 4: Remotivation/Reminiscing and Level 5: Resocialization. Level 3: Validating Activities is for your participants who are very disoriented, whose goals are not focused on orientation but on feelings and emotions. Level 4: Remotivation/Reminiscing is for your participants who benefit from a stepping-stone to and from sensory awareness. The participant is aware of self and motivated to seek out others. Level 5: Resocialization is for your participants who have the skills to socialize and would benefit from being with others in a structured group. These groups are geared toward maintaining an awareness of person, time and place.

Level 3: Validating Activities

The goal of validating activities is to validate the memories and feelings of individuals who are very disoriented. They do not focus on orientation but rather on the individual's perception of what happened in the past and his/her memory of this at the present time (correct or incorrect — it doesn't matter). For more on validation see Naomi Feil, 1993, *The Validation Breakthrough*, Health Professions Press.

Use these activities with residents who have the following characteristics:

- Moderate disorientation
- Time/place confusion
- Unawareness of environment
- Lack of rational thinking
- Locked into fantasy (as if to embrace a safer, happier time)

- Feelings mirrored in body movements
- Distractibility

Some of the things you need to do to make these activities work include:

- Use touch with approval
- Maintain eye contact
- Communicate with clear and repetitive conversation
- Acknowledge feelings
- Mirror movements
- Validate verbally both their feelings and fantasy
- Use active listening. If s/he needs to go home to feed the children:
  1. acknowledge his/her thought
  2. acknowledge his/her experience as a father or mother
  3. state: "You must have very special children" or "What is your son's name?"
- Use age appropriate themes
- Unravel the meaning behind the responses you receive in conversation and body language
- Use simple creative/expressive program ideas
- Encourage laughter and humor
- Be yourself

Some programming ideas that promote the validating process include:

- Name Games — to increase identity and sense of self
- Music — can be used as an opening and closing of group for structure
- Movement — body awareness and identification activities
- Hand/eye coordination exercises
- Parachute games
- Hand gesture games
- Ball games
- Trivia, simple matching games
- Pet programs
- Show-and-tell to stimulate feelings
- Visual cues
- Intergenerational programs
- Discussion groups which rekindle fond memories of different themes (kids, work, school, home, pets, food, holidays, travel)

Another program idea is shown on the following pages.

What's in a Name?

Giving someone back the memory of his/her name — *especially if s/he has forgotten it* — is giving the gift of self. Our name not only represents ourselves, but the history of our family and a personal interest story about the people who named us.

Purpose of Activity:

1. To provide reality
2. To introduce each participant by name
3. To stimulate reminiscence of family and self
4. To encourage social contact within group
5. To learn the history behind different names
6. To provide a discussion-oriented group to participants who can respond successfully to direct questions regarding their names
7. To feel pride in oneself
8. To be recognized for yourself as the accomplishment
9. To be part of an enjoyable and sometimes humorous experience
10. To respond to the expectations of others
11. To reduce feelings of being disenfranchised

Type of Appropriate Participant: This group has been successfully offered to both alert and responsive participants as well as a group comprised of participants with cognitive losses.

Duration: 30 to 40 minutes

Supplies Needed: Name tags (optional)
Library resource books: *What to Name Your Baby, Origin of Names, Popular Names According to Years*
Famous First Names — Quiz
Family stories of names/nicknames
List of nicknames
Pictures of famous people (optional)
Well-known records (to name famous singer) (optional)
Who Am I?

Procedures:

1. Place your participants in a circle facing one another.
2. You should be seated with the group, but able to move about and directly assist or respond to any of the participants.
3. Begin the activity with yourself — state your name and give a personal story about your name, family names, nickname, etc.
4. It is recommended that you add humor to your story since this will set a playful mood for the group.
5. After you share the story of your own name, go around the circle to each person.
6. One by one have the participants state their names, ask if they ever had a "special" name that their parents called them, etc.
7. Mention their last name and country of birth.
8. If one of the participants, upon hearing his/her name, becomes anxious and hesitant to respond, reaffirm the name and mention that you find it to be especially pretty or unique. This will help decrease his/her anxiety regarding the need to respond to you.
9. Depending on how well the activity is received, you may begin the Famous First Name quiz. You name a first name and ask the participant's to call out a last name that comes to mind.

10. Using all the names of the group members, the leader may also design an art project displaying the names on a mural, a poem or a picture as a closure to this group or a future group.
11. To close this group the leader could go around the circle stating all the names and have each individual hear his/her name being spoken one last time.
12. Go around the circle and while stating each name, have the group member write the name in the air as an exercise.
13. End with a round of applause for the group.

Other related program ideas:

- Use this group as a progression towards a "beginning writing" group — where the participants write their signatures as a first exercise.
- When leading adults through any group process, add the element of education and human interest. This piques their interest in the topic and provides a sense of pride and dignity to the participants.
- Once an individual feels respect for you as facilitator, s/he will be more receptive to respond appropriately because *you* have that expectation of them.

Level 4: Remotivating/Reminiscing Activities

Remotivation is a bridge between the time a participant is concerned only about his/her own problems and the time when s/he is ready once again to help others in the community. It is important for each of us to think of ourselves as an important, contributing member of a community. These activities are designed to help the participant see that s/he has contributed by looking at past achievements. The activities also help to point out that even if the participant has lost some level of functioning, s/he is still able to make a contribution.

The goals of remotivation activities are to:

- Start the process of bringing the individual back into the community
- Stimulate thinking about the real world
- Stimulate and revitalize individuals who have shown interest or involvement in the present or future
- Increase a sense of reality
- Begin practicing healthy roles
- Maintain present functional level

Use these activities with participants who have the following characteristics:

- Fearful of decreased cognition
- Short term memory loss
- Forgetful
- Passive
- Able to follow directions
- Good potential for progress

Some of the things you need to do to make these activities work include:

- Consistency
- Clarity of communication
- Encouragement
- Ability to facilitate responses
- Reinforcement of strengths and abilities
- Reinforcement for individuality and life
- Humor and laughter
- Touch and eye contact
- Giving immediate feedback for involvement and response
- Being yourself

The activities in this section are usually done one-on-one or with small groups, but notice that it is very possible to have both people in the one-on-one session be participants. The activities for remotivating and resocializing work together. A participant who is remotivated and is now working on resocializing can help you with another participant who is ready for remotivation activities.

With the right group of people you can create activities that run themselves with little effort on your part. Just make sure that each of these activities is documented to explain how and why it was beneficial to each of the participants.

Some ideas that are appropriate for Remotivation Groups include:

- Name game
- Sharing stories of yourself with another participant or a group
- Gardening
- Cooking
- Pet programs
- Familiar themes (family, pets, work, food)
- Creative writing
- Exercise/movement/breathing
- Trivia
- The question book
- Life review

An interesting idea is shown on the following page.

Food and Culture Class

Description:	Food and Culture is a class emphasizing social interaction and reminiscing, utilizing culture and food as a theme.
Materials:	Food to be prepared Music, slides and visual aids to enhance the cultural theme
Content:	Use geography and culture as the basis for the class. Discuss: 1. music 2. dances 3. geography 4. memories
Set Up:	Have food, music and decorations set up in the activity or dining room. Also be sure to include participants who are confined to their rooms by taking decorations and food to them. Perhaps participants could have nametags with their names both in English and Italian.

Activity Process:

1. Welcome.
2. Introduction to theme "ITALY."
3. Movement to Italian music.
4. Geography and description of life in this country (slides, maps, photos, costumes, flags, weather, houses, families, customs).
5. Reminiscing/discussion. Discussion topics may include; travel, vacations, family heritage, people we know who are Italian, famous people who are Italian.
6. Class participants receive some token to wear which represents the country (flag, paper flower in country colors, name tag, copy of familiar setting in that country).
7. Social exchange with conversation to complement theme.
8. Food preparation or cooking experience (after lunch so as not to decrease appetite). Example: Bring in a pasta machine, explain how it works, and pass out lengths of fresh pasta for tasting.
9. Discuss other Italian food experiences such as prosciutto ham and melon. Slice melon with a hint of ham for taste. Talk about where the melons are grown, etc. This section can be very adventurous and fun.
10. *Closure of class.* Using a few Italian phrases, thank participants and look forward to next week's class on: Morocco — exotic land of spices.

Level 5: Resocializing

When an individual has participated and met the goals as a member of a remotivation group, s/he will be encouraged to build onto these social skills and continue to successfully interact with others. This is known as Resocialization. Resocialization can be considered step two in the process of bringing the individual back into the facility community.

The participants who are able to participate in resocialization activities are also likely to be able to engage in other thoughtful activities. The activities in this section encourage the participant to explore his/her feelings, as well as interact with others in a meaningful way.

The goals of resocializing activities are to:
- Finish the process of bringing the individual back into the community
- Stimulate and revitalize interest in other people
- Practice healthy roles
- Promote greater level of independence
- Encourage social interaction
- Build social skills
- Increase ease in social encounters with others
- Build relationships with other participants

Use these activities with participants who have the following characteristics:
- Able to follow directions
- Interested in socializing
- Interested in the concerns of other participants
- Good potential for progress

Some of the things you need to do to make these activities work include:
- Consistency
- Clarity of communication
- Encouragement
- Ability to facilitate interactions
- Reinforcement of strengths and abilities
- Reinforcement for individuality and life
- Humor and laughter
- Touch and eye contact
- Being yourself

Some ideas that are appropriate for Resocializing Groups include:
- Sharing stories of yourself with another participant or a group
- Problem solving groups, "What would happen if … "
- Resident Council or other decision-making group for participants
- Creative expressive experiences
- Drama/role playing
- Life review
- Creative writing
- Helping others
- "Who Am I?" quiz
- Dear Abby

You will also need to coordinate groups of participants who are willing to work together to help each other regain the ability and desire to socialize with others.

Other ideas follow. Many of these ideas are considered social services groups, often run by social services professionals. There is no requirement about who should be in charge of them. As with all team situations, the person with the time and understanding of the goals and concerns should be responsible for creating and supervising the groups.

One good thing about these groups is that they involve participants who are able to function well enough cognitively to be part of a group. In many cases these groups provide a pleasant change of pace for the leader. In a well-functioning group, you will be able to have fun, as you explore the past and present through the eyes of people with significantly different experiences than your own.

There are five important aspects to the design of a resocialization group:[44]

1. "Climate of Acceptance" Use introductions to create accepting environment.
2. "Bridge to Reality" Read article aloud to develop a group theme.
3. "Sharing — The World We Live In" Develop topics through questions and visual aids to encourage responses.
4. "Appreciation of the Work of the World" Think of work in relation to selves.
5. "Climate of Appreciation" Take time to express pleasure with group and plan next meeting.

Let's Talk! [45]

Fifty Topics Guaranteed to Get Discussion Started

Do you want to improve your participants' self-image, decrease their boredom, increase interaction among staff and participants, decrease negative participant behaviors and reinforce positive ones, plus stimulate verbalization? Group socialization sessions may be the answer. Conducting weekly group sessions just takes a little planning. Limit meetings to 30–45 minutes, have a definite structure and only include participants who are not disruptive in a group. Begin each meeting by asking participants to give the date. Next have members recite the names of others (to encourage memory and socialization). Then introduce new participants.

Now you're ready to move on to the topic. The session topics listed here are varied and have all been used successfully at a veterans' nursing home. They are designed to stimulate the senses. This is important because the elderly, whether institutionalized or at home, can become progressively nonverbal as the aging process diminishes vision, hearing and mobility. These 50 topics are general. By personalizing them you can boost your participants' verbalization and feelings of self-worth. Plus, leading a weekly group can be challenging and rewarding for you.

Sensory Sessions

1. Colors: Have participants name the colors of construction paper as you hold up the sheets. Ask if the color makes them feel hot or cold, sad or happy. Then name objects indoors and outside that are this color.

2. Puppets: Ask participants to tell stories, express feelings and portray fears, using the puppets.

3. Wildlife: Borrow stuffed animals from a museum or arrange for an animal expert to come to talk. Discuss habitats, mating, foods, pets and nature facts.

4. Famous Lady For A Day: Distribute wigs, hats and scarves to female participants and have each devise a costume and talk about whom she is portraying.

---

[44] Robinson, A. M. "Remotivation Techniques."

[45] This section is by Harriet Berliner, RN-C, MSN, ARNP, geriatric nursing service at Harborview Medical Center, Seattle, WA.

5. Barnyard Visit: Arrange with a local animal shelter or youth group to bring in various animals. Then have the participants discuss proper care for the animals; allow hands-on contact.

6. Surprise Bag: Give each participant a shopping bag containing a variety of small, common objects. Ask the participants to select an item and discuss how it is used.

7. Botany: Bring in fresh leaves or flowers. Ask participants to touch and smell them. Then talk about gardens and favorite plants.

8. Halloween: Let the participants "dress up" pumpkins with paint, glue and glitter. They can reminisce about dressing up as a child and maybe read aloud Washington Irving's *Legend of Sleepy Hollow.*

9. Stuffed Animals: Have participants give the animals names and tell where they might be found in nature or fiction. Discuss the toys the participants had as children.

10. Ladies' Day: Arrange with a cosmetics company to demonstrate products geared for elderly skin care. Discuss how participants used to dress up when they were young, fashion changes and different hairstyles.

11. Fashion Show: Ask a local clothing store or specialty shop for the disabled to put on a fashion show. The participants can act as models and you can discuss fashions from powdered wigs to grunge.

12. Art Critique: Bring in sculptures and artwork in different media. (These can often be borrowed from a library or museum.) Discuss different art forms, likes and dislikes and favorite artists and their works. Let the participants touch the artwork and discuss the different textures and effects.

13. Touch Stimulation: Have each participant reach into a bag, close his or her eyes and try to match samples of various fabric swatches and sandpaper by touch.

14. Architecture: Using large sheets of paper and markers, draw simple house types and discuss them.

Music Sessions

15. Favorite Music: Get a tape player and cassettes of music from different time periods like the Big Band era. Participants can sing or clap to the music and reminisce about dates and dancing and favorite singers and groups.

16. Sing Along: Have someone play piano or guitar and then you can all sing "old favorites."

17. Percussion "Jam": Borrow instruments or make them using common items like combs. Let the participants "play along" to piano or taped music. This is especially fun at holiday times.

Reminiscence Sessions

18. War Stories: Talk about wartime job changes, hardships, rationing and loss of loved ones.

19. Birthdays: Discuss the ages of participants, who's the oldest and who's the youngest. How did they celebrate in the past? How would they like to celebrate now? Ask what age they would like to be again and why. How old would they like to live to be?

20. Holidays: Each month, discuss holidays and how participants used to celebrate them.

21. Memories: Use tapes or videos of old radio or television comedies and humorous old commercials. Have the participants name all of their favorite comedians and programs, tell some old jokes and discuss vaudeville versus the comedians of today.

22. Home Cooking: Bring fresh homemade bread. Then talk abut the participants' favorite meals, their own best recipes and helpful hints and their special cooking talents.

23. Advertising: Borrow old newspapers or magazines from a library and discuss old versus new products. How have things changed? Compare old and current prices.

24. Home Remedies: What did their mother give them when they were sick? Discuss advances in medicine, country doctors and home remedies.

25. Presidents: Have the participants name all of the presidents, then discuss old campaign slogans and different parties and platforms.

26. Sports: Show old sports films and talk about the participants' favorite athletes, "superstars," the Olympics and artificial turf.

27. School Days: Ask participants about their favorite teachers, schools, types of discipline, grading systems and best subjects.

28. Occupations: Discuss careers and jobs and how they've changed over the years, salaries, equal pay, women in the job market. Ask if they would work for a woman boss.

29. Idols: Have the participants talk about the most influential people in their life. Then ask: Do you think you have emulated them? Whom do you feel you have had an effect upon? Can you name some famous world leaders?

30. Old Cars: Pass around photos of old automobiles. What was the participant's first car? What part has the auto played in their lives (weddings, rushing to the hospital to give birth)?

General Discussion

31. Astronomy: Hang up a large poster of the solar system. Then participants can name planets, describe their sizes and compositions and discuss space travel, astronauts and inventions. Ask if they would like to be astronauts and where they would go. What will future life in space be like?

32. Geography: Use a large map of the US or the world. Have participants show where they were born and have lived. Tell travel stories.

33. Favorite Dinner: Ask participants where they would go. With whom? What would they eat if they could go anywhere in the world?

34. Let's Make a Meal: Use pictures from diet or nutrition posters. Serve sliced fruit and iced tea or punch during discussion. Talk about proper nutrition, the food pyramid and plan a full day's menu. Have participants comment on how they feel about the food pyramid versus the four (or seven) food groups.

35. Love: What does love mean? Should everyone marry? Discuss weddings and families and today's morals versus the past.

36. At The Movies: Have the participants name all the cowboys, comedians, male and female stars, animal stars, villains, movie monsters and silent film stars they can.

37. Plan a Picnic: Plan the menu, date and time and enlist volunteers to barbecue or arrange for box lunches indoors. Discuss past family picnics.

38. Ethnic Day: Talk about ethnic souvenirs, photos and costumes brought by participants or their families. With the help of families and staff, this can be expanded to include ethnic music, food and decorations.

39. Politics: Use current events materials like newspapers and magazines. Discuss present world and national events. Talk about different political systems and how they're changing.

40. Travel: Choose a specific country and use slides, posters or film to start a discussion of dress, customs, foods, products and travel. Staff can also show vacation films.

41. Guest Speakers: Use the local college and hospital speakers' bureaus, which are often free.

42. Values: Ask the participants what beliefs and values are important to them. If they had their life to live over, what would they do differently?

43. Shipwrecked: Ask what three things the participants would pack in their suitcase if they knew they were going to be shipwrecked on a desert island.

44. Literature: Discuss favorite authors and books, story types and forms of writing the participants like best. Taping their stories to start a "living library" might be a good idea.

45. Poetry: Choose a poem and read it as a group or have a member read or recite one of his or her favorites. Discuss what it means, other poems remembered and poems they had to memorize as a child.

46. Clowns: Put up posters of clowns or circuses. Talk about the types of clowns they remember, their favorites and circus memories. What makes people laugh?

47. Life After Death: What are the participants' religious beliefs, concepts of heaven and hell? Do they fear death? Do they believe in reincarnation?

48. Inventions: Discuss the first inventions made by man, the most significant ones, and the most harmful. What would the participants like to see invented? Is man's life easier or harder today and why?

49. Pen Pal Club: Contact the local school or Scout troop and ask that they send letters and photos to the participants to be read and answered as a group.

50. Alphabet Soup: As you say each letter of the alphabet, have participants call out people, places and things that begin with that letter.

Creating a Living History Group

One of the most difficult tasks of a leader working with people who are frail is to spark interest, generate conversation and discussion and keep them involved and curious in the events of the day.

Why is Living History Important?

"No one wants to be a footstep planted in the sand near the rushing sea, a footprint to be washed away into eternal waters, a sign seen for an instant and then erased forever. The sense of identity with other loving creatures, a sense of belonging to the human endeavor or being a part of creative movement, a realization that one's life has counted to someone else have to be realized by persons growing older."   — author unknown

Realizing that one's life has counted to someone else by having experienced something, shared this with others and made their lives richer and easier is giving life purpose. This purpose is important at all ages, but especially for people who are in the process of life review.

How to Develop a Living History Group

The most important elements are personal interest, thought-provoking questions and topics that can be "brought home." An example would be a headline of an air disaster. Instead of referring to this event as frozen in time, personalize the event with other events that some of your group may have experienced. "Do you recall when the Hindenburg blew up in 1937? How about the problems with the Apollo 13 flight to the moon? How did those affect you and your family?"

Then bring the group back to the present event. Now they have shared personal experiences and the facilitator should direct this energy into a discussion of current events. By incorporating the past and present, you are validating the importance of personal experiences and acknowledging that we all play significant roles, not only in our own lives, but in the lives of those around us.

How to Begin a Living History Group

Begin with a small group of approximately seven to eight individuals. It would be ideal to combine some people who are avid news readers and television watchers with those less involved but curious. This creates a good mixture.

Start off the class with a few items on the news or in the paper. Also mention the dates and weather conditions in your city and the hometowns of group members.

Take the theme that you started the group with, such as, "The unemployment rate is increasing across the United States." Then bring the national issue closer to the group with: "What was your first job and how much did you make? How did Roosevelt's CCC program assist those troubled years?"

The group should now be in discussion, remembering years past and connecting them to events taking place today. It is rewarding for someone to feel proud in sharing personal anecdotes, taking pride in his/her citizenship and feeling that s/he is still involved in his/her world.

Responsibilities of the Living History Instructor

Be aware of your group member's special interests and backgrounds. Refer to this information and to the individual to acknowledge his/her accomplishments or experiences.

Have your materials prepared with at least three topics to work around. Avoid reading from the newspaper itself. If one topic shows little response, leave it and start another one immediately. Any lapses of time create distance with your group.

Feel comfortable in directing specific questions to a group member and asking for his/her opinion.

Encourage the group to get involved with voting issues and writing letters to the local Congressional Representatives regarding pertinent issues.

Take topics of interest from the group and incorporate these into future classes.

Share personal experiences that are taking place in your life and within the day-to-day confines with your class. Have them get involved with solving dilemmas that you are experiencing. This type of interactive problem solving and discussion among the group creates the ultimate goal of all groups: concern and involvement in a continually changing world.

Pen Pals

Goal: To provide a structured opportunity for participants to write to participants in another facility.

Objectives:

1. Establish a relationship with participants in a similar, yet distant, environment.
2. Compare emotional and physical likenesses in lifestyles in the two facilities.
3. Relieve the isolation created by living in a self-contained environment.
4. Re-use social skills (letter writing) not often employed after entrance into an assisted living or long term care facility.

Participants' needs/problems:

For many participants the world outside seems to fade away as their world becomes more and more centered in the facility. Many also forgo the social skills they had used routinely. Even shopping and church going provided some outlets for these skills. This group will provide an opportunity for the expression of social needs which an enclosed community cannot meet and will, hopefully, stimulate the ability to "reach out." It will also be a forum for comparing coping skills with others who are experiencing similar life changes.

Number of participants involved: 3 to 7

Number of sessions: Optional

Length of sessions: 30 – 40 minutes

How often: Weekly

Agenda ideas:
1. How do we initiate new friendships?
2. What is it about our everyday lives that we wish to communicate through letters?
3. Can we become interested in someone that we will never see and only know by way of written communication?
4. What can we say that will offer comfort/support to a new friend who is reaching out to us?
5. Do we really have the energy and need to expand our environment?

Using Relaxation to Address Anxiety

Goal:　　To learn relaxation techniques in response to anxiety produced by living in a community environment and to share relaxation techniques that work for individuals who are participants in the group.

Objectives:
1. Offer a quiet, stress-free environment that will allow maximum participation in this activity.
2. Provide visual and word cues for use as personal focal points to initiate the relaxation process.
3. Exchange personal coping mechanisms with other group members.

Participants' needs/problems:

The group will begin each session with a series of exercises to relax the participants. Individuals will be given attention to ensure that everyone participates. After this portion of the class is completed, there will be group discussion and experimentation with ideas elicited from group members.

Number of participants involved:　　6 to 12

Number of sessions:　　Optional

Length of sessions:　　20 – 30 minutes

How often:　　Weekly

Agenda ideas:
1. What visual/auditory images do you use to separate yourself from your surroundings and begin to relax?
2. What are the barriers to relaxation that you currently experience?
3. What is the most effective way to create a stress-free environment in your present situation?
4. Drawing from your past, paint a verbal picture for the group of the most relaxing memory you can think of.
5. What relaxation techniques have you used successfully in the past?

Living in an Institutional Setting

Goal: To provide a special time in the week for participants to express feelings regarding loss of autonomy, to discuss replacements for losses and to provide a support network for participants by allowing them to share experiences.

Objectives: 1. Stimulate discussion regarding issues of life change.
                     2. Discuss coping mechanisms that have been adapted to a changing life style.
                     3. Share feelings of loss and restructuring.
                     4. Support change as an enabler.

Participants' needs/problems:

The basic group method will be discussion/sharing. Participants will give feedback each week, especially if anyone has tried a new coping skill.

Number of participants involved: 3 to 8

Number of sessions: Optional

Length of sessions: 20 – 30 minutes

How often: Weekly

Agenda ideas:
1. List the range of feelings you have experienced since you started living here.
2. What facet of your previous life do you miss the most?
3. What things can be brought from home to give you a feeling that you are living in a place that is more like you want it to be?
4. Has there been any substitute person or thing in your current environment to help you cope with your lost autonomy?
5. Do you find solace in accepting the fact that you are receiving care that you need?

Life and Times in a Long Term Care Facility

Goal: To provide a structured opportunity for participants to express their feelings and concerns about living in a closed society, i.e. the long term care facility.

Objectives:
1. Discuss loss of personal freedom: what is the most significant loss for your?
2. Explore choices/options that are available in the long term care facility.
3. Relate successful/unsuccessful coping skills to others in the group.

Participants' needs/problems:

When living in our own homes, totally independent or with help, we are in control. Options are taken away when hospitalization becomes necessary. Some may never fully adjust to this lack of independence and limited choices. This group may provide a forum for involving participants more fully in their environment and giving them an opportunity to problem solve some of the obstacles to freedom of choice.

Number of participants involved: 3 to 7

Number of sessions: Optional

Length of sessions: 30 – 40 minutes

How often: Weekly

Agenda ideas:
1. What loss has been the most significant for you?
2. What do you do when the facility staff wants one thing and you want another?
3. What coping mechanism do you use to make it okay for you while you're here?
4. How do you assert your right to choice as provided by federal regulations?
5. What gain has been the most significant for you?

The leader may want to modify this activity for individuals in different situations. This modification would require little more than the substitution of the phrase "long term care facility" for "assisted living facility" or "adult day program."

About Music and Memories

Goal: To provide a structured opportunity for participants to reminisce about music and the part it has played in their lives.

Objectives: 1. Divide the decades between 1920 and 1960 into segments and focus on the most popular music of each era.
                     2. Provide historical information that coincides with the music being presented.
                     3. Identify memory associations of the music and history for each person who is able to express this.
                     4. Interact within the group to stimulate memory and orientation.

Participants' needs/problems:

This group was formulated as an outgrowth of the weekly sing-along sessions, which attracted a cross section of participants, probably because of the high energy it provided and also because of the memories it seemed to stimulate. Participants who are not communicative and/or oriented in other areas are often able to sing along with the old songs or even dance. This group is an intellectual extension of that emotional experience.

Number of participants involved: 5 to 10

Number of sessions: Optional

Length of sessions: 45 – 60 minutes

How often: Weekly

Agenda ideas:
1. What is it about music that stimulates your emotions?
2. Which music memory has the most significance for you?
3. How does music influence your mood?
4. Is there an era in music that reflects the time in your life when you were happiest?
5. Have you created any music memories since you became a participant here?

Cooking Class — Incredible Edibles

Goals:
1. Provide an opportunity for involvement in a familiar pastime
2. Achieve success in a short term activity project
3. Encourage socialization and team effort in a group
4. Reminiscing
5. Rekindling a past interest
6. Opportunity to achieve success
7. Provide a time of enjoyment
8. Provide a nutrition-related activity to meet needs of participants and enhance self-care skills

Equipment Needed:
- Recipe
- Handiwipes or wet towels
- Big bowls
- Plates
- Measuring cups and spoons
- Electric skillet, toaster oven or convection oven
- Potholders and hot pads
- Supply of spices, sugar, flour, etc. (these really enhance the group)
- Blender
- Utensils to serve and eat the finished product
- Some of these supplies may already be available through the Dietary Department. Be sure to plan these classes with the Dietary Supervisor to schedule times that work out for both departments.

Length of Activity: 1 hour

Number of Participants: 8 to 12

Precautions and Adaptations:

1. Be sure to place participants according to equipment proximity and helpful partners (i.e. a participant who is blind should be next to someone who will be willing to help him/her).
2. Check the bowl sizes so the participant will be able to reach inside easily.
3. Use utensils that are large and easily manipulated by hands with arthritis.
4. Be careful of all electrical wires, hot pans and placement of oils, liquids, etc.
5. CHECK SPECIAL DIETS BEFORE THE ACTIVITY BEGINS!
6. Create jobs for participants that will be success oriented, choice producing and achievable.
7. Be sure to praise each participant's efforts.
8. As often as possible, have the participants be responsible for making decision on choices of recipes and procedures.

Procedures:

1. Be sure that all participants have clean hands before beginning.
2. Pass Handiwipes to each participant to clean hands before each session begins.
3. Have the room all ready and prepared to begin. All ingredients, pictures of finished product and recipes should be on the table.
4. Explain the recipe and procedures to the group. Detail special jobs that you will be delegating.
5. Be sure that the recipe entails jobs for many hands. (If the recipe is made for individual servings, this is not a problem.)
6. Find a recipe that can be completed within an hour's time.
7. If this involves cooking/baking time, have something planned for the interim.

8. Include nutrition and a discussion of the ingredients involved. Try to cook and make things that are nutritious and a supplement to the diet, if possible.
9. Have the cooking group share favorite recipes with the group and try to schedule some of these into future classes.
10. When they are experienced enough, have the group make special hors d'oerves for a Happy Hour or prepare treats for staff recognition.
11. Don't forget your camera!

Cooking Class Ideas

1. Miniature pizzas (English muffins, cheese, mild sauce)
2. Guacamole and chips
3. Finger sandwiches (bread, cream cheese, olives)
4. Blender fruit drinks (bananas, milk, yogurt, vanilla)
5. Cookies and hot chocolate
6. Melons, their history and differences
7. Cold blender soups (tomato, cucumber)
8. Pita bread with a variety of stuffing (taco style)
9. Pigs in a blanket (small Hormel sausage in white bread)
10. Coleslaw
11. Club sandwiches
12. Quiche
13. Stir fried vegetables

A fun variation is to provide the participants with all of the ingredients that go into chocolate chip cookies but hold back the recipe! Have the group work together to try to remember the recipe for chocolate chip cookies. These cookies take such a short time to bake that the group can try out a couple batches from "memory" and then vote on the best memory recipe.

Men in a Women's World — Discussion[46]

When a man enters a facility, he may suddenly become aware of an unusual phenomenon. For the most part, he has entered into a world of women, where less than 30% of the population are men. That in itself is unusual, but what is more unusual is the fact that 80% of the staff are women, the majority of visitors appear to be women and the main group of volunteers are again, women. It is not that he doesn't like women; it's a problem of being so grossly outnumbered and not represented in his male differences.

Another consideration for the new male participant would be the limited ability of other males to relate to him. More than 1/3 of the 30% of male participants appear to be mentally incapable of communicating or relating because of their medical and/or mental conditions.

It is interesting to note that the number of boys born makes for a greater population of males than females until the age of 18. The shift begins at this age, due to accident, suicide, war, lung cancer, emphysema and industrial accidents. By the time middle age is reached, the trend is to a greater female population.

For a professional whose responsibility is to meet the needs and interests of each participant and to develop individual activity care plans, it has become an ever-increasing problem to plan successfully for men in long term care facilities. The majority of activities offered are oriented towards the majority population of women and it is women who attend the predominant number of activities offered.

One experience with a facility planning for a men's activity consisted of an afternoon special event where 15 men were brought into a small dining room. A woman wearing a coat entered the room, set down a tape recorder, removed her coat and began to belly dance for the men. The dancer was well endowed and wore enough veils to create a suggestive appearance. The veils were slowly removed. For some men, the movement and closeness of the dancer offended their religious beliefs. Others were well entertained. The staff was entertained, too, peeking in to see the men's reactions. After 15 minutes and 3 dances, the music stopped, the dancer was thanked, beer and chips were served and the men were taken quietly back to their areas. The belly dancer was the only program offered to the men.

Our planning and scheduling of men's activities has got to involve more depth, consideration, balance and variety. Here are some basic concepts and recommendations for your consideration in planning activities for the men in your facilities.

The first step is vital and involves assessment of leisure interests. Without an individual assessment of each man's interests, you are not doing justice to their special needs. Review your assessment and activity check sheet and note the types of activities you review with the male participants. Most of the assessments being used have detailed and specific female-oriented activities. An approach to a male-oriented assessment is to include activities where you need to probe for more detail and specifics in discussing both likes and dislikes. For example, following the questions of whether a man enjoys fishing there should be details of what kind, where, when, with whom and how often. It would be most important in the interviewing and assessment process to concentrate on the individual and his background, rather than the content of your prepared activity program. (Besides, you are not meeting the requirements of the federal laws for nursing homes if you gear your assessment to activities that you offer instead of activities that the participants are interested in.) There will be plenty of time to orient the participant to the existing activity program. Discussing only the existing program may act as a barrier to his opening up to express his particular interests and background.

---

[46] **Men in a Women's World** is by Michael Watters, CTRS. Used with permission.

The lack of leisure skills or mastery of specific activities in earlier life can cause problems in involvement later. Men are embarrassed to start a new skill with the fear of not being competent or appearing to be unsuccessful. Professionals will need to consider the fear of failure, self-consciousness or public showing of self with a disability as deterrents to a man's participation. Any one of the above mentioned situations can be enough to cause withdrawal or resistance to participation. It was also found that if a person had a positive view of himself earlier in life, it has generally carried over to later life skills. The same is true of a negative view of self and feelings of low self-esteem.

Another interesting fact appears to be that the blue-collar worker engages in fewer leisure activities than those in white-collar jobs and professions. The white collar and professional tended to work outside the home, in the community and with many different people. Their leisure activities tend to be more diverse and of an active nature. The blue-collar workers tend to engage in more family-centered, home-based activities. Reasons were based on income, educational level, home locations, peer expectations and access to leisure areas. There appears to be a definite relationship between the man's job role and his use of leisure time. Consideration needs to be given to the elements of technical work, selling, manual labor, the number of hours worked, job isolation, the reading required for a job, the use of tools and specialty tools used, sociability on the job and overall responsibility which can be useful in developing a creative care plan.

Another major area of concentration and interest appears to be a man's family, especially the children. In a California facility, the activity professional asked a group of men meeting for the second time, what they were most proud of and each individual responded with glowing stories about his family. Men appear to talk a great deal about how proud they are of their families and can go into detail of the history of each child and grandchild.

Professionals should begin to make a concerted effort to recruit male volunteers, both group and individual, to provide the meaningful relationships which are otherwise lacking in other areas of the facility.

In one San Francisco facility there was a man who had been a union organizer for the garment industry. After entering the facility, he had reduced his activities to staying in his room and wearing only his bathrobe. Due to his long history as a San Francisco resident, he was asked to make a presentation for a special earthquake survivor party. He arrived, wearing his blue suit with a flower in his lapel and made a warm and sincere welcome to the gathering. This was the beginning of his continued role as the host and emcee at parties and special events for the facility.

If you search your facility, you will find duties, responsibilities and roles which give male participants some of those roles that have been lost or re-invest them in duties and activities which they have long since put aside.

For example: The Adopt-a-Grandparent program plays into the role of confidant, friend and family member which many have lost as their own family has diminished. Maintenance personnel may become involved by supplying ideas, materials and leadership for tinkering with projects that many of the men used to enjoy. Adapted setups for tools and workbenches can give back a sense of work and productivity. Barbershop quartets, choirs, sports events and discussion groups can give some of the camaraderie which has been lost with the reduction of male social contacts.

In summary, although men represent a small minority in a world of women, their needs and interests should be given careful consideration, planning and timely involvement in the overall program. Being left out of the activity program services should not have to be another loss in the series of life's disappointments. Sincere efforts, specific programming ideas, recruitment of volunteers and groups, plus a commitment to involve men in dynamic programming can make a change in the life of a facility.

Some specific program ideas include:

- Making or repairing toys and children's furniture
- Construction of wooden animals
- Coin collecting
- Animal care and feeding
- Bone and horn polishing and engraving art
- Brass crafts
- Bonsai
- Printing
- Rope tying
- Contests and non-cash gambling
- Story telling of special events in history
- Cooperation games and events
- Films of famous men who may have had an effect on their lives
- Sport quizzes, trivia, records and events, personalities
- Men's group singing
- Activities sponsored by men's groups (social clubs, fraternities)
- Debate, Toastmaster speaking groups
- Mime and theater groups
- Walking club — wheelchairs included
- Metalsmith work
- Wire work — soft wire sculpture
- Electrical work — tinkering with small appliances
- Soap carving
- Sawdust craft — relief maps
- Monthly breakfast speakers
- Speakers and visits to service equipment: fire station, ambulance, police station, farms, construction sites
- Hardware store owners who show the latest in tools
- Tournaments
- Liar's contest
- Lunch at a local men's club
- Fishing outings
- A day at the races
- Big Brothers sponsorships
- Adopt-a-Grandparent programs
- All male play readings
- Talent show
- Wood making projects
- Readers for the blind
- Teaching specialized subjects — computers
- Pool and billiards
- Bocce ball
- Bird watching — field identification
- Men's fashion show
- Rock collecting
- Stamp collecting
- Radio equipment
- Gold panning

Men in a Women's World — Activity

Goal: To provide a structured opportunity for men to discuss their lives in a community of women.

Objectives: 1. Compare and contrast life in your facility and life in society as a whole: Who is in control — men or women?
                     2. Discuss individual adaptations to dependence on women for most care.
                     3. Interact in a group of mostly men to provide relief from the women's society.

Participants' needs/problems:

The men now in facilities have, for the most part, lived their lives with the assumption that men are dominant in society. It is assumed that they are the decision makers, the ones in control of their life situations. When care becomes necessary due to physical limitations, however, the status of men changes, as does the amount of their perceived control.

What effect does this have on the male ego, this loss of control and this entry into a society dominated and controlled and mostly populated by women? This group explores these issues with men.

Number of participants involved: 3 to 5

Number of sessions: Optional

Length of sessions: 30 – 60 minutes

How often: Weekly

Agenda ideas:
1. What is it like to be in a matriarchal society?
2. How do you see your role?
3. How has this changed since you were "out in the world?"
4. What have you learned to do in this environment to enable you to assert yourself as an individual?
5. Is there any way you could have prepared yourself to live in this new "society?"

Chapter 9
Rehabilitation Focused Groups

Many of the individuals you work with will have the potential to regain function. This group will want more than activities meant to keep the skills they have, provide entertainment and ensure a reasonable quality of life. Individuals who have the real potential to improve their function are likely to want to work hard to recover what they can. In many cases an improvement in function will move the individual to a less restrictive setting — and hopefully closer to the ones s/he loves.

Building upon the five levels already discussed in Chapter 7: Programming for Low Function (Levels 1 and 2) and Chapter 8: Programming for Moderately Impaired Function (Levels 3-5), this chapter covers work done with individuals who would benefit from cognitive stimulation (Level 6), short term rehabilitation (Level 7) and community integration (Level 8).

Level 6: Cognitive Stimulation/Cognitive Retraining includes techniques used with individuals suffering from trauma to the brain and showing cognitive disorganization. Level 7: Short Term Rehabilitation includes programming which enhances personal goals worked on in physical therapy, occupational therapy, recreational therapy and speech therapy. Level 8: Community Integration includes individuals who are preparing for discharge; focusing on skills, resources and independence when back at a previous living situation.

Level 6: Cognitive Stimulation and Retraining Activities

Cognitive Stimulation is a term coined for techniques used in therapy to stimulate cognitive function and assist in retraining an individual to his/her optimum level of function. These techniques may also give an individual memory tools and strategies to compensate for a memory loss s/he has experienced.

There are many excellent resources in this field to draw from. Activity ideas may vary from concentration games, completion of simple tasks such as puzzles, color and shape sorting, connecting dot-to-dot puzzles, hand water games which involve sensory motor skills, analogies, trivia games, problem solving situations, etc.

Other valuable resources for memory retention and cognitive stimulation activities are the speech therapist, occupational therapist, recreational therapist and psychologist under contract with your setting. Each of these specialties will offer ideas specific to the immediate needs of the participant.

Memory and cognitive function techniques can also be utilized with participants who are there for short term rehabilitation even though they are generally focused on therapy goals and not interested in most of the other programs that are offered.

Brain Function

The types of cognitive stimulation and retraining activities that are required depend on the diagnosis of the participant. Sometimes there is known damage to some part of the brain (as with a stroke). The chart on the next page provides a brief summary of the functions of different areas of the brain and should help you understand which skills have been lost.

Memory

In nearly all of the cognitive stimulation programs offered through activities, memory techniques and interventions will play an integral part.

Memory loss can occur for many reasons. Some of these may be related to depression, nutritional imbalance, medications and changes, emotional losses and significant transitions. Other reasons for memory loss are more organic such as a head injury, stroke, cerebral tumor or a progressive degenerative disease such as Parkinson's disease, Alzheimer's disease and other dementia disorders.

Memory takes place as three separate processes:

1. From our earliest experiences, we not only explore and learn new things — but, in addition, our brain registers this information. This is the first process of memory — Input.

2. The next function of memory is to store this new information in such a way that it relates to the experience. This is the second process of memory — Storage.

3. The final and most important function is the ability to retrieve and use the information experienced and learned before. In the retrieval process, the brain is able to dip into its bank of information and retrieve information specific to the current need. This is the last process of memory — Retrieval.

Memory is quite a miraculous feat and, of course, there are things that can go wrong in all three processes.

In addition to the three processes of memory there are also three types of memory:[47]

1. **Sensory Motor Memory:** From the physical and sensory experience, we use visual, auditory, tactile, proprioceptive, olfactory and gustatory senses. An example of this would be a smell that brings back a memory associated with it, the proprioceptive experience or whole body experience of walking on sand at the shore. This sensory motor memory seems to predate all other memory and leaves an imprint on us forever. Sensory stimulation is an intervention to restimulate and remember through this process.

2. **Short Term Memory:** The short term memory is the ability to experience and replay new information. Short term memory is exactly as stated, short term. If we read a map and go in that direction, we have processed the new information and applied it to the current task. If we are learning a new card game, we need to understand the rules and process them in order to successfully participate in the game. This is our working memory.

---

[47] Atkinson, R. C. and Shiffrin, R. M., 1971, "The control of short-term memory and its control processes," *Scientific American*, 225, 82-90.

Brain injuries and their effects

The brain controls more than our ability to think. Most of the brain's higher functions are located in the dome-shaped cerebrum, which is divided into four lobes. The cerebellum regulate subconscious activities such as coordination. The brainstem connects the cerebrum with the spinal cord. The diagram below explains what happens when different areas of the brain get injured.

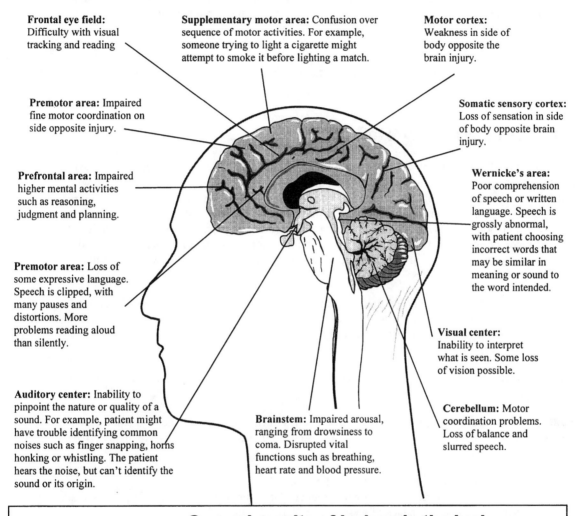

Frontal eye field: Difficulty with visual tracking and reading

Supplementary motor area: Confusion over sequence of motor activities. For example, someone trying to light a cigarette might attempt to smoke it before lighting a match.

Motor cortex: Weakness in side of body opposite the brain injury.

Premotor area: Impaired fine motor coordination on side opposite injury.

Somatic sensory cortex: Loss of sensation in side of body opposite brain injury.

Prefrontal area: Impaired higher mental activities such as reasoning, judgment and planning.

Wernicke's area: Poor comprehension of speech or written language. Speech is grossly abnormal, with patient choosing incorrect words that may be similar in meaning or sound to the word intended.

Premotor area: Loss of some expressive language. Speech is clipped, with many pauses and distortions. More problems reading aloud than silently.

Visual center: Inability to interpret what is seen. Some loss of vision possible.

Auditory center: Inability to pinpoint the nature or quality of a sound. For example, patient might have trouble identifying common noises such as finger snapping, horns honking or whistling. The patient hears the noise, but can't identify the sound or its origin.

Brainstem: Impaired arousal, ranging from drowsiness to coma. Disrupted vital functions such as breathing, heart rate and blood pressure.

Cerebellum: Motor coordination problems. Loss of balance and slurred speech.

The four major lobes

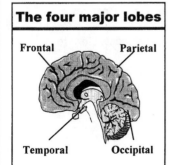

Frontal   Parietal

Temporal   Occipital

General results of lesions in the brain

Frontal: Impaired motor skills, speech, intellectual functions, emotional status. Patient may be apathetic, impulsive, irritable or provocative. Also may have trouble starting, sustaining or ending a specific behavior. For example, a patient sitting in a car might not get up unless told to.

Temporal: Difficulty discriminating and sequencing what is heard. Memory problems. Seizures. Partial loss of vision in upper field of each eye.

Parietal: Loss of sensation in half the body opposite brain lesion. Loss of sense of touch. Patient can have trouble telling what is in hands without looking. Impaired sense of place. Trouble taking things apart and putting them back together. Fifty percent loss of vision in left or right half of visual field.

Occipital: Patient may seem blind since he or she can't identify things by sight alone. Though vision loss is partial, patient needs to touch to identify things.

3. **Long Term Memory:** Long term memory is information that was stored a long time ago. It is our secondary memory. Some participants may not remember who you are or what their own names are, but they will be able to sing all the words of an old song. A similar example would be the ability to recite, word for word, a poem that was learned 60 years ago.

The more that one has memorized in their lives, the stronger the memory. In the early 1900's, education was based on memorizing material and reciting it in class. Because of this method, many of the individuals in care settings can successfully recite and engage in activities that focus on long term memory skills.

Programs we develop need to include all three types and processes of memory. According to the individual's health issues, you can determine what type of memory intervention is most needed.

Treatment for Memory Deficits

The professional will find that s/he is likely to have better results if s/he works on attention span and sensory exercises instead of just working on improving an individual's memory. Working with participants who have memory problems can be tough. However, without attention span, memory is not likely to improve, or even stay at the same level of ability. Also, sensory memory and sensory stimulation seem to be a more basic activity than verbal memory. There are many different types of memory, including verbal memory, kinesthetic memory and auditory memory. Work with your participant to see how well his/her short term memory in all three areas is working. Zoltan[48] suggests the following exercises:

Visual: The participant is asked to reproduce simple geometric figures, which are presented for 5 to 10 seconds and then covered. Note: if a person's perceptual abilities are impaired, it is likely that this will affect memory for visual material and the ability to use visually based solutions to assist in memory problems. - like cermaces, might forget but repatove brings back.

Kinesthetic: The participant is asked to reproduce a series of hand positions presented to him or her. Remembering how to do it

Auditory: The participant is asked to reproduce a series of rhythmic taps. Note: if the participant has aphasia, verbal memory and the ability to use verbal memory solutions are likely to be affected. Short verbal cues,

Some important things for the professional to determine:
- Can the participant continue to learn with practice? Or is the inability to complete a task due to a lack of skill instead of a lack of memory?
- Is the participant's memory loss always a problem, or does there seem to be a pattern to memory loss (e.g., more problems at night)?
- What types of cues help the participant remember better? It is best to give the cue as close to the time the participant needs to remember something as possible.
- Question the participant about what s/he is doing during the activity and wait for a response. If the participant talks about what s/he is doing and gives the activity professional feedback during the activity, the participant will tend to remember more about the activity later.

---

[48] Barbara Zoltan (1996). *Vision, Perception and Cognition, Third Edition*. Page 140.

Memory Book

This activity is for an alert participant interested in documenting his/her life for family and friends in a life review process. The use of a memory book is valuable for individuals who remember, recall and reminisce; and also for individuals who can use these memories and reinforcers to feel safe, enhance long term memory, reduce anxiety and promote safe, acceptable social responses.

A memory book highlights the individual and increases a sense of self and self-esteem. This book can be experienced both on a one-on-one basis and in a small group setting. Family and friends are invited to share stories and memories of this individual and perhaps bring in photos to bring the stories to life.

There may be pages with reinforcement statements. Many individuals dealing with memory loss issues become easily agitated and upset with the loss of words and memories. Each person needs his/her own pages of reminders that will be individualized to specific needs and concerns.

The book can be filled with art and writings from its owner. This book should always be available and accessible for the individual to find or keep around.

Goal:	Opportunities for participant to reminisce about his/her life; to reexamine past experiences, beliefs, values; to recall happier times; to socialize with others.
Equipment Needs:	Memory Book — blank book with questions from master list. (See the following page for a sample Memory Book.) Photos, drawings and stories from the participant or his/her family and friends, which can be placed in the memory book. Pen.
Length of Activity:	30 – 45 minutes
Number of Participants:	1– 6
Adaptations:	Move chair up close to bed; possibly use tray table to write on.

Procedures:
1. Greet participant; catch up on recent events (briefly).
2. Sit down; ask participant next question from the list below or other questions that have been suggested for this participant. (You can briefly review last session if you like.)
3. Be patient — give participant plenty of time to answer. Ask helpful questions to stir memory.
4. Do not be too aggressive — this is not a quiz! Be kind, helpful. Keep an open mind — you will hear all kinds of things — funny, heart-warming, aggravating, very sad.
5. Thank participant; read next 1–2 questions for next time.
6. Participant presents completed book to loved one(s).

Questions For A Memory Book About Your Family:

1. From what country or countries did your family ancestors emigrate? When was this and where did they settle?
2. What are your parents' names?
3. When and where were they born?
4. What was your mother's maiden name?
5. What do you remember most about your mother from your childhood?
6. What do you remember most about your father?
7. What work did your parents do?
8. What is your birth date?

9. Where were you born?
10. Was there anything unusual about the circumstances of your birth?
11. Were you born in a hospital or at home?
12. What is your full name and how was it chosen? Does it have a special meaning?
13. Who in your family do you most look like?
14. How many brothers and sisters did you have? (List them in the order they were born and include children who may have died early in life or at birth.)
15. Where did you fit among them?
16. To whom did you feel closest?
17. How did you spend your time together?
18. Did you ever take trips or vacations with your family? Where did you go? Tell about a favorite one.
19. Was another language besides English spoken in your home? What was it?
20. Did your family attend a church or synagogue? Was religion an important part of your family life?

The table below gives examples of pages that you might want to place in a participant's memory book. Each section of the table should be its own page within the memory book. Your participants will have an easier time reading what is written if you use **Bold Arial Type** about 24 point in size.

The Idyll Arbor web site has a full-sized sample of a memory book available at www.IdyllArbor.com/memory.pdf.

Elements of a Memory Book

My Memories by _____	My name is My spouse's name is
I was born on My home town is Places I lived	My past occupations were My hobbies, interests I currently live at
My favorite photos	Family Stories I have _____ children Their names are:
My favorite memories to share	My room number is _____ My roommate's name is _____
Lunch is served at _____ Dinner is served at _____	Some reminders: My purse is in my room. My children know where I live so I don't have to worry. When I smile, I feel better.
I don't have to worry because all of the bills for staying here are taken care of. Everyone here knows my name and who I am. I am very safe here with people who care for me.	Some of my favorite things to do are:

Attention Flexibility

Attention Flexibility Tasks[49]

The ability to maintain one's mental flexibility requires regular practice. The activities listed below are divided into three levels to better match the individual's current ability.

Purpose:	To maintain and/or increase the participant's ability to pay attention to a sequence of events.
Skills Necessary:	Ability to tend to a task and to demonstrate the mental flexibility to switch attention as needed.
Goal:	To be able to successfully execute change of attention.
Objectives:	To be able to successfully execute one change of attention. To be able to successfully alternate between two different sequences or responses. To be able to alternate responses between multiple tasks.
Materials:	Index cards with the following typed on them in 24 or 32 point **Arial Bold**: <ul><li>mmmmmmnnnnn</li><li>mnmnmnmnmn</li><li>2 4 5 6 7 3 (first line) 5 5 9 3 7 3 (second line)</li><li>2 4 7 3 6 7 9 2 (first line) 12 4 11 6 13 5 15 3 (second line)</li><li>"If you had $9.85, tell me all the different lunches you could order."</li><li>"Tell me all the different coin combinations that will make 1.05"</li><li>"Tell me all the different card combinations that add up to 21"</li></ul>A deck of playing cards with easy to read numbers Menus from various restaurants like Denny's or Cracker Barrel Paper and pencil
Process:	Follow the instructions in the table below depending on the participant's ability.

---

[49] The idea for this activity is from Toglia, J.P. (1992) "Cognitive Rehabilitation" in *Vision, Perception and Cognition, Third Edition.* By B. Zoltan. 1996.

Attention Flexibility Tasks

Level	Activity Professional	Participant
Level 1 Follows one change	Copy the following:	mmmmmmnnnnnn
	Add these pairs of numbers.	2 4 5 6 7 3
	Now subtract these numbers.	5 5 9 3 7 2
	Using a deck of playing cards, spread face up all over the table.	Turn over the even-numbered cards. Now turn over the odd- numbered cards.
Level 2 Alternates between two different sequences or responses	Copy the following:	mnmnmnmnmn
	Add the first 2 pairs of numbers. Subtract the next 2 pairs of numbers and continue alternating.	2 4 7 3 6 7 9 2 12 4 11 6 13 5 15 3
	Using a deck of cards placed in rows on the table, face up.	Turn over the odd cards, but as soon as you get to a J, Q or K card, switch to turning over even cards. When you get to the next J, Q, or K card, switch back to odd cards and so on.
Level 3 Generates alternate responses or ideas	Give the participant a piece of paper, pencil and restaurant menu. Ask the following:	If you had $9.85, tell me all the different lunches you could order.
	Give the participant a piece of paper and pencil. Ask the following:	Tell me all the different coin combinations that will make $1.05.
	Give the participant a deck of playing cards. Ask the following:	Tell me all the different card combinations that add up to 21.

Map Test

Purpose:	To maintain and/or increase the participant's ability to pay attention to task for a short period of time.
Skills Necessary:	To scan a document in all directions. To attend to a task for two minutes. To distinguish between different symbols.
Goals:	To exercise the participant's mental flexibility. To exercise the participant's attention to task.
Objectives:	To attend to the task for 60 seconds. To visually distinguish between symbols found on a map.
Materials:	Large map with symbols depicting locations on the map. Maps from the parks or cities with large symbols work well. We suggest that you have between four and six maps that measure about three feet by three feet and which are laminated (for infection control). Use an erasable magic marker.

This timed activity requires that the participant search a map for a total of two minutes and circle a particular symbol on the map each time s/he locates one. Some people have the participant use one color marker for the first minute and a second color marker for the second minute. Show the participant the key that contains the symbols that can be found on the map. Indicate which one symbol you want the participant to circle. This helps the professional know how long the participant can attend to a task. On-going practice with different maps helps the participant stay "mentally sharp."

Popular Games for Cognitive Stimulation[50]

The following is an alphabetical list of games that are commercially available which could be used in a cognitive stimulation program. This list is by no means comprehensive. The manufacturer of the game is provided after each entry (unless the game is available through several manufacturers) along with a listing by number of the cognitive skills required. The number coding of cognitive skills is as follows:

1. Perceptual accuracy — All games require perceptual (usually visual) accuracy to some extent but some focus on accuracy as a goal.

2. Spatial organization — Games requiring, as a basic focus organization of material in two or three dimensions are given this designation.

3. Perception-motor functioning — This entails fine motor functioning or motor speed when it represents a primary component of the game.

4. Verbal skills — Games addressing the generation of words or other verbal material.

5. Math skills — Games in which basic arithmetic plays a central role, including the handling of money.

---

[50] Williams, J. M., 1987, "Cognitive Stimulation in the Home Environment," *The Rehabilitation of Cognitive Disabilities*, Center for Applied Psychological Research, Memphis State University, Plenum Press, New York, NY.

6. Convergent problem solving — The emphasis here is on piecing together solutions in a step-wise fashion, an essential component to effective strategy.

7. Divergent problem solving — Flexibility in approach is the hallmark. In other words, diverging from step-by-step solutions to generate new strategies.

8. Sequencing — This is often a component of convergent and divergent problem solving but, in some cases, is a goal in itself.

9. Memory — All games require ongoing monitoring and recall as part of the game process but some games focus on memory itself, that is, the ability to retrieve information from long-term storage.

The complexity of the games varies a great deal and is very difficult to rate in a consistent fashion. However, even complex games can be made simpler by altering rules, such as by removing special cards and liberalizing time constraints. For instance, the game Uno (International) can be simplified by removing all special cards, such as Draw Four and Reverse.

Games for Cognitive Stimulation

Aggravation (Lakeside) — 6
Backgammon — 2,5,6
Bargain Hunter (Milton Bradley) — 5,6
Battleship (Milton Bradley) — 2,6
Bed Bugs (Milton Bradley) — 3
Bingo — 2
Boggle (Parker Brothers) — 4,7
Checkers — 2,6
Chess — 2,6,7
Clue (Parker Brothers) — 6
Connect Four (Milton Bradley) — 1,6
Dominoes — 1,2
Erector Sets — 2,3,6
Etch-A-Sketch (Ohio Art) — 2,3
Foursight (Lakeside) — 2,7
Gridlock (Ideal) — 1,2,6
Lego — 1,2,3
Life (Milton Bradley) — 5,6
Lincoln Logs (Playskool) — 1,2,3
Lite-Brite (Hasbro) — 1,2,3
Lotto (Edu-Cards)
Farm Lotto — 1,6
Object Lotto — 1,6
Go-Together Lotto — 1,6
The World About Us Lotto — 1,6
Zoo Lotto — 1,6
Luck Plus (International) — 1,5
Mastermind (Pressman) — 2,6
Memory Original (Milton Bradley) — 2,9
Animal Families (Milton Bradley) — 2,9
Fronts & Backs (Milton Bradley) — 2,9
Step by Step (Milton Bradley) — 6,8

Mhing (Suntex) — 6,7,8
Models, plastic replica — 1,2,3,8
Monopoly (Parker Brothers) — 5,6
Mystery Mansion — 6
Othello — 2,6
Paint-by-numbers — 1,2,3
Parcheesi (Selchow & Righter) — 6
Password (Milton Bradley) — 4,6,9
Pay Day (Parker Brothers) — 5,6
Pente (Parker Brothers) — 2,6
Perquacky (Lakeside) — 4,7,9
Picture Tri-Ominoes (Pressman) — 1
Pic Up Stik (Steven) — 3
Racko (Milton Bradley) — 8
Rage (International) — 6,8
Risk (Parker Brothers) — 2,6,7
Sabotage (Lakeside) — 6,7
Scotland Yard (Milton Bradley) — 2,6,8
Scrabble — 2,4,7,9
Smath (Pressman) — 2,5,6
Sorry (Parker Brothers) — 6
Think & Jump (Pressman) — 2,6
Toss Across (Ideal) — 3
Tri-Ominoes (Pressman) — 1
Tripoley — 1,8
Uno (International) — 1,8
Verbatim (Lakeside) — 4,7,9
Whodunit (Selchow & Righter) — 6
Word War (Whitman) — 4,6,7,9
Word Yahtzee (Milton Bradley) — 4,7,9
Yahtzee (Milton Bradley) — 5,6

Level 7: Short Term Rehab Activities[51]

One of the current issues of professionals is how and what to do with people who are here for short-term or acute rehabilitation who prefer not to get involved in activities and who have very specific and different needs.

This section will look at working with participants who are in your facility for rehabilitation treatment, especially for those admitted to a nursing home. Some of the important questions include:

- What is rehab? What is the team? Who are the players?
- How do you help rehab succeed?
- How do you work with consultants vs. facility employees?
- How do you coordinate care after specialized therapy (PT, OT, RT, Speech Therapy) has occurred and the participant needs to stay in the facility?

The goal of rehab activities is to help the participant get back to the target level of functioning as quickly and easily as possible.

Some of the things you need to do to make these activities work are

- Realize the differences between the individual admitted for rehabilitation and the individual admitted for long term care.
- Provide activities that are coordinated with the goals of other members of the rehab team.
- Understand if the participant is too tired to participate in your activities.

Trends

The profile of the participant in a long term care facility is as diverse as the services provided. What once was a setting created for individuals who were frail or elderly has evolved into a setting that provides for a profoundly differing participant population. Today a participant may be young or old. S/he may be receiving treatments such as chemotherapy, wound care, IV therapy and head injury treatment, previously offered only in acute care settings. Along with these specialized treatments, we may be seeing participants needing special care from ventilator dependent services and tracheostomy units. There will also be an increase in the numbers of participants of all ages who are HIV positive.

As the acuity level increases, so does the need to clearly understand medical diagnoses and how professionals play an integral role in quality of care and quality of life issues.

The Rehab Team

The Team Players
Working in rehab in a long term care facility may include working with the following members of the rehab team: doctor, nurses (licensed and aides), physical therapist, occupational therapist, speech pathologist, respiratory therapist, recreational therapist, hospice workers, clergy, dietitian, social services professional, activity professional, psychologist, psychiatrist, administrator.

Each facility addresses the participant on rehab in a team approach. Facilities hold meetings on a regular basis to design a specific plan for each individual. The content of these meetings may be participant progress, discharge planning, coordination of services, eligibility for current insurance

---

[51] This section is by Lauren Newman, OTR. Used with permission.

coverage, eligibility for programs, services in the future, planning for family conferences, participant care plan and sharing of information and techniques that may or may not be working.

It is important to get to know the therapists in your facility and their individual roles as part of the team. Some therapists are consultants under contract and are in the facility specifically to work with an individual participant. They need to be approached directly so that they can understand your role and willingness to help follow through with their treatments. On the other hand, some therapists are full time employees within the facility. They may be available for additional support for the activity and social services departments regarding specific participants and their therapy.

With the new Medicare PPS (Prospective Payment System), the rehab team needs to very closely monitor a participant to ensure they are meeting the criteria to receive specific rehab services according to their diagnosis and rehab potential. Review the PPS guidelines in Chapter 12: Resident Assessment Instrument.

The Role of Professionals

When the Resident is Actively Involved in Therapy

When a participant is newly admitted to a long term care setting and is receiving therapy on a daily basis, his/her primary goal is to regain strength and independence and be discharged. Because the focus is short term and centers on returning home, this individual is usually not interested in activities that are offered. For some, the experience of socializing with participants who are confused and disoriented is a hard and constant reminder that they may also need to remain long term and possibly begin to experience further declines in function. Because of this, their choice is often to go to therapy and then spend the majority of the day in their room. Some participants in rehab will seek out other participants in rehab programs for support and contact because of their common challenges and goals.

The professional needs to listen closely at the rehab meetings so that s/he understands clearly what the therapy goals are and how the participant is progressing with them. At this stage, you should discuss with the therapists how activity staff or social services staff can reinforce and align themselves with the current therapy goals. If the therapist encourages the participant to work with you, there is a greater chance for either involving the participant in a group or in working with them on a one-on-one basis. Therefore, it is important to make agreements with the therapists regarding the non-therapy time the participants may have.

When Assisting with the Therapist's Treatment Goals

The following set of goals show examples of ways that activities can help participants make progress toward their therapy goals:

When the therapist has given approval for independent ambulation, the activity professional can assist with "*increasing endurance of walking.*" This can be done with the help of a walker or other device. Activities such as mail delivery and assistance with participant transportation to and from activities may be appropriate.

"*Increase endurance in time out of bed in wheelchair from 1 to 2 hours per day.*" The activity professional can find activities that will not only challenge but also engage the participant in meaningful activity, which can at the same time be enjoyable.

"*Increase strength in upper extremity.*" This could be incorporated into an exercise group, beanbag toss, balloon volleyball, parachute game and movement to music.

"*Increase endurance and accuracy in upper extremity.*" This could be stacking and sorting activities, sewing or weaving, bingo, checkers, puzzles and many other activities.

"Improve visual scanning skills." This could be done through bingo and flashlight tag.

"Improve conversational skills: auditory comprehension, intelligibility of speech, word finding." This could be done in social services discussion groups or as part of an activity where conversation goes on between the participants.

"Improve reading and writing skills." This could be done with current events groups, through discussions of literature or by writing down life histories.

"Improve skills in ADLs: grooming and dressing." This could be helped with various grooming activities (including fixing nails or hair) and activities involving period clothes.

When the Participant Stays after Formal Therapy Has Ended

When participants are discharged from formal therapy services and need to stay in the facility for additional convalescence or long term stay, the need for activity involvement becomes crucial. Many participants feel a sense of failure and loss when they have not been able to achieve their therapy goals. They often develop close and significant relationships with the therapist. This therapist plays a pivotal position in refocusing the participant's goals and establishing a new framework. By encouraging work with the professionals with goals similar to the ones previously established, the therapist assures the participant a better chance of not "giving up" and continuing his/her work towards a higher functional level.

In determining the best and most realistic discharge plan for a participant, the interdisciplinary team works closely with the physician to assess the participant's level of independence. The activity professional can help assess this level of independence and orientation by including the participant in a "helper" or a volunteer role and closely observing him/her in group settings and projects. Things such as mail delivery or requesting the participant's assistance with special projects and events help not only to assess abilities, but also to give him/her a sense of usefulness and self-esteem, which are paramount to continued progress.

When the Participant is in Need of Long Term Stay

The activity and social services professionals may be the most helpful staff members facilitating the transition to long term care and daily routine. After acute rehab is completed, there is usually a room change for the participant. This means new roommates, new orientation to the area of the facility and, sometimes, different staff members attending to his/her needs. The activity and social services staff may be *the* point of stability for these participants.

When the Participant is in Need of Recreational Therapy Services

The types of rehabilitation treatment provided by a recreational therapist are different than the types of interventions offered by the activity professional (even if the activity professional is a recreational therapist). So the question is, what types of special treatments or procedures fall within the scope of recreational therapy practice, which are not already considered to be part of expected and required activities listed under Tag F248? (Tag F248 is the section of the US OBRA nursing home law which outlines the type of services required by the recreational therapist/activity professional/occupational therapist/certified occupational therapy assistant who is in charge of ensuring that each resident's needs related to activities are being met.) To understand what falls outside of the expected and required activities, it is best to understand what types of activities are expected and required. These can be found at Tag F248 under both the regulation and the guidelines for surveyors. Tag F248 states:

Tag F248 "(Regulation) The facility must provide for an ongoing program of activities designed to meet, in accordance with the comprehensive assessment, the interests and the physical, mental and psychosocial well-being of each resident.

(Guideline) Because the activities program should occur within the context of each resident's comprehensive assessment and care plan, it should be multi-faceted and reflect each individual resident's needs. Therefore, the activities program should provide stimulation or solace, promote physical, cognitive and/or emotional health; enhance, to the extent practicable, each resident's physical and mental status; and promote each resident's self-respect by providing, for example, activities that support self-expression and choice. Activities can occur at any time and are not limited to formal activities being provided by activity staff. Others involved may be any facility staff, volunteers and visitors.

(Probes to Surveyors) Observe individual group and bedside activities. Are residents who are confined or choose to remain in their rooms provided with in room activities in keeping with life-long interests (e.g., music, reading, visits with individuals who share their interests or reasonable attempts to connect the resident with such individuals) and in-room projects they can work on independently? Do any facility staff members assist the resident with activities he or she can pursue independently? If residents sit for long periods of time with no apparently meaningful activities, is the cause: resident choice, failure of any staff or volunteers either to inform residents when activities are occurring or to encourage resident involvement in activities; lack of assistance with ambulation; lack of sufficient supplies and/or staff to facilitate attendance and participation in the activity programs or program design that fails to reflect the interests or ability levels of residents, such as activities that are too complex?"

Some of the key words and phrases found under expected and required activities are 1. interests and well-being of each resident, 2. provide stimulation/solace, 3. promote health, 4. enhance status and 5. promote self-respect. For the recreational therapist, the ability to determine if the treatment provided is enhancing and providing well-being and health or if it is a treatment intervention that goes beyond is often very difficult. Most of the treatment provided which allows the resident to maintain his/her status (or to slow decline) and which allows the resident to engage in leisure/free time activities is considered to be part of the required and expected services. Required and expected activities would include reality orientation; exercise group; almost all adaptation of supplies and activities to allow the resident to engage in activity; modifying activities/providing activities which are culturally, age or gender appropriate; cognitive stimulation; reminiscing; remotivation; resocializing; solace; generalized relaxation techniques; most in-room activities; range of motion through activity; activities to increase self-esteem/self-respect; teaching new leisure skills; and providing structure to modify behavior. Other activities, generally outside what is traditionally thought of as the activity professional's job, relate to general resident safety and well-being. These activities would include infection control; ensuring that residents have adequate skin protection including pressure releases, changing positions and appropriate padding; maintaining a safe environment; and ensuring a respectful environment.

Most of the work that a recreational therapist does in a long term care setting that is different than the work of an activity director relates to community integration, improved function through the use of aquatic therapy, increased independence through adaptive computer equipment and cognitive exercise through cognitive retraining/cognitive therapy. Greater detail can be found in Chapter 3: The Work We Do under the section Recreational Therapy Services.

Level 8: Community Integration Activities

At times it may be vital, prior to discharge from our services, for the participant to be escorted into the community on short outings. Not all participants can adjust immediately to a new (usually lower) health status. They may need the professional to venture into the community with them, helping to solve problems along the way. Such help from the professional (and the rest of the team) involves preparatory activities, which take place both inside and outside of the facility.

Some of the activities involve the use of standardized integration programs such as the *Community Integration Program (CIP)*[52]. Others involve the use of activities in the facility for the development of skills such as working, communicating and the basic ADLs. One important element of community integration activities is to never let the community get too far away from the participant's day-to-day life.

Professionals work with the interdisciplinary team's goal of discharging participants to their next level of care. Some of the ways that professionals can assist in this process are
- Identify and list community resources for leisure activities in the community.
- Assist participant in contacting support groups or recreational groups s/he has expressed interest in joining.
- Create a "map" of the community with names and addresses attached to the map for reference.
- Offer participant the name of an individual or staff person to call if s/he has any questions or needs to talk after discharge and during integration into community.
- Identify transportation systems which participant may need to contact in community.
- Touch base with family briefly by phone or during discharge to offer them support in and after discharge.

As a step toward a return to the community, you can establish programs such as the Intergenerational Program (in Chapter 6) to reconnect your participants with the community outside the facility. Even if the participants need to stay in a long term care facility for medical reasons, they can still be an integral part of the community outside.

Recreational Therapy Services in Community Integration Programming

Using a pre-established set of community integration treatment protocols such as the *Community Integration Program (CIP)* (Armstrong and Lauzen, 1995) helps the therapist ensure that the treatment provided is likely to have positive outcomes based on the participant's actual level of ability. An example of one of the *CIP's* treatment protocols is the *Module 1A: Environmental Safety* protocol. The purpose of the protocol is to first determine how safe the participant will be in the community and second, to provide training in the community safety areas which will limit the participant's safe use of the community after discharge. This is important information for the entire treatment team to know as they plan the participant's discharge. The therapist takes a 3 x 5 card with instructions written on one side of the card. The instructions take the participant from one of the doors of the facility and uses five turns along sidewalks, driveways and other areas to have the participant get to a spot where s/he can no longer see the door from which s/he started. At this point the therapist asks for the card back and then instructs the participant to return to the door from which s/he started. *Module 1A* provides the therapist with a series of questions related to participant knowledge, endurance, safety of ambulation/locomotion, speed of both gross motor and cognitive actions, problem solving, personal safety, awareness of his/her own needs for

---

[52] Armstrong, Missy and Sarah Lauzen, 1994, *Community Integration Program, 2nd Edition*, Idyll Arbor, Inc., Ravensdale, WA.

assistance, appropriateness of grooming and clothing for situation, and ability to tolerate stimulation in the environment.

It is a common practice for the recreational therapist to use a standardized program for community integration interventions. Another of the programs that is commonly used is *Out in the World* by Johnson and Orichowskiyj (1999). The section on Consumer Buying provides the therapist with over 20 different types of consumer oriented training programs and forms. There are also many other commercially available programs that help teach advanced activities of daily living. The therapist should have a variety and use the ones appropriate for a particular participant.

Chapter 10
Documentation

What is a health record? Why are health records kept? Who owns the health record? Are there rules to follow when making an entry in a health record? Are there mandated forms and content to the health record? These questions and more will be answered in this chapter. While the specifics found in this chapter apply to nursing homes, the general principles will apply to all settings.

First, an introduction to the basic requirements of clinical record keeping as defined in the federal regulations (483.751 1–5, Tag F514 Clinical Records). The health record is owned by the long term care facility and kept for the benefit of the resident (or his/her legal guardian) and the health care team. The record is used for primary resident care, continuity of care, quality assurance, proof of care given, research and reimbursement or billing. The health record must be protected from loss, destruction or unauthorized use. The record must be kept for the period of time required by state law or five years from the date of discharge if there is no requirement in state law; for a minor, three years after the resident reaches legal age under state law.

All information in the health record must be kept confidential. No information may be released without authorization from the resident except when it is required by law. The resident's records may not be released, even to his/her insurance company or to a facility to which s/he is being transferred, without prior, written consent. The facility must permit the resident to inspect his or her records within 24 hours of request and must provide copies no later than two working days after notice from the resident. All records are kept in accordance with accepted professional standards and practices. Records must be complete, accurately documented, readily accessible and systematically organized. These are the minimum requirements for record keeping.

Every state will have requirements as well and facility and corporate policy may also require additional record keeping practices. The wise practitioner will be familiar with all regulations and policies. If copies of the federal and state regulations are not readily available in the facility, they may be reviewed at the local county law library or the Internet. (To find the federal health care regulations on the Internet go to <http://www.cms.gov/> or use a search engine like *Google* and ask for "State Operations Manual.")

Let's look again at the purposes of the health record.

1. *Primary Care.* The record gives the information the health care team needs to deliver direct care — orders for medications, treatments, diet and nursing care as specified in the treatment plan.

2. *Continuity of Care.* The record provides a means of communication among members of the health care team and gives a report of assessments, interventions, evaluations of the individual's progress and response to the treatment plan.

3. *Quality Assurance/Proof of Care.* The record documents care and services provided. The record can be examined by outside reviewers for evidence of appropriate care and intervention. The record is a legal document and can be used as evidence in defense of claims of providing inadequate care and intervention. (If a treatment *isn't* documented in the health record, the legal assumption is that it *wasn't* given.)

4. *Research.* The record can be used by health care professionals for research in many fields.

5. *Billing/Reimbursement.* The record is reviewed by third party payers for proof that services, supplies and equipment were provided as claimed.

Because there are so many purposes for the record, including that of evidence in legal proceedings, standard documentation principles have been established. Following these principles assures that the record can be used for all of the purposes listed above. Failure to follow the principles may render the record useless.

Documentation Principles

Entries into the record must be permanent, legible, timely, accurate and authenticated. Let's examine each of these principles.

1. *Permanent.* All entries must be made with an indelible ink pen. Do not use pencil, erasable pen or a felt tip pen, which may run when wet. Your entry should not be erasable or alterable once in the record. Pages of the record should never be destroyed before the legal time requirement nor should the record be modified by crossing over or using correction fluid.

2. *Legible.* Write clearly. If your penmanship is poor, try printing. You and others must be able to easily interpret what you write. Do not use short hand or other personal abbreviations. (A set of generally recognized abbreviations can found in Appendix A.) Use a pen dark enough that the entry is capable of being photocopied or faxed. Black ballpoint pen is best.

3. *Timely.* Document as events occur noting the complete date: month, day, year and time. Don't rely on your memory and don't document actions in advance. Never backdate, tamper with or add to notes previously written. Never write between lines or squeeze in words after the fact. It should never appear that the record has been altered with the intent to mislead.

4. *Accurate.* Entries should be factual and describe only events that you know to be true through direct observation. Entries should be objective, describing what you can see, hear, smell or touch. Subjective entries — hearsay, statements from others, opinions or feelings — should not be used unless they are documented in the form of a direct quote from a resident or family member.

   It is also important that the entries are within the scope of your education, training and, if applicable, your professional credential. Entries should be specific to your discipline and appropriately express your clinical opinion. Use only words that you understand. Don't attempt to diagnose or assess an individual's psychological or physical condition unless you have the appropriate training. Never speculate about possible causes or interpret behavior unless it is your legal responsibility as a credentialed therapist or social worker to do so. For an example, weeping may be caused by many factors, both internal and external. Unless you are trained to assess the causes with assessment tools or observation, you must wait for the individual to tell you what is causing the weeping before you state a reason. Even then the reason should be documented as a quote from the individual.

Document only what you do. Do not document actions of other members of the health care team. Do not document actions or interventions that you aren't legally allowed to perform (and don't perform them in the first place!).

5. *Authenticated.* Sign all entries with your name and title. First initial and full last name with title is acceptable. Example: M. Smith, AC. In signing with your title, you let the other members of the health care team know your background and training.

All of this may make the documentation process look intimidating. You may be saying to yourself, "But I'm only human! Humans make mistakes!" You're right. Because you are only human, there are methods for correcting honest mistakes. It is important that corrections look like corrections and not deliberate attempts to mislead or defraud. Simple errors in charting, the wrong word, date or name, may be corrected by drawing one line through the error, dating and initialing it. The time is sometimes recommended.

Example:

The first part of an entry was correct but then ~~the words that were here originally were not correct.~~   error SW 1/16/99

Omissions in charting, forgetting to record an event, may be made as late entries to the record. The current date and time is entered, then the phrase "late entry for _____" entering the date and time for the missed event.

Example:

1/5/99 2:00 PM Late entry for 1/4/99 10:00 AM.

Late entries should not be made long after the event and are generally recommended to be made no longer than 48 hours after the missed event. Some states will only allow late entries if they are made in 24 hours or less. Check with your medical records professional or legal counsel. If a late entry is not allowed and the information is felt to be important to the record of resident care, an addendum may be made. This is done on a separate page of the record. The current date and time is entered, then the phrase "Addendum to the record for _____" entering the date and time for the missed event.

Both late entries and addenda to the record should be used sparingly. The impression created (and it is an accurate impression) is one of inaccuracy and lack of timeliness in record keeping. Late entries and addenda cast doubt on the reliability of the entire health record. In all documentation, remember that many people, including the person we serve and his/her family, may look at the record.

Claims for slander and defamation of character may be avoided by describing events factually, by avoiding blaming and finger pointing and by avoiding personal opinions. Do not document an observation in the record that you would not support in public. Entries into the record should be objective as stated above. Instead of describing a resident as a "nasty old man," the description could be a "99-year-old male dissatisfied with facility routine."

Be aware of the individual's rights when documenting and remember that the individual and the family should be a part of the decision making process. Statements of problems and concern about the individual and family behavior should be discussed openly and should not be discovered by the individual or family only upon reviewing the record.

Introduction to Required Documentation

Non-medical/non-nursing professionals are responsible for five types of documentation about the resident. Each one must be written carefully to be sure that it reflects the actual state of the resident and meets all federal and state regulations. The documents include the initial assessment, the care plan, the discharge plan, ongoing monitoring and reassessment and updates.

Initial Assessment

Each department is responsible for completing an initial assessment of the individual who is newly admitted. Although state law and facility policy will determine the time frame for completion, it should be completed prior to completion of the *Minimum Data Set* (MDS). The MDS is the name given to the nursing home assessment used by every nursing home in the United States. All of the different professionals who work with residents in nursing homes have some part of this interdisciplinary form to fill out.

The initial assessment is the first step in getting to know the individual. Although it is not required, most facilities use an assessment form to gather this information.

The activity assessment includes identification of past and present interests, previous lifestyles, and functional limitations and sensory deficits that need to be accommodated. The assessment will also identify individualized programming plans.

The social services assessment includes identification of personal history, family relationships, psychosocial needs, mood and behavior problems and concrete needs. The assessment will indicate whether or not social services interventions are needed.

The recreational therapy assessment includes information about the individual's functional ability as it relates to advanced activities of daily living: 1. Basic environmental/community safety skills, 2. Community mobility skills, 3. Consumer skills, 4. Community resource identification, 5. Advanced dressing skills, 6. Time management skills and 7. Social interaction skills. (The scope of the assessment is often determined by the physician's order for recreational therapy services.)

Resident Assessment Instrument (RAI)

Completion of the Resident Assessment Instrument is required for all residents residing in a nursing home for 14 days or longer. The RAI is a comprehensive assessment that includes the Minimum Data Set (MDS) and the Resident Assessment Protocols (RAPs) and is the first step towards care plan development. Resident Assessment Protocols (RAPs) is the name for a set of decision-making tools that help team members know if a specific, standardized intervention should be used. The RAPs do not cover all interventions, just the most common ones. The MDS identifies real or potential problem areas, which are then further assessed by using the RAPs. This in-depth assessment determines whether or not identified problems need to be addressed in the care plan.

The RAI establishes a baseline functional status for each resident, which is reassessed quarterly with an abbreviated MDS. Improvements or declines in status are tracked through this process to maintain the residents at their optimal level of functioning. The RAI process is completed at least yearly, more often if a resident experiences a significant change of condition.

The RAI's main purpose is to improve the quality of care and quality of life for each resident. It is also used for reimbursement and monitoring of care issues by state and federal regulatory agencies.

Care Plan

A care plan is required for all residents residing in the nursing facility. The care plan is started on admission to manage the resident's immediate needs. The comprehensive care plan, including all of the resident's identified needs, is completed within 21 days of admission. Both the RAI and the initial assessments are used to develop the comprehensive care plan.

The purpose of the care plan is to provide a "road map" to resident care. The care plan identifies a resident's needs and strengths and establishes goals to maintain a resident at the optimal level of functioning through aggressive staff interventions.

Care plans are developed with the resident's and family's participation. Resident rights require that the resident or his representative is "afforded the right to participate in care planning and is consulted about care and treatment changes." The resident is to be afforded the "opportunity to select from alternative treatments" and to refuse treatment. The social services professional needs to be very proactive in promoting the resident's participation in the care planning process and act as an advocate when the resident cannot represent himself/herself.

Discharge Planning

Discharge planning begins at admission. The initial interview determines the potential for discharge. The resident's and family's expectations regarding discharge, resources available and level of care needed upon discharge are examined. For residents with the potential for discharge, a care plan is initiated and the steps required to facilitate a successful discharge are outlined as part of the care plan. Periodic progress notes document the progress toward discharge and a final note is written summarizing the outcome of process.

For residents without the potential for discharge, a quarterly or annual update may be required by state regulation or by facility policy.

Monitoring

The resident's progress and response to care interventions are monitored on an ongoing basis. The activity professional documents daily participation in activities to track the effectiveness of the individualized activity program and the care plan. The daily attendance log will also track refusals to participate in the activity plan. This can be used to modify the plan to meet resident's interests. It can also be used as proof that activities are offered to residents when surveyors question why a resident appears not to be involved in activities or when residents state that no activities are offered.

For some residents a bedside log will be maintained. This should document the type, frequency, length of visit and resident response to the visit. Again, this serves as proof that the care plan interventions are being carried out.

A social services log is kept in an easily accessible location to allow all staff to communicate resident needs to the social services professional. The assessment of the problem, the interventions and the outcome are documented in the log or in the progress notes. If the problem is affecting the resident's functioning or psychosocial well-being, a care plan should be initiated. The resident will then be monitored to determine if the problem is temporary or represents a significant change in condition.

The recreational therapist maintains documentation for each treatment session. This would include the treatment offered, the individual's response to the treatment offered, and plans for the next treatment session.

Reassessment and Updates

At a minimum, the resident is reassessed on a quarterly basis when either the quarterly or annual MDS is due. At this time, the professionals review the resident's progress over the last three months. The monitoring logs are reviewed; staff, resident and family are interviewed; and the chart is reviewed.

After the MDS is completed, a quarterly progress note is written summarizing the resident's progress, identifying any new or unresolved problems and establishing goals for the next quarter. The care plan is then reviewed and updated as necessary.

The discharge plan is updated at this time if required by state regulation or facility policy.

During the resident's stay slight changes in functioning may occur. These may be transitory, resolving with immediate staff interventions. In some cases, the changes may be major and more permanent. These will require review by the interdisciplinary team to determine the need for a new RAI and revision of the care plan. Professionals should document their assessment of the change in condition in the progress notes. The note should include an assessment of the impact of the change on the resident's psychosocial well-being, activity participation and functional ability.

More detailed information about each of these types of documentation will be found in the following chapter. A summary of documentation, in flow chart form, is shown on the next three pages.

Activity Documentation

1. Initial Assessment Form
Assessment of the newly admitted resident. Identifies needs, strengths, and lifestyle. Leads to development of an individualized activity program. Completed prior to the MDS.

2. Resident Assessment Instrument (RAI) = MDS+RAPs
Comprehensive interdisciplinary assessment of the newly admitted resident by day 14 of admission. Activity professional is responsible for completion of Section N and, if triggered, the Activity RAP and the information on the RAP Summary Form. Quarterly MDS completed every 90 days thereafter and a full MDS annually and on significant change in condition. Additional MDSs may be required for billing purposes.

3. Care Plan
Started on admission to address immediate needs. Comprehensive, interdisciplinary care plan based on assessments and the RAI completed within 21 days of admission. Sets goals for resident to measure progress each quarter.

4. Attendance
Daily documentation of activity attendance. Proof that activities were offered to each resident. Bedside log to be used for room-bound residents reflecting type, frequency, length of visits and response to visit. Resident refusals to be documented with each occurrence.

5. Quarterly Progress Note
Completed with the MDS review. Documents overall progress and response to programming for the previous quarter. Addresses any changes in coding on the MDS and the need to revise the activity care plan interventions in response to these changes. The rationale for decision to revise or not revise the care plan is documented in the progress note.

6. Change in Condition Progress Note
Completed with a change in level of activity participation or ability to participate. Changes may be temporary, due to an illness like the flu, or may be permanent. Progress note addresses the need for a revised activity plan and the care plan is updated. Permanent changes due to a decline in physical, mental or psychosocial functioning are assessed by the interdisciplinary team for the need for a new MDS.

Social Services Documentation

1. Initial Assessment Form
Assessment of the newly admitted resident. Identifies psychosocial needs, concrete needs, interests, strengths and lifestyle. Leads to development of the resident care plan. Completed prior to the MDS.

2. Resident Assessment Instrument (RAI) = MDS+RAPs
Comprehensive interdisciplinary assessment of the newly admitted resident by day 14 of admission. Social services professional is usually responsible for completion of Sections AC, E, F and Q and if triggered, the related RAPs and the information on the RAP Summary form. Quarterly MDS completed every 90 days thereafter and a full MDS annually and on significant change in condition. Additional MDSs may be required for billing purposes.

3. Care Plan
Started on admission to address immediate needs. Comprehensive interdisciplinary care plan based on assessment and the RAI completed within 21 days of admission. Identifies mood, behavior or psychosocial problems that need resolution or management. Sets goals to measure effectiveness of interventions.

4. Social Services Log
Ongoing documentation of services and counseling provided to the resident. May be documented in a separate log or in the resident's health record. Follow up note is required to document resolution or outcome of the interventions.

5. Quarterly Progress Note
Completed with the MDS review. Documents overall progress for the previous quarter. Assesses the resident for any unmet needs. Addresses any changes in coding on the MDS and the need to revise the care plan interventions in response to these changes. The rationale for decision to revise or not revise the care plan is documented in the progress note.

6. Change in Condition Progress Note
Completed with any changes in mood or behavior problems, including starting or stopping use of a psychotropic drug or a physical restraint. Changes may be temporary, due to an illness or changes in environment, or may be permanent. Progress note addresses the need for a revised interventions and the care plan is updated. Permanent changes due to a decline in physical, mental or psychosocial functioning are assessed by the interdisciplinary team for the need for a new MDS.

7. Discharge Plan and Progress Note
Started on admission to assess potential for discharge. A care plan is initiated for the resident with a potential for discharge to a lesser level of care. Periodic progress notes track the progression of the discharge planning. A final note must show that sufficient preparation and orientation have been provided to assure a smooth transfer. The note summarizes the outcome of the plan and post discharge planning. Resident/family training, resident counseling and post discharge referrals are documented.

Recreational Therapy Documentation

1. Initial Assessment Form
Assessment of resident after receiving prescription for recreational therapy services from resident's physician. Identifies needs and strengths within the scope of the prescription.

2. Resident Assessment Instrument (RAI) = MDS+RAPs
Comprehensive interdisciplinary assessment of the resident by day 14. Recreational therapist (CTRS) is responsible for completion of Section T concerning TR services. Subsequent MDSs completed depending on length of prescription received from physician and/or significant change in resident status.

3. Care Plan
Started when prescription for recreational therapy services received from physician. Set goals for resident to measure progress for duration of prescription, or quarterly time period, whichever is shorter.

4. Chart Note for Each Treatment Session
Recreational therapy to document resident's performance and feelings after each treatment session.

5. Progress Note
Complete weekly or quarterly note. Quarterly notes are completed with the MDS review. Documents overall progress and response to programming for the previous quarter. Addresses any changes in coding on the MDS and the need to revise the recreational therapy care plan interventions in response to these changes. The rationale for decision to revise or not revise the care plan is documented in the progress note.

6. Change in Condition Progress Note
Completed if there is a change in level of function within the scope of the prescription. Changes may be temporary, due to an illness like the flu, or may be permanent. Progress note addresses the need for a revised treatment plan and the care plan is updated. Permanent changes due to a decline in physical, mental or psychosocial functioning are assessed by the interdisciplinary team for the need for a new MDS.

Chapter 11
Designing the Treatment Plan

Planning an individual's care is a five-step process. It starts with the initial assessments that you and the rest of the treatment team make. After all of the assessments have been made, the team meets to create a care plan that is designed to meet the needs of the individual, the goals you will be working on for the next quarter and the progress you expect to see. The third step is implementing the care plan and monitoring the progress the individual is making. The fourth step is updating the care plan based on your observations of the individual or because the individual's condition changes. The final step, which may not be appropriate for all of the people you serve, is discharge planning. The discharge plan summarizes the current condition of the person, the care s/he has received and the continuing care that will be needed.

This chapter will look at what needs to be done in each of these steps, especially showing the documentation required to demonstrate that each of the steps was done correctly.

Initial Assessment

The first step in an individual's care is to assess the person. Assessment is the process of discovering who the person you will be serving is and what his/her physical and psychosocial needs are in terms of optimum care and functional status. You use that information to create the care plan.

The assessment process begins with the first information that you receive about the individual. During the first few days after admission, you should introduce yourself to this individual in an informal visit. At this time you will be making observations in areas such as appearance; understanding and comprehension; orientation to person, time and place; understanding of diagnoses; and any personal possessions or items in his/her room, which give information on past lifestyle and interests. You may or may not have had a chance to review this person's medical chart before meeting him/her the first time. With the information gathered from this initial visit, you proceed to the medical chart for more information specific to past social and medical history, primary and secondary diagnoses, rehabilitation issues and goals, etc.

There are some basic concepts to remember as you move through the assessment process. First, people do not perceive themselves as their chronological age. The spirit of adventure and the child within is always much younger. Find the key to this real age of the person to open an understanding of who they really are. Look less at age and more at the individual. Help identify

215

potential. Regardless of limitations, there are many strengths, abilities and talents to discover about this person. Additionally, consider:

- Individual leisure interests and hobbies
- Customary routine — what is or was an average day like?
- Educational background
- Community involvement and volunteer work
- Family, children, grandchildren
- Previous travels
- Hopes and goals/aspirations
- Leadership experiences
- Spiritual/religious affiliations, needs and interests
- Special talents and strengths
- History of physical activity and current level of fitness
- Mobility issues
- Adaptive equipment needs and sensory aides
- Functional abilities/independence in activities of daily living
- Special requests for programs or resources

As you get to know the individual better, you will make updates to your assessment. The original assessment and the updates provide important information for making program plans. Planning programs for individuals requires making plans based on what the person is like now and making adaptations when the individual has a change in ability or situation. That is what the ongoing care plan process is designed to let you do.

Assessing a New Individual

The assessment process employs a variety of techniques to reveal as complete a picture as possible of an individual's situation and condition. On the following pages are forms for gathering the information you need on a new admission.

Usually there is an initial assessment or screening form. The information you gather using this form will be used to fill out the MDS and the RAPs. Some state requirements are for a seven-day assessment period and others allow up to fourteen days. Whatever your state mandate is, use the maximum amount of time to assess the person. This will give the individual time to more fully present to you a picture of who s/he is. Initially there is pain, disorientation, often depression and sometimes delirium — all of which will color your assessment.

The assessment of new individuals is the key to individualizing and understanding individual needs. Meet with him/her informally to introduce yourself. Offer support and welcome him/her without too many questions during this first visit. Make your visit short unless s/he asks you to stay longer.

During the first informal visit, you are in the first stage of the assessment process. Keep your eyes open and listen carefully to the conversation. There is some factual information that you need to find out during the initial assessment process. Some you will be able to get from talking to the individual and his/her family. Other information will come from the medical chart. The information includes:

• date of birth	• lifestyle	• level of alertness
• marital status	• leisure interests	• orientation
• children	• hobbies	• hearing
• religion	• talents	• vision
• occupation	• political interests	• adaptive devices
• physical history	• social history	• compensatory skills
• language(s) spoken	• voter registration	• language
• communication skills	• communication deficits	• discharge plan

- allergies
- special diets
- grooming issues
- diagnoses

- emotional health
- dependency issues
- mental attitude
- prognosis

- attention deficits
- short term memory loss
- long term memory loss

But what is more important to creating an appropriate care plan is understanding the individual as a person, not as a set of facts. When you complete this part of the assessment form, do it away from the individual so this person will not feel anxious about the answers that s/he gives you.

- Discover who this person is!
- Be aware of cognitive and functional levels.
- Be aware of sensory deficits.
- Be aware of ability to communicate needs and interests.
- Be aware of personal possessions in the room.
- Be aware of previous lifestyle issues and interests.

We have included forms that you can use to gather information about new individuals. The forms, as they are presented, include information that we feel is most important, but you may need to modify them to meet the needs of your facility. Following the forms are some additional tools and techniques to help you gather information for the initial assessment.

Activity Assessment

The activity assessment form in this section is designed for the activity professional completing the initial activity assessment. This is an example of an assessment (intake) form. There are many variations and styles available. The form will be completed before the MDS and used in conjunction with the MDS assessment process. This intake form may be used in a variety of settings.

Background Information

Background information, such as the person's name, date of birth, educational background, etc., can be found in the medical chart. It might be a good idea for the activity professional to fill this part of the form out (as much as possible) *before* interviewing the new participant. This allows the professional to check the individual's answers to these questions against what is in the medical chart. (Remember, a "wrong" answer by the person you are interviewing could be a mistake in the medical chart and not problems with dementia!)

Voting Status

Is the individual registered to vote? Is s/he interested in voting? Does s/he have an absentee ballot? This question is not asking for political party preference but whether an individual is interested in registering or completing a change of address form.

Mobility Information

This area addresses any mobility issues, assistive devices or transfer information regarding an individual who can ambulate but also spends a certain amount of time in a wheelchair. Add any information that assists you in the assessment process. Mobility is important in addressing how functional and independent an individual may be. You also need to know whether this person needs assistance to and from activities or whether their therapist will be encouraging them to propel themselves to and from groups.

Identified Leisure Interests

List any leisure and lifestyle information that has been gathered by family, staff or previous medical notes. Only list interests that have been identified. Do not add areas that you think would be of interest to this person.

Previous Leisure Interests and Information Related to Previous Lifestyle and Customary Routine

In order to better understand a new person, it is important to know his/her previous interests. They give you clues as to what you might attempt to offer him/her in terms of one-on-one interventions or programs. What did a typical day in his/her life look like? How can we assist in maintaining the normalcy of routine and interests?

Levels of Programming

When you reach this part of the assessment, you have not only reviewed the medical record, but also interviewed and possibly observed the person on a one-on-one basis or in a group activity. This is your assessment of what level of activity programming s/he needs. Circle the types of programs from the list. If you need to add to the list, be sure to do so. Remember: for each level circled, you must document involvement and response to this type of program. So, when you circle two areas, you must also document on these two areas in the progress notes.

Sensory Stimulation

For the person who is regressed. Sensory stimulation is a therapeutic intervention and program that provides multi-sensory experiences for individuals who otherwise would not reach out or respond to stimuli. Although all of us need stimulation, this specific program is for an individual with minimal to no response unless the stimuli are presented in a structured program.

Assessment Comments and Treatment Plan

This section of the form is to be completed for every assessment. If an individual is identified as having sensory deficits, specify what *type* of sensory stimulation you will be starting with: auditory, tactile, gustatory (taste), visual, olfactory (smell).

If there are any identified behavioral issues that need to be addressed, indicate specifically what they are. Some examples would be hitting, screaming, eating inappropriate objects, poor judgment skills that may be safety issues, etc.

This section should also be used to record any other areas that you feel need to be addressed. Be specific about the treatment plan and goal.

Remember — the individual has the right to know about and agree with all aspects of his/her care before it is written into the care plan.

Activity Assessment

Resident Name: _____ **Admit Date:** _____

Date of Birth: _____ **Place of Birth:** _____

Educational Background: _____ **Former Occupation:** _____

Religion: _____ **Marital Status:** _____

Diagnosis: _____

_____

Medications: **Antidepressants** **Antipsychotic** **Antianxiety** **Hypnotics**

Voting Status: **Interested in voting Y N** **Registered Y N** **Absentee Y N**

Diet: _____ **Diet/Fluid Restrictions:** _____

Mobility Information: _____

Identified Leisure Interests: (Information gathered by interview, family, previous history)

_____

Previous leisure interests and information related to previous lifestyle and customary routine:

_____

According to this activity assessment and in addition to the MDS, the following level of programming is identified as appropriate for this individual's leisure needs and interests: (Circle)

Social Interaction Activities   Religious Activities   Creative/Expressive Activities
Relaxation and Solace Activities   Group Games and Projects   Physical Activities
Community Outings   Outdoor Activities   Resident Council
Intellectually Stimulating Activities Task Oriented Activities   One-on-One
Rehab Oriented Activities   Work Related Activities (with physician's orders)
Structured Sensory Stimulation Program

Assessment Comments and Treatment Plan for Resident:

_____

_____

_____

_____

_____

_____

_____

_____

_____

_____

_____

_____

Date plan reviewed with resident _____

Date: _____ **Activity Professional:** _____

Assessment Box: Assessing the Less Responsive Individual

There are many reasons why an individual may not be as responsive to some facets of the assessment processes as you might wish. The assessment box is a therapeutic tool to assist the individual in taking a more active role — to participate more fully in the initial assessment process.

The box should include both familiar and unusual items. Some of these items should be leisure related. Some should be orientation objects. Others should be unique and unexpected in order to stimulate the senses.

Some items found in an Assessment Box could be

- paint brush and paints
- various types of small balls
- sandpaper
- camera, view finder
- whistle
- pictures of familiar things
- sheet music

- wallet
- deck of cards
- sports equipment
- binoculars
- egg beater
- maps
- music box, tapes

- potpourri
- newspaper
- mirror, lotion, make up
- gardening tools
- scarves, gloves, ties
- coins, keys
- silverware

Assessment Procedures:

1. Eliminate as many distractions as possible.
2. Sit across from the individual at a distance where there is close eye contact and s/he does not need to strain to hear you.
3. Place the objects either on the table in front of the individual or leave them in the box and place the box on the table.

At this stage of the assessment, the goal is to create curiosity about the objects and then to assess the individual response to the objects. The goal is for the individual to identify items that appear familiar to him/her. This tells you what is familiar to the individual from his/her long term memory. These may become leisure activities or games created for this individual because of *his/her* response to them.

There are a multitude of observations you can make. You are most often looking for response of either familiarity or interest. For example, if there is positive and immediate response to a picture of a dog, this could indicate a past and also present interest and affection. If further indications confirm this observation, animal related programming would be a good idea. Remember, curiosity can initiate involvement and growth.

Puzzles with more than one shape that require the individual to place a piece in the correct outline, could indicate that s/he recognizes and processes the steps necessary to engage in this leisure pursuit.

Some individuals have experienced cognitive and sensory losses. Visual cues may assist them in participating more fully in the assessment process. Regardless of the functional level, you should strive to make the assessment experience an empowering one and the Assessment Box is an ally in this effort.

Some specific questions you may seek to answer through observation include:
- Does individual seem most interested in bright objects? small objects?
- Does s/he appear to recognize the object presented?
- Does s/he use the objects as intended (e.g., does not try to eat the photograph)?

- Can s/he repeat the name of the object or acknowledge recognition with a yes/no or a nod of the head?
- Is there any differentiation between positive or negative responses?
- Does s/he look for an object that has been removed?
- Is s/he unwilling to return an object to you?
- Does s/he refuse to respond to this entire experience?
- Is s/he able to use small motor/fine motor movements to pick up and examine objects?

Focus on task and success in involvement can hopefully be nurtured and expanded with information gained through this assessment activity.

Social Services Assessment

The social history of the individuals: who they are and were, where they lived, who they lived with, their occupations and the kinds of community support they received prior to joining your facility describe the patterns of previous lives. These patterns help you tailor treatment plans to match each individual's unique needs.

Typically, gathering this information for the rest of the team is the responsibility of the social services professional. That person should ensure that an accurate picture of the individual's social history is presented as inaccuracies could lead to inappropriate treatment goals. Ideally you will create a biography of the resident: begin at the beginning and make logical progress through his/her life. However, do not limit yourself to facts; assess also what you see. Mood is often worn on one's face, in one's affect. It takes more than words to assess mood; use your skills of observation for a complete picture of the individual. When you are finished, you may have the data for a social history. If you are unable to obtain biographical information (because the individual is unable and there is no one else to act as historian), you will need to "see" the individual to produce a psychosocial assessment. Hopefully, you will have access to both forms of information.

Two methods of obtaining the information are presented. The next two pages have a set of questions you can ask to help you write a narrative social history. The two pages after that show a more structured form for gathering much of the same information. Adapt the forms as required to meet your particular needs.

A note of caution: do not allow yourself to be constrained by these intake forms. These forms are simply tools to provide a skeleton of selections to be used during the assessment process. Also, some corporations have specific policies related to the forms you must use. Check this out before you begin.

If you are inclined to write a narrative note, take a blank progress note and develop your statement based on what you have seen and what you have heard about the individual. This kind of note will allow you to focus freely on the personality of the individual: describe actions and reactions and important relationships. Use anecdotes relayed to you by the individual and his/her family.

Narrative notes are fun to write and interesting for the staff to read (isn't that our goal?). You will develop your own story-telling style and can more fully depict the individual. Remember that you must use your skills every day. No one's assessment is ever finished; even the most ill individual continues to evolve within the boundaries of the facility.

Identify changes because change is what we must be alert for; it drives our care interventions. Do not stop with the identification of change. Chart it. Make sure that the rest of the care team also knows about the change. Be assertive; be proactive; do not wait to react. Act on behalf of the individual every day by assessing, documenting and keeping all information current.

Social Services Assessments for New Admissions

1. Reason for Admission to a Long Term Care Facility at this Time
- Where was individual living previously/now?
- What were precipitating factors for this change?
- How was admission decision made? Was the individual involved in the decision?
- Were family or friends involved in the decision? Did they help with the moving or the transition?
- Who is primary contact person for the individual?

2. Social History
- Where did the individual live?
- Where was the individual born?
- What was his/her occupation?
- Why did s/he stop working?
- Was s/he married? Length and quality?
- Did s/he have children?
- What other important relationships did s/he have in the past or present?
- What were the most significant life events and/or losses? How did s/he react to these events?
- How does s/he feel about them now?
- What is the ethnic, cultural and religious background? How important to the individual?
- Has s/he seen a psychiatrist or other similar professional? Why? How long?
- What are his/her current relationships with family or friends like?
- Who provided this information?

3. Current Psychosocial Functioning
- Does the individual have the capacity to make decisions regarding individual needs and wishes?
- How does the individual present herself/himself to other people?
- Is s/he well groomed? Is there anything striking about his/her appearance?
- Does s/he have any idiosyncratic mannerisms?
- What is his/her general behavior like (e.g., nervous, clingy, sad, quiet, content, etc.)?
- What is his/her cognitive functioning like? Is s/he oriented to person, place and time?
- Is s/he forgetful of recent or remote events?
- What does s/he talk about most of the time?
- What are his/her fears?
- How does s/he cope with physical and emotional losses?
- What is his/her sense of humor like?
- What achievements is s/he proud of?

4. Psychosocial Care Plan Recommendations
- What difficulties is this individual likely to experience in adjusting to the program?
- What can be done to ease his/her adjustment?
- How can specific departments in the facility be of help?
- Will family members also need assistance? How?
- Will family members participate in the individual's care? How?
- Should this individual be encouraged to attend group activities or be left alone?
- Should this individual be referred for social work assessment?

5. Discharge Planning Assessment
- Why is this level of care required?
- Under what conditions will this individual be able to go to a less structured environment?
- What social or environmental supports would be required?
- What is the projected timetable?
- Does the individual agree with discharge plan?
- Does family agree with discharge plan?
- What difficulties can be anticipated in implementing this plan?

Social Services Assessment

Medical Record # _____ Admission Date _____

Room # _____ Admitted From _____

Readmit   Yes _____No _____   Date of Birth _____

I. Identifying Information

Name: _____ Age:_____   Sex: M ____ F ____

Religion: _____ Contact:_____

Diagnosis: _____

Marital status: Never Married _____ M _____ W _____D _____ Sep. _____

Financial Resources: Medicaid _____ Medicare _____ Private _____ Other _____

Responsible Party or Conservator: _____ Relationship: _____

II. Mental Status

		Yes	No	At Times
1.	Oriented to:			
	Person	_____	_____	_____
	Place (Facility/Room)	_____	_____	_____
	Season	_____	_____	_____
	Staff	_____	_____	_____
2.	Long Term Memory Problem	_____	_____	_____
	Short Term Memory Problem	_____	_____	_____
3.	Problem Behavior:			
	Wandering	_____	_____	_____
	Verbally Abusive	_____	_____	_____
	Physically Abusive	_____	_____	_____
	Socially Inappropriate	_____	_____	_____
	Indication of Delirium	_____	_____	_____
4.	Quality of Life:			
	Makes Own Decisions	_____	_____	_____
	Uses Telephone	_____	_____	_____
	Manages Own Money	_____	_____	_____
	Takes Own Medication	_____	_____	_____
	Sets Own Goals	_____	_____	_____
5.	Has Verbal Expression of Distress	_____	_____	_____
6.	Has Observable Signs of Mental Distress	_____	_____	_____
7.	Receives Psychoactive Medication	_____	_____	_____

	Yes	No	At Times
8. Emotional Status:			
Moods Interfere With Daily Activity	_____	_____	_____
Aware of Diagnosis	_____	_____	_____
Participates in Care Plan	_____	_____	_____
Accepts Facility Placement	_____	_____	_____
Expresses Upset Over Lost Roles/Status	_____	_____	_____
Unsettled Relationships:			
Family Member	_____	_____	_____
Other Residents	_____	_____	_____
Staff	_____	_____	_____

III. Personal Data:

A. Family Relationships/Emotionally Supportive Persons:

Name	How Related	Phone
_____	_____	_____
_____	_____	_____
_____	_____	_____
_____	_____	_____
_____	_____	_____
_____	_____	_____
_____	_____	_____

B. Birthplace_____Education _____
Lifetime Occupation(s) _____

C. Cultural Background _____
Interests/Hobbies _____

D. Adaptive Aids Used/Needed:
Hearing Aid _____ Glasses _____ Dentures _____
Clothing _____Special Eating Equipment_____
Ambulation Equipment _____

E. Information Received From_____
_____

IV. Identified Psychosocial Problems/Needs/Concerns:
Areas include: psychosocial, family, financial and social

_____
_____
_____
_____

Date Plan Reviewed with Resident: _____
Discharge Plan: _____
_____

Social Services Professional _____ Date of Assessment _____

Recreational Therapy Assessment

The recreational therapy assessment in a nursing home setting is limited in scope and must reflect measurement of the specific areas prescribed by the physician. The prescription from the physician (along with a physician's signature) should indicate the frequency, scope and duration for treatment of the functional skill area to be addressed.

If the physician wants the recreational therapist to make sure that the patient can use public transportation to reach his/her outpatient appointments, then the recreational therapist will need to assess the patient's skills related to public transportation and not leisure interests. The recreational therapist will want to use a standardized assessment such as *Module 4B (Taxi/Taxi Vans)* or *Module 4E (City Bus)* from the *Community Integration Program* (Armstrong & Lauzen, 1994). For patients with less physical impairment but large deficits in executive function the *Bus Utilization Skills Assessment* (BUS) (burlingame, 1989) may be more appropriate.

If the physician wants to increase muscle strength and to increase range of motion for a patient who is so weak that hydrotherapy is the best choice, then the therapist may want to use the *Oxford Scale for Muscle Power Modified for Water* (Skinner and Thomson, 1983). The Oxford Scale is a modification of the standard 0 (zero) through 5 scores given for muscle strength on land. When the patient is able to increase his/her Oxford Scale up to 4 or 5, s/he may be ready to work on muscle strengthening exercises on land.

As our communities and population become more computer literate we will find that using information technology will greatly enhance the independence of our patients. A recreational therapist might get a prescription to help an older patient "get on line" so that the patient can be more independent and return home. The therapist can increase the technology's usability by understanding the needs and characteristics of individuals who are older. As an example, age-related changes in visual functioning, including a "reduction in light sensitivity, color perceptions, resistance to glare, dynamic and static acuity, contrast sensitively, visual search, and pattern recognition." (Kosnik et al., 1988)[53] Making sure that the patient has a computer system that will work for him/her, such as a large screen monitor that allows high contrast, is important. The patient will also need to be taught how to use the various web pages to shop on line, communication with others via e-mail and to keep up with daily events through the Internet.

Standardized Scales and Assessment Tools

One of the standards of practice for almost every health care profession is the standard to measure the individual's functional (skill) level before any type of intervention or activity is taken to modify that function. This standard requires that some kind of measurement be taken that not only measures the individual's ability but, when reported, the report can be understood by the other members of the health care team. For this reason health care professions have developed "standardized" testing tools and scales. A *scale* is a type of measurement that goes from the least to the most, usually using numbers (e.g., 1 to 5). An assessment is a tool to gather information that may or may not use scales to record the information gathered. Because the measurements are standardized, they can be taught to students all over the world, developing a common language. This section provides you with an introduction to a few of the standardized scales and tools. The

---

[53] Kosnik, W, Winslow, L, Kline, D. (1988). Visual changes in daily life though adulthood. *Journal of Gerontology: Psychological Sciences, 43,* 63-70.

next chapter covers one specific standardized tool, the Resident Assessment Instrument that is used in every nursing home in the United States.

Scales

There are three primary scales used by the professionals who work with the people we serve. These three scales are the Functional Independence Measure (FIM), the Likert Scale and the Manual Muscle Evaluation. Other scales frequently seen by the professional include the vital signs (blood pressure, pulse and respiratory rate).

The FIM Scale

The Functional Independence Measure, or "FIM," scale is a standardized, seven-point scale that measures the degree of independence an individual is able to demonstrate for any type of task. The professional may take any skill attempted by the individual s/he is assessing and use the FIM scale to show how independent the individual was in completing the task. The FIM Scale is shown below.

Functional Independence Measure (FIM)™
© Copyright 1987 Uniform Data System for Medical Rehabilitation — State University of New York

Independent — Another person is not required for the activity (No Helper).
  7 **Complete Independence** All of the tasks described as making up the activity are typically performed safely without modification, assistive devices or aids and within reasonable time
  6 **Modified Independence** Activity requires any one or more than one of the following: an assistive device, more than reasonable time or there are safety (risk) considerations

Dependent — Another person is required for either supervision or physical assistance in order for the activity to be performed or it is not performed (Requires Helper).
  Modified Dependence — The subject expends half (50%) or more of the effort. The levels of assistance required are
  5 **Supervision or Setup** Subject requires no more help than standby, cueing or coaxing, without physical contact. Or, helper sets up needed items or applies orthoses
  4 **Minimal Contact Assistance** With physical contact the subject requires no more help than touching and subject expends 75% or more of the effort.
  3 **Moderate Assistance** Subject requires more help than touching or expends half (50%) or more (up to 75%) of the effort.
  Complete Dependence — The subject expends less than half (less than 50%) of the effort. Maximal or total assistance is required or the activity is not performed. The level of assistance required are
  2 **Maximal Assistance** Subject expends less than 50% of the effort, but at least 25%.
  1 **Total Assistance** Subject expends less than 25% of the effort.

The Likert Scale

The Likert Scale is a numerical scale developed by Rensis Likert to be used when measuring someone's attitude or values and not someone's functional ability. Likert scales usually have five levels but may also include three or seven levels. Likert scales are used to measure an individual's satisfaction with the services provided, his/her feelings of happiness or other types of "feelings." The standard Likert scale using five levels is shown to the right.

1	Strongly Disagree
2	Disagree
3	Uncertain or Neutral
4	Agree
5	Strongly Agree

The book *Quality Assurance for Activity Programs, Second Edition* by Cunninghis and Best-Martini (1996) contains some examples of questionnaires that use the Likert scale. The sample below is a part of a larger *Family Questionnaire* in the book. This provides you with a sample of a questionnaire using the Likert scale.

	Please rate:
	Respect and kindness shown your family members by the staff.
	Care taken to protect your family member's privacy.
	Encouragement given your family member to make full use of the center and its programs.
	Extent to which your family member feels comfortable with the staff at the center.
	Extent to which you feel welcome when visiting your family member.
	Your ability to communicate (phone, mail, visit) with your family member without limitations set by staff.
	Accessibility of staff by phone or in person to meet with you and address your concerns about your family member.
	Extent to which the staff keeps you informed about your family member.

Manual Muscle Evaluation

One important measurement to be aware of is muscle strength. By knowing how much strength the individual has, the professional should also be able to understand how far the individual can walk, how long s/he can physically engage in activity and what modifications to equipment (that might be too heavy) will be required. While the activity, social services and recreational therapy professionals do not usually measure strength, it is important that they understand the meanings of the numbers used in the manual muscle strength evaluation. The table below shows the five levels of the manual muscle strength evaluation.

Manual Muscle Evaluation — Strength

100%	5	N	Normal	Complete range of motion against gravity with full resistance
75%	4	G	Good	Complete range of motion against gravity with some resistance
50%	3	F	Fair	Complete range of motion against gravity
25%	2	P	Poor	Complete range of motion with gravity eliminated
10%	1	T	Trace	Evidence of contractility
0%	0	0	Zero	No evidence of contractility
S			Spasm	If spasm or contracture exists, place S or C
C			Contracture	after the grade of a movement incomplete for this reason.

Assessments

Some professionals may decide to use a standardized testing tool in addition to the forms shown above to obtain more information about an individual. Some assessment tools have been written using ideas and information obtained from rigorous research. An example of a standardized testing tool, the *Checklist for Nonverbal Pain Indicators*, is shown below.

Two books that provide greater information on the subject are *Assessment Tools for Recreational Therapy and Related Fields, 3rd Edition* by burlingame and Blaschko, 2002 and *Assessing the Elderly: A Practical Guide to Measurement* by Kane and Kane, 1984. A widely used assessment, the *Therapeutic Recreation Activity Assessment* (*TRAA*), 1994, measures fine motor skills, gross motor skills, social behavior, expressive communication, receptive communication and cognitive skills. The *TRAA* may be used with individuals who range from very impaired and on bed rest to individuals who have only slight impairments. Another standardized testing tool is the *Leisure Assessment Inventory* (2002), which measures the leisure behaviors of adults using laminated color photographs. The *LAI* has four subscales: 1. the Leisure Activity Participation Index, reflecting the person's leisure participation, 2. the Leisure Preference Index, measuring activities in which the individual would like to increase participation, 3. the Leisure Interest Index, measuring the degree of unmet leisure involvement, and 4. the Leisure Constraints Index, assessing the degree of internal and external constraints that inhibit participation.

Checklist of Nonverbal Pain Indicators

Measuring pain in residents with cognitive impairments is a challenge. Because of this difficulty with measurement, residents with cognitive impairment are significantly more likely to be undermedicated for pain than clients who exhibit little or no cognitive impairment (Geriatric Video Productions, 1998). Feldt (2000) developed a tool to measure pain in residents with cognitive impairment called the *Checklist of Nonverbal Pain Indicators* (*CNPI*). The *CNPI* is best used when the resident is moving about and engaging in activity, so this test is very appropriate for the activity professional to use.

Checklist of Nonverbal Pain Indicators

Date: _____ Patient Name: _____

Write a "0" (zero) if the behavior is not observed, and a "1" (one) if the behavior occurred even briefly during activity or rest.

	With Movement	Rest
1. **Vocal Complaints: Nonverbal** (Expression of pain, not in words, moans, groans, grunts, cries, gasps, sighs)		
2. **Facial Grimaces/Winces** (Furrowed brow, narrowed eyes, tightened lips, dropped jaw, clinched teeth, distorted expression)		
3. **Bracing** (clutching or holding onto side rails, bed, tray table, or affected area during movement)		
4. **Restlessness** (Constant or intermittent shifting of position, rocking, intermittent or constant hand motions, inability to keep still)		
5. **Rubbing** (Massaging affected areas, in addition, record verbal complaints)		
6. **Vocal Complaints: Verbal** (Words expressing discomfort or pain — "ouch," "that hurts" occurring during movement, or exclamations of protest — "stop," "that's enough")		
Subtotal Scores		

Total Score (Movement + Rest)

©1998 K. Feldt. From K. Feldt (1996). *Treatment of pain in cognitively impaired versus cognitively intact post hip fractured elders.* (Doctoral dissertation, University of Minnesota, 1996). Dissertation Abstracts International, 57–09B, 5574 and Feldt, K. S. (2000). Checklist of Nonverbal Pain Indicators. *Pain Management Nursing, 1*(1), 13–21. Used with permission.

Discharge from the Nursing Home

The process of planning for discharge begins at the time of admission to the nursing home. At that time the treatment team will use the medical database and the resident/family goals to begin the process of discharge planning. This includes an assessment of the change in medical status that has necessitated admission, an assessment of the home situation (from resident/family interview) and discussion with the rehabilitation staff concerning the possibility of improvement.

Then progress itself must be monitored. To do so, it is essential to attend weekly rehab meetings; in fact, in terms of any successful determination of discharge potential, this may be the most important meeting of the week. At this session, you will have available to you all of the resources which are acting in either a rehabilitative or a supportive role with the resident. You will be able to examine his/her daily pattern from every aspect: dietary to therapy to activity level to nursing. From this comprehensive overview, you will be able to note progress (if any) and to inform the resident and the family of the consensus opinion so that: 1. neither becomes unnecessarily discouraged nor encouraged and 2. they can begin to plan and prepare the home environment if this seems feasible.

Meanwhile, the social services professional uses the interdisciplinary team's assessments to continue to evaluate the resident for home care needs. With this information, s/he will make referrals, under the doctor's orders, for follow-up care to be initiated at the time of discharge.

Many residents and families regard admission to the long term care facility as final but it is actually possible for many residents to return to a lesser level of care, either as a result of rehabilitative service or a change of condition toward — not away from — wellness.

Although some residents may not be able to go home due to the constraints of care needs or lack of support, other options exist in most communities and you can explore the choices with the resident while s/he is in the facility.

When home is the best answer, enlist the assistance of the occupational therapist for a home visit to assess the safety and accessibility of the home. S/he can make valuable recommendations about removing hazardous rugs and other obstacles, and suggest ramps and safety bar placement (especially in bathrooms). The responsible party should be able to follow up on these suggestions, using parts that can be found in most hardware stores, to improve the safety of the home.

Once the environment has been made safe, follow up care can be arranged. Home care agencies, some hospital-based, some private, are a rich source of assistance. They can provide physical therapists, occupational therapists, recreational therapists, skilled nurses and home health aides. The social services professional makes the initial contact after receiving the doctor's order. The agency will then review the case, frequently meeting with the resident and/or the responsible party before the discharge to make the transition as easy as possible.

If there is a Meals on Wheels program in the community, which can bring at least one hot meal a day, check to see if the resident would like to have the service. We like to recommend it for the first two weeks at home. It must be ordered by the doctor.

For the actual discharge, arrange transportation. Can the family transport? If not, check with your local resources to determine what will work best. Usually a private car or van service will suffice.

If the resident wants a homelike setting, but does not want all of the responsibilities that entails, you can look into assisted living complexes in the community.

There are several variations on this theme. Some include well care, supervised care and skilled nursing. Some have only the first two options. Some are only for those who are independent. Research the possibilities to find the best match for the resident.

Assisted living facilities will allow the individual to have all the possible amenities in his/her apartment, including his/her own furnishings and kitchen facilities. S/he will be able to use congregate dining facilities and planned activities within the complex, too. This is often a good transitional environment from total independence to the beginnings of supervised care. It is an excellent option if the individual is still able to be independent and manage his/her own personal and health care needs.

The next step toward supervised care is a board and care facility. Most board and care facilities pride themselves on being homey but the sizes vary considerably and it is important to visit them to find the one that will best suit the resident's needs. Look for the availability of supervised care: medication administration and personal needs such as bathing and dressing. Then assess the match between the facility and the personal style of the resident:
- Does s/he prefer social settings or quiet and privacy?
- Are there grounds for strolling (and does the resident care)?
- Are there animals?

If there is family to help with this, they can usually be relied upon to provide accurate assessments. If there is not, perhaps you can take the resident for a visit. If this is not a possibility, ask the board and care facility operator to meet the resident and bring photographs of the facility.

Board and care facilities will allow the resident to bring personal possessions such as a favorite chair. This will help the move seem more like a return home rather than like being a guest in someone else's home.

For both assisted living and board and care facilities, home care agencies will follow residents who have a doctor's order for follow up. Take advantage of these resources since they provide an excellent bridge between long term care facility dependence and the next level of independence.

As exciting as the prospect of a discharge might seem to the health care workers, do not forget that the time leading up to the long term care facility placement may have been extremely traumatic for the resident and the family and they may be reluctant to accept a discharge plan, seeing it as another opportunity for failure. In fairness to everyone, the social services professional should make every effort to give progress reports to all concerned parties at appropriate intervals, assuring them always that a support system (usually home care) will be built into any discharge plan and that they, as the major components of the plan, must be honest and forthcoming with their input and their anxieties. Involving them at all levels of planning and organizing the discharge will give the discharge the best chance of success.

In anticipation of the discharge, the interdisciplinary team must complete an interdisciplinary discharge summary. In this way, resident and family will be given some of the tools needed to insure that successful return "home."

All of those involved in a discharge, from the resident to the CNA, wish for a successful homecoming, one that will "stick." Communication among all members of the health care team, especially at rehabilitation meetings and ongoing communication with the resident and the family, are the key factors for a successful discharge from the long term care facility.

Writing the Discharge Summary[54]

A discharge summary is a report that the professional writes when s/he will no longer be treating the patient. This report may be seen by another health care professional the same day that the report is written or it may be reviewed by a health care professional years later. To help make the discharge summary useful and easy to understand, it is recommend that:

---

[54] This section is used with permission from *Idyll Arbor's Therapy Dictionary* (2001). Idyll Arbor, Inc.

- Whenever possible, refer to the specific instead of the general; be concrete instead of abstract.

- Take care with what you say and how you say it. Avoid fancy or obscure words, abbreviations or words that overstate. Avoid qualifiers such as "rather, very, little, pretty."

- When you write, be clear, document sequentially; be brief but do not take short cuts, which might leave out key information.

- Whenever possible, write your statements in the positive, e.g., "patient was able to ambulate 45 feet between stores before needing to rest" versus "patient was not able to ambulate between stores before needing to rest." The second sentence leaves the reader wondering if the patient had no functional ambulation skills or if the patient could go 50 feet before needing a rest – two very different cases. While being positive, do not be reluctant to provide realistic or negative findings.

- If the treatment was as a result of a referral, make sure that all issues addressed in the referral are answered in the discharge summary.

- It will not be helpful to future readers of the discharge summary if you include just raw data from your assessments. Include a concise interpretation of all data presented.

- Whenever you make a recommendation, make sure that the justification for that recommendation can be found in your discharge summary.

- Without being long-winded, include an alternative recommendation or an alternative course of action, if it is appropriate for the situation.

- Make your recommendations realistic for the patient, his/her cultural, social and economic background and for his/her discharge destination.

- Remember that the discharge summary is just that, a summary. All of the information presented should be brought together in a way that presents the entire picture of all the pertinent information. (Armstrong & Lauzen, 1994 and Zuckerman, 1994)

Chapter 12
Resident Assessment Instrument

Every facility in the United States accepting Medicare and Medicaid funds is required to complete a comprehensive assessment using the Resident Assessment Instrument (RAI). The information placed on this assessment comes from the intake assessments completed by the various professionals who work in the nursing home. Each state must use a standardized form that is approved by the Centers for Medicare and Medicaid Services (CMS). It must cover required core items and may include additional approved items individualized to each state. It is a functionally based assessment tool designed to establish a baseline for each resident. It is then used to track changes in a resident's status throughout his/her stay. The RAI provides a holistic view of each resident by assessing both quality of life and quality of care issues.

There are three components of the RAI: the Minimum Data Set (MDS), the Resident Assessment Protocols (RAPs) and the Resident Assessment Protocol Summary (RAP Summary). The comprehensive care plan is the end result of the assessment process and may be thought of as the fourth component.

The *RAI User Guide* — MDS Version 2.0 explains each of these components in great detail, and has numerous examples and case studies to make the instructions very clear. Every professional should have a copy of this manual for his/her department and refer to it often when learning the RAI process.

Appendix B in the back of this book contains the full MDS form. Referring back to the form while you read the various sections of this chapter may help you better understand the RAI assessment process. At first this whole process may seem daunting — but don't give up hope. After you run through it a few times it becomes fairly easy to understand.

MDS — the Minimum Data Set

The Minimum Data Set (MDS) forms the foundation of the comprehensive assessment. It is a core set of screening questions that identify real or potential problems in quality of life or quality of care. Actual or potential problem areas will "trigger" (identify) the need for further assessment. This further assessment is completed using the Resident Assessment Protocol (RAP). Completion of the MDS is an interdisciplinary process involving chart review; observation; and staff, resident and family interviews.

Purposes of the Assessment

The primary purpose of the RAI is to improve the quality of life and care for the nursing home resident. It facilitates assessment, decision making and care planning as well as implementation and evaluation of care.

The MDS is also used for reimbursement. The Prospective Payment System (PPS) bases payment on the MDS coding for all residents who have part or all of their nursing home bill paid for through Medicare Part A. Some states also use the MDS for Medicaid payment.

The last purpose of the MDS is to monitor quality of care in the nursing homes. Each time a MDS is completed, it is electronically submitted. Because of built-in quality indicators, the surveyors are able to monitor how well each facility is doing without even going to the facility. Quality indicators based on MDS items will allow the federal and state survey agencies to track nursing home performance between survey visits.

Two Types of MDS

There are two types of MDS assessments. The first is a comprehensive assessment. This is sometimes also referred to as a "full MDS." The full MDS is completed for any resident residing in the facility 14 days or longer, annually and upon a significant change in condition. Completion of the RAP summary form and the RAPs is required with the comprehensive assessment.

The second type of assessment is a quarterly assessment. This is a shortened version of the full MDS and a new one is required every 90 days. The quarterly assessment tracks the resident's status in key areas to monitor for declines and improvements.

Timing of Assessments

A typical resident will have a full assessment completed within 14 days of admission, three quarterly MDSs completed every 90 days thereafter, and an annual full assessment completed by the 365th day of residency. Additional assessments will be completed if the resident experiences a significant change in condition or if the resident is receiving Medicare Part A benefits.

To calculate the next assessment date, two sections of the MDS are referred to — Section R2b, the last Section of the MDS and Section VB2, found on the RAP summary form. These are the dates that the MDS is signed off as being complete. Which section is used depends on the type of assessment that was last done. When the full MDS was the last MDS done, Section VB2 is used. When the quarterly MDS was the last MDS done, Section R2b is used.

SECTION R. ASSESSMENT INFORMATION

MDS Section R

When completing the assessment it is important that all persons involved use the same observation period. This is accomplished by setting an assessment reference date. This establishes the last day of the observation period. Commonly referred to as the "look back date" this date is recorded in Section A3a, shown on the next page.

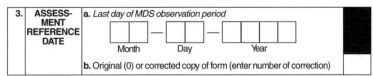

MDS Section A3a

RAI Completion Date Schedule

Assessment Type	Requirement	Assessment Reference Date (A3a Date)	Grace Day Period	Completion Date (R2b Date)	Payment Dates For Medicare
Medicare 5 day	PPS billing	Days 1-5 of admission	6-8	No later than day 14	Days 1 -14
Admission assessment +	Regulatory compliance	Days 1-14	not applicable	No later than day 14	not applicable
Medicare 14 day	PPS billing	Days 11-14	15-19 unless used as admission assessment	No later than day 14 or 14 days from A3a date	Days 15-30
Medicare 30 day	PPS billing	Days 21-29	30-34	14 days from A3a date	Days 31-60
Medicare 60 day	PPS billing	Days 50-59	60-64	14 days from A3a date	Days 61-90
Medicare 90 day	PPS billing	Days 80-89	90-92	14 days from A3a date	Days 91-100
Quarterly	Regulatory compliance	No later than 90 days from R2b date	not applicable	No later than 90 days from R2b date	not applicable
Significant change + PPS	Follow definitions for significant change**	Within 5-7 days of noted change	not applicable	14 days from A3a date	pays days from A3a date to next assessment
Significant change +	Follow definitions for significant change**	Within 14 days of noted change	not applicable	No later than 14 days from the noted change	not applicable
Annual review +	Regulatory compliance	No later than 365 days from Vb2 date	not applicable	No later than 365 days from Vb2 date	not applicable
Other Medicare required assessment (OMRA)	When all therapies are discontinued and no significant change in condition	8-10 days from discontinuation of therapies	not applicable	14 days from A3a date	pays days from A3a date to next assessment
Significant correction of prior assessment	follow definitions for significant correction	not applicable	not applicable	not applicable	adjusted prospectively from A3a date

+ requires completion of the RAPs and the care plan
** refer to the **RAI User Guide** for definitions of significant change

The schedule on the previous page lists all of the types of assessments that are required with time frames for assessment reference dates and completion dates. The shaded assessments are required for Medicare Part A residents only. In calculating assessment reference dates and the completion dates, the day of admission is counted as day one.

The MDS must be encoded and locked within seven days from the date that the MDS is signed as being completed by the Resident Assessment Coordinator (the VB4 or R2b dates). It is then electronically transmitted within 31 days of the final lock date. Failure to lock and transmit on a timely basis can result in federally mandated sanctions.

Prospective Payment System (PPS)

The Balanced Budget Act of 1997 created widespread payment and regulatory reform for many health care providers. CMS's goals were to enhance access to care, improve equity and predictability of payment amounts, streamline the payment processes and improve quality of patient care.

The payment reform moved nursing home reimbursement to a capitated Prospective Payment System (PPS) for Medicare skilled nursing facility reimbursement over a three-year phase-in period beginning on July 1, 1998. The Prospective Payment System is a type of insurance reimbursement system that reimburses facilities based on the diagnosis or MDS category the resident fits into instead of being reimbursed for the actual costs of treatment. If a facility can deliver the necessary treatment for less than the reimbursed rate, it can make money. If a facility can't deliver the necessary treatment for less than the reimbursed rate, it loses money. This payment system is based on a patient classification system known as the Resource Utilization Group system version III or RUG-III. It is a case-mix system that uses Minimum Data Set (MDS) assessment data to classify residents into different payment groups — RUG categories. A set dollar amount per day—or per diem rate—is assigned to each RUG category, which is determined by how much care the resident needs and uses. If more care if required, the payments are higher.

Briefly the process is as follows: an MDS assessment is completed for the appropriate billing period and the MDS is entered into the facility MDS software program. A feature of the software, referred to as the grouper software, "groups" the resident into a RUG-III category based on how the MDS was coded. Grouper software is specially designed computer software that takes the information written on the resident's MDS assessment and, after analyzing the information, assigns the resident to a RUG (or payment) category. The RUG-III code, which can be found at the bottom of Section T of the MDS, is entered on the Medicare UB 92 billing form, and the MDS is electronically transmitted to the state repository.

To have Medicare pay for the nursing home stay, the resident is required to have a three day qualifying hospital stay, admission within 30 days of the hospital stay or last covered nursing home stay, and the resident must need daily skilled inpatient service. The resident must have not used up all of his/her benefits under Medicare to have Medicare pay for the admission. It is most likely that the first four major RUG categories will qualify for Medicare reimbursement beyond the basic room rate because the system recognizes that residents in these categories require extra services from nursing, CNAs and therapists. Extensive and ongoing documentation to demonstrate complex need would be required to gain extra funds for a resident falling in the last three categories because skilled services are not usually indicated for these conditions.

Timing of PPS Assessments

For the Medicare resident there is a potential for completion of as many as seven assessments in the first three months of his/her stay. The setting of the assessment reference dates and completion dates are critical for reimbursement. Failure to meet the completion dates will result in receiving the default rate, the lowest reimbursement rate. It is important that the interdisciplinary team meet daily to review the time frames for the assessment reference dates and completion of each MDS.

A full MDS must be submitted for each Medicare billing period, on discontinuation of all therapies if the resident continues to meet skilled coverage requirements and for significant change in condition. Refer to the RAI Completion Date Schedule for calculating specific completion dates. Note that completion of RAPs and the care plan is not required for each assessment.

The RUG-III System

The RUG-III (Resource Utilization Group version III) classification consists of seven major categories. Each resident must be placed in one of these categories. The software that each facility uses "scores" the resident's MDS and assigns each resident to the appropriate "category." It is the resident's medical condition that determines in which category s/he is placed. The categories represent the different levels of insurance payment to the facility. They are
- Rehabilitation
- Extensive Services
- Special Care
- Clinically Complex
- Impaired Cognition
- Behavior Problem
- Reduced Physical Function

The seven major categories are subdivided by patient groupings, which are determined by the degree of Activities of Daily Living dependency, referred to as the ADL index score. The following describes the conditions a resident would need to meet to qualify for each of the RUG categories.

Rehabilitation Category (14 patient groupings)

The resident qualifies for this category if:
- Therapy services are provided
- The number of therapies, days and minutes provided and the ADL score determine the grouping

Extensive Services (3 patient groupings)

The resident qualifies for this category if services are provided for:
- IV medications, IV feeding, suctioning, tracheostomy care, ventilator/respiratory care
- And ADL index score is seven or greater

Special Care (3 patient groupings)

The resident qualifies for this category with:
- A diagnosis of multiple sclerosis, cerebral palsy or quadriplegia and an ADL index score of at least ten

Lacking one of the above diagnoses, the resident must have an ADL index score of seven or more and one of the following items: (ADL index score of < 7 qualifies for clinically complex)
- Fever with vomiting, dehydration, pneumonia, tube feeding or weight loss
- Tube feeding with aphasia and 501 ml of fluid and 26% of daily calories through the tube
- Two or more pressure or stasis ulcers with treatments
- Radiation therapy
- Respiratory therapy seven days a week
- Surgical wound or open lesion

Clinically Complex (6 patient groupings)

The resident qualifies for this category if s/he has:
- Comatose with total dependence in ADLs and no time awake for activities
- Hemiplegia and an ADL index score of 10 or more
- Pneumonia
- Septicemia
- Dehydration
- Internal bleeding
- End stage disease
- Feeding tube and parenteral/enteral intake level count is 1
- Burns (second or third degree)
- Infection of foot or open lesion of foot and application of dressings
- Chemotherapy
- Dialysis
- Oxygen therapy
- Transfusions
- Diabetes with injections and two or more days of order changes
- Four or more days of physician order changes and one day or more of physician visits
- Two or more days of physician order changes and two days or more of physician visits
- In addition, signs of depression will further group the resident. If three or more items in section E1 of the MDS are checked, the resident is determined to be depressed.

Impaired Cognition (4 patient groupings)

Resident qualifies for this category with:
- Score of 3 or more on the Cognitive Performance Scale

Behavior (5 patient groupings)

Resident qualifies for this category with four or more days per week of exhibiting:
- wandering, physical or verbal abuse, inappropriate behavior
- resisting care, combativeness
- hallucinations or delusions and documentation of skilled nursing service

Physical Function Reduced (10 patient groupings)

Resident qualifies for this category with:
- Documentation of skilled nursing and nursing rehab and an ADL index score of four or greater

Completion of the MDS

Ideally the interdisciplinary team completes the RAI assessment. Whenever possible, the resident, family and direct care staff should be primary sources of information. The coordination of the RAI is assigned to an RN, known as the Resident Assessment Coordinator (RAC). The RAC is responsible for assuring that all sections of the MDS and the RAPs are completed on a timely basis.

Often certain sections are assigned to an individual discipline for completion. If this is the case, the MDS should be reviewed as a group after each discipline has completed its section. This allows the interdisciplinary team to get a holistic view of the resident before proceeding to care planning.

For a detailed explanation of completion requirements including the assessment reference date and signature requirements see Chapter 2 of the *RAI User Guide*.

Suggested responsibility for completion for each section:

MDS Section		Designated Discipline
Section AA.	Identification Information	Admitting, signatures for all people filling out parts of the form
Section AB.	Demographic Information	Admitting and Social Services
Section AC.	Customary Routine	Social Services
Section AD.	Face Sheet Signatures	Signatures of people filling out sections AB and AC
Section A.	Identification and Background	Admitting and Social Services
Section B.	Cognitive Patterns	Nursing and Social Services
Section C.	Communication/Hearing Patterns	Nursing and Speech Therapy
Section D.	Vision Patterns	Nursing
Section E.	Mood and Behavior Patterns	Social Services
Section F.	Psychosocial Well-being	Social Services
Section G.	Physical Functioning and Structural Problems	Nursing and Therapies
Section H.	Continence	Nursing
Section I.	Disease Diagnoses	Medical Records and Nursing
Section J.	Health Conditions	Nursing
Section K.	Oral/Nutritional Status	Dietary and Speech Therapy
Section L.	Oral/Dental	Nursing
Section M.	Skin Condition	Nursing
Section N.	Activity Pursuit Patterns	Activities
Section O.	Medications	Nursing
Section P.	Special Treatments and Procedures	Nursing and Therapies
Section Q.	Discharge Potential and Overall Status	Social Services and Nursing
Section R.	Assessment Information	Social Services and RN Coordination
Section T.	Therapy Supplement	Nursing, Therapies, including Recreational Therapy (CTRS)

Filling out the MDS

The *RAI User Guide*, Chapter 3 gives item-by-item instructions for completion of the each section of the MDS. It should be used side by side with the MDS form when an assessment is being completed to avoid errors in interpretation of the intent of the questions. The following information is an introduction to the parts of the MDS most important to Activity and Social Services Professionals.

Section E of the MDS

Section E1: Indicators of Depression, Anxiety, Sad Mood

Note that Section E1 is to be coded for indicators observed over the last 30 days.

The intent of this section is to record indicators of distressed mood *irrespective of the assumed cause*. The indicators are divided by verbal expressions and nonverbal expressions of distress. For residents who cannot express their feelings, the manual instructs the evaluator to observe residents carefully for any indicator and to consult with direct care staff *over all shifts*. Chart review and family interview are also recommended. Parts of the chart to be reviewed include ADL flow sheets, licensed nurses' progress notes, MD progress notes and past history, any psychologist or psychiatrist evaluations and progress notes and behavioral monitoring sheets.

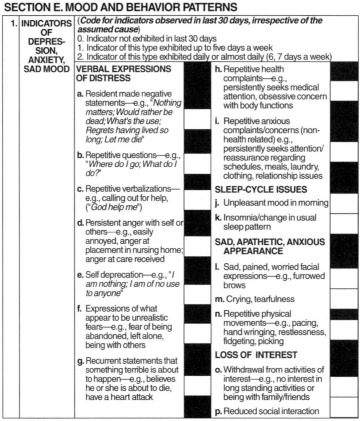

MDS Section E1

Section E4: Behavioral Symptoms

Note that Section E4 is to be coded for indicators observed over the last seven days.

Again the coding for this section focuses on the *resident's actions, not intent*. Are the behavioral symptoms present or not? Often common behaviors such as yelling or hitting are accepted as the "norm" for residents who are confused. The direct care staff may not think to record these because it is not a problem for them or because the behavior is just considered normal for the resident. It really is important to record these behaviors because they are important to consider in the care plan (and because they will often be worth extra income for the nursing home to help them deal more effectively with the resident's difficult behavior). Careful interview of staff and family members is key in coding this section correctly.

The definitions for wandering and for resisting care should be read carefully. Wandering (E4a) does not include pacing. Pacing should be coded under "repetitive physical movements." Resisting care (E4e) does not include purposeful refusal of care, when the resident is exercising his right to free choice. The instructions also state that these "behaviors are not necessarily positive or negative." The cause of these behaviors and whether or not they impact the resident's functioning should be investigated in the RAP and care planning process.

As with Section E above, parts of the chart to be reviewed when completing this section include the ADL flow sheets, licensed nurses' progress notes, MD progress notes and past history, any psychologist or psychiatrist evaluations and behavior monitoring sheets.

4. BEHAVIORAL SYMPTOMS	(A) *Behavioral symptom* **frequency in last 7 days** 0. Behavior not exhibited in last 7 days 1. Behavior of this type occurred 1 to 3 days in last 7 days 2. Behavior of this type occurred 4 to 6 days, but less than daily 3. Behavior of this type occurred daily (B) *Behavioral symptom* **alterability in last 7 days** 0. Behavior not present OR behavior was easily altered 1. Behavior was not easily altered	(A)	(B)
	a. WANDERING (moved with no rational purpose, seemingly oblivious to needs or safety)		
	b. VERBALLY ABUSIVE BEHAVIORAL SYMPTOMS (others were threatened, screamed at, cursed at)		
	c. PHYSICALLY ABUSIVE BEHAVIORAL SYMPTOMS (others were hit, shoved, scratched, sexually abused)		
	d. SOCIALLY INAPPROPRIATE/DISRUPTIVE BEHAVIORAL SYMPTOMS (made disruptive sounds, noisiness, screaming, self-abusive acts, sexual behavior or disrobing in public, smeared/threw food/feces, hoarding, rummaged through others' belongings)		
	e. RESISTS CARE (resisted taking medications/ injections, ADL assistance, or eating)		

MDS Section E4

Section N: Activity Pursuit Patterns

Section N is designed to capture the ratio between the time available for activities and the time involved in activities. This can help identify residents who might not be participating at their optimal level. In order to complete this section accurately the definitions of time awake and time involved must be clearly understood.

N1 — Time awake: the time when resident was awake all or most of the time, with no more than a one hour nap during any period. The morning period is from 7 a.m. until noon. Afternoon is from noon to 5 p.m. and evening is from 5 p.m. until 10 p.m. (or bedtime if earlier).

N2 — Time involved: this is the percentage of the free time available spent in activities and independent pursuits. To calculate this answer the following formula can be used:

$$\frac{\text{total hours spent in facility and independent activities}}{\text{total number of hours awake} - \text{time involved in daily care}} \times 100 = \text{average time}$$

Section N has three levels of participation: most (more than 2/3 or 67%), some (1/3 to 2/3 or 33% to 66%) and little (less than 1/3 or 33%). Code the participation you calculate in the correct box.

A resident who is awake 15 hours per day and spends 5 hours per day in ADL care and receiving treatments has 10 hours of free time available for activities and independent pursuits. The resident spends 8 of these hours visiting friends, watching TV and going to group activities.

$$\frac{8}{15 - 5} \times 100 = 80\%$$

This would be coded as N2 most — more than 2/3 of time involved in activities. A totally dependent resident will have less free time available than the independent resident, but they both may participate most of the time.

N5 — Prefers change in daily routine: the intent of this section is to identify residents who may want a change in existing activities or may want to pursue a new activity not available in the facility. Also coded here are residents who resist attendance or involvement in activities offered. Pay special attention to the coding instructions for this section.

SECTION N. ACTIVITY PURSUIT PATTERNS

1.	TIME AWAKE	(*Check appropriate time periods over last 7 days*) Resident awake all or most of time (i.e., naps no more than one hour per time period) in the:			
		Morning	a.	Evening	c.
		Afternoon	b.	*NONE OF ABOVE*	d.

(If resident is comatose, skip to Section O)

2.	AVERAGE TIME INVOLVED IN ACTIVITIES	(*When awake and not receiving treatments or ADL care*) 0. Most—more than 2/3 of time 2. Little—less than 1/3 of time 1. Some—from 1/3 to 2/3 of time 3. None		
3.	PREFERRED ACTIVITY SETTINGS	(*Check all settings* in which activities are *preferred*)		
		Own room	a.	
		Day/activity room	b.	Outside facility d.
		Inside NH/off unit	c.	*NONE OF ABOVE* e.
4.	GENERAL ACTIVITY PREFER-ENCES (adapted to resident's current abilities)	(*Check all PREFERENCES* whether or not activity is currently available to resident)		
		Cards/other games	a.	Trips/shopping g.
		Crafts/arts	b.	Walking/wheeling outdoors h.
		Exercise/sports	c.	Watching TV i.
		Music	d.	Gardening or plants j.
		Reading/writing	e.	Talking or conversing k.
		Spiritual/religious activities	f.	Helping others l.
				NONE OF ABOVE m.
5.	PREFERS CHANGE IN DAILY ROUTINE	Code for resident preferences in daily routines 0. No change 1. Slight change 2. Major change		
		a. Type of activities in which resident is currently involved		
		b. Extent of resident involvement in activities		

MDS Section N

Section T of the MDS[55]

Section T's purpose is to gather information about the amount and types of therapy services provided to residents of nursing homes which are outside the definition of expected and required treatment or activities. In this case, expected and required means expected and required by the federal government and not by the therapist's standards of practice or scope of practice. Section T measures only the number of days and the total minutes of special treatments or procedures therapists administered during a specific time period.

There are two parts to Section T. The first deals with Special Treatments and Procedures. Section 1.a has been added to the MDS for a CMS study that will be in progress for four years. The study is trying to determine how much recreational therapy is being offered nationally in skilled nursing facilities for Medicare residents. The study hopes to determine if recreational therapy should be added to the therapy mix reimbursed by Medicare. This section cannot be completed by anyone other than a CTRS (Certified Therapeutic Recreation Specialist). This therapist must not only be a CTRS, but must also have physician's orders to provide this therapy. The orders must include frequency, scope and duration along with a physician's signature.

To count for this section the recreational therapy treatment provided must also be outside of the expected and required activities and inside the scope of practice for the recreational therapist. Section T is in no way indicating that a CTRS has priority for the position of the activity director. Section T services are a totally different scope of service than what is expected and required of the activity director. (See the flow diagram following Section T, which shows how the decision to use recreational therapy services is made.)

This is a unique opportunity for the recreational therapy profession as Centers for Medicare and Medicaid Services has determined that there is quite a significant percentage of recreational therapy currently being provided nationally in skilled nursing settings and they wanted to literally "take a closer look." If the facility does not have a CTRS on staff or under contract with the facility, this MDS area is coded "0."

---

[55] This section is modified from the web article written by joan burlingame, 1998.

Section 1.b looks at the amount of therapy provided by physical therapy, occupational therapy and speech pathology services. The second part of Section T deals with the resident's ability to walk when specific forms of treatment to regain walking ability were provided for the resident.

SECTION T. THERAPY SUPPLEMENT FOR MEDICARE PPS

1.	SPECIAL TREAT-MENTS AND PROCE-DURES	**a. RECREATION THERAPY**—*Enter number of days and total minutes of recreation therapy administered (**for at least 15 minutes a day**) in the last 7 days (Enter 0 if none)* **(A) = # of days** administered for 15 minutes or more **(B) = total # of minutes** provided in last 7 days	DAYS (A) / MIN (B)

Skip unless this is a Medicare 5 day or Medicare readmission/return assessment.

b. ORDERED THERAPIES—*Has physician ordered any of following therapies to begin in FIRST 14 days of stay—physical therapy, occupational therapy, or speech pathology service?*
0. No   1. Yes

If not ordered, skip to item 2

c. Through day 15, provide an estimate of the number of days when at least 1 therapy service can be expected to have been delivered.

d. Through day 15, provide an estimate of the number of therapy minutes (across the therapies) that can be expected to be delivered?

2.	WALKING WHEN MOST SELF SUFFICIENT	*Complete item 2 if ADL self-performance score for TRANSFER (G.1.b.A) is 0,1,2, or 3 AND at least one of the following are present:*

- Resident received physical therapy involving gait training (P.1.b.c)
- Physical therapy was ordered for the resident involving gait training (T.1.b)
- Resident received nursing rehabilitation for walking (P.3.f)
- Physical therapy involving walking has been discontinued within the past 180 days

Skip to item 3 if resident did not walk in last 7 days

(FOR FOLLOWING FIVE ITEMS, BASE CODING ON THE EPISODE WHEN THE RESIDENT WALKED THE FARTHEST WITHOUT SITTING DOWN. INCLUDE WALKING DURING REHABILITATION SESSIONS.)

a. Furthest distance walked without sitting down during this episode.

0. 150+ feet	3. 10-25 feet
1. 51-149 feet	4. Less than 10 feet
2. 26-50 feet	

b. Time walked without sitting down during this episode.

0. 1-2 minutes	3. 11-15 minutes
1. 3-4 minutes	4. 16-30 minutes
2. 5-10 minutes	5. 31+ minutes

c. Self-Performance in walking during this episode.

0. *INDEPENDENT*—No help or oversight
1. *SUPERVISION*—Oversight, encouragement or cueing provided
2. *LIMITED ASSISTANCE*—Resident highly involved in walking; received physical help in guided maneuvering of limbs or other nonweight bearing assistance
3. *EXTENSIVE ASSISTANCE*—Resident received weight bearing assistance while walking

d. Walking support provided associated with this episode (code regardless of resident's self-performance classification).

0. No setup or physical help from staff
1. Setup help only
2. One person physical assist
3. Two+ persons physical assist

e. Parallel bars used by resident in association with this episode.

0. No   1. Yes

3.	CASE MIX GROUP	Medicare						State					

MDS Section T

Determining if a Medicare Resident is a Candidate for Recreational Therapy

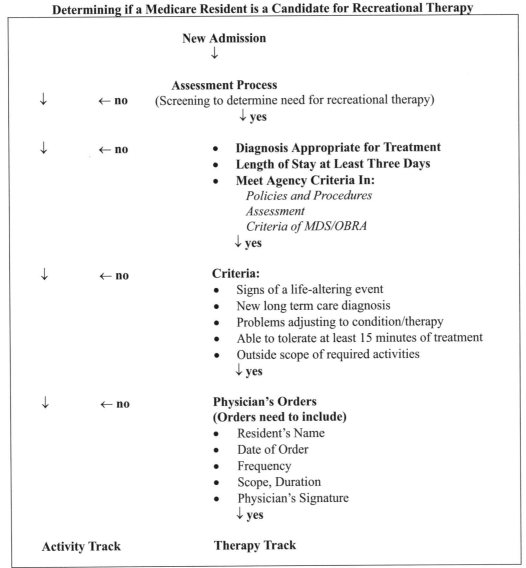

by Elizabeth Best Martini, MS, CTRS, ACC and B. J. Grosvenor, CTRS

Section B: Cognitive Patterns

Section B of the MDS evaluates the resident's cognitive patterns. While a professional other than the activity professional or recreational therapist usually fills out this section, these two professionals frequently help address functional loss in this area. The percentage of residents with some level of cognitive impairment has a great impact on the one-on-one therapy provided by the recreational therapist. It also has an impact on the programs designed by the activity professional. The team needs to assess the level of individual impairment and design interventions and groups that are appropriate for levels of ability and interest. Consider using the MDS assessment process to not only assess but to determine what level of programming is appropriate. You are completing Section N and, with doctor's orders for recreational therapy, parts of Section T. As you review the entire MDS document and its coding, be sure to review how Section B, Cognitive Patterns is coded.

Target Section B4, "Cognitive Skills for Daily Decision Making" as your assessment base for the resident's level of ability to make good decisions regarding recreation and leisure. There are four possible areas listed: Independent in Decision Making (0), Modified Independence (1), Moderately Impaired (2) and Severely Impaired (3).

The higher the coding on Section B, question #4, the greater the need for the recreational therapist and activity professional to identify meaningful and therapeutic interventions for both a one-on-one and group interaction. For example:
- Residents who coded independent to modified independent in decision making have potential for orientation and many times are receiving therapy.
- Residents who coded modified independent to moderately impaired in decision making have potential for reality orientation and improvement in functional skills.
- Residents who coded moderately impaired but most likely severely impaired in decision making have little or no potential for reality orientation but have many other abilities and multi-sensory needs.

Additional information on cognitive loss and the Dementia RAP can be found later in this chapter. Programming ideas for residents with cognitive loss can be found in Chapter 9: Rehabilitation Focused Groups.

RAPs — the Resident Assessment Protocols

The RAPs provide further assessment of "triggered areas" from the MDS. Just as the MDS provides a broad screening for real or potential problems, the RAPs provide a finer screening to determine actual needs and possible interventions. Completing the RAPs is the first step in developing a comprehensive care plan.

The RAP process can seem overwhelming. It helps to remember that the RAPs are the second screening process to determine whether or not a potential problem requires further follow-up. There are 18 RAPs (shown on the next three pages) developed to provide more clinical information, understanding of problems, their possible causes and their impact on the resident.

A review of the triggered RAPs is required for new admission, significant change and the annual MDS. Completion of RAPs is not required for the quarterly MDS.

RAP Descriptions

RAP NAME	FOCUS OF RAP	CARE PLAN GOALS
Delirium	• detect signs and symptoms of delirium • review the major causes of delirium and treat any found.	1. prevent cycle of worsening symptoms (e.g. infection, fever, dehydration, confusion syndrome). 2. resolve delirium.
Cognitive Loss or Dementia	• enhance quality of life. • sustain functional capacities, minimize decline and preserve dignity. • identify potentially reversible causes for loss in cognitive status. • identify and treat acute confusion.	1. provide positive experiences for the resident. 2. define appropriate support roles for each staff member in the resident's care. 3. lay the foundation for reasonable staff and family expectations.
Visual Function	identify two types of residents: 1. those who have treatable conditions that place them at risk for permanent blindness.	1. proper use of eye medications. 2. examination and follow-up by a vision consultant.
	2. those who have impaired vision whose quality of life could be improved through use of visual appliances.	1. appropriate use of vision appliances. 2. modification of environment to meet individual's needs.
Communication	identify three types of residents: 1. those with serious communication deficits who have retained some decision-making ability.	1. restorative communication treatment program.
	2. those with serious communication deficits in addition to no ability to make decisions but no underlying CVA or neurological problems.	1. address behavioral, mood, environmental limitations that complicate communication.
	3. those with hearing deficits and some ability to make decisions.	1. restorative hearing program. 2. compensation strategies for communication loss (e.g. nonverbal communication skills).
ADL Functional Rehab Potential	• identify residents who either have the need and potential to improve or the need for services to prevent decline.	1. restore function to maximum self-sufficiency. 2. replace hands-on assistance with a program of cueing and task segmentation. 3. restore abilities to a level that allow functioning with fewer supports. 4. shorten time required for providing assistance. 5. expand the amount of space in which self-sufficiency can be practiced. 6. avoid or delay additional loss of independence. 7. support the resident who is certain to decline to lessen the likelihood of complications (e.g. ulcers and contractures)

RAP Descriptions

RAP NAME	FOCUS OF RAP	CARE PLAN GOALS
Urinary Incontinence and Indwelling Catheter	• improve incontinence either by bladder training or by detecting reversible causes of incontinence such as infections, medications, situationally induced stress incontinence. • identify harmful conditions such as bladder tumors or spinal cord diseases. • consider the appropriateness of catheter use.	1. improve incontinence. 2. resolve incontinence. 3. discontinue use of indwelling catheter.
Psychosocial Well-Being	• identify distressing relationships and concern about loss of status. • identify situational factors that may impede ability to interact with others. • focus on areas where resident may lack the ability to enter freely into satisfying social relationships. • identify lifestyle issues.	1. develop treatment for mood/behavior problems. 2. develop staff interventions to change environmental and situational problems without "changing the resident."
Mood State	• determine if an altered care strategy is required (e.g. sad mood, feelings of emptiness, anxiety or unease, weight loss, tearfulness, agitation, aches and pains which persist with current care strategy).	1. resolve mood problem.
Behavior Problems	• draw a distinction between serious behavior problems and others that can more easily be accommodated. • identify potential reversible causes or factors involved in the manifestation of problem behaviors. • develop a management plan to avoid the use of restraints.	1. resolve causes and factors manifested by behavior problems. 2. adapt environmental and staff responses. 3. involve resident in psychological treatment plan. 4. limit use of restraints.
Activities	• focus on cases where the system has failed the resident or where the resident has distressing conditions that warrant a revised activity plan. • identify factors that impede resident involvement in activities.	1. help resident overcome distressing conditions. 2. remove factors that impede involvement in activities.
Falls	• identify and assess those who have fallen and those who are at risk for falls.	1. identify and address risk factors. 2. manage risk factors and/or eliminate.
Nutritional Status	• focus on signs and symptoms that suggest that the resident may be at risk of becoming malnourished. • early detection is the key.	1. identify and address risk factors. 2. adjust feeding patterns. 3. compensate or correct food intake problems.

RAP Descriptions

RAP NAME	FOCUS OF RAP	CARE PLAN GOALS
Feeding Tubes	• focus on reviewing the status of the resident using tubes. • assess risks vs. benefits of tube use.	1. remove tube. 2. prevent complications and serious negative consequences.
Dehydration and Fluid Maintenance	• identify any and all possible high-risk cases. • early intervention with hydration programs to prevent the condition from occurring.	1. restore normal fluid volume. 2. identify and resolve risk factors for dehydration. 3. avoid consequences of dehydration.
Dental Care	• identify compounding problems that may prevent a resident from adequately removing oral debris. • identify residents who may benefit from dental treatment.	1. resolve compounding problems. 2. promote good oral health. 3. obtain appropriate dental services.
Pressure Ulcer	• ensure a treatment plan is in place to treat actual pressure ulcers. • identify residents at risk for pressure ulcers.	1. resolve ulcers following specified treatment plan. 2. prevent development of pressure ulcers.
Psychoactive Drug Use	• evaluate the need for the drug. • start low, go slow. • evaluate side effects and interaction with other medications. • consider symptoms or decline in functional status as a potential side effect of medication.	1. reduce or eliminate use of drug. 2. assess and prevent side effects of drug use. 3. assess and prevent decline in functional status.
Physical Restraints	• evaluate the need for the physical restraint. • evaluate needs, problems, risk factors that if addressed could eliminate the need for the restraint. • evaluate side effects of restraint use.	1. reduce or eliminate use of physical restraint. 2. assess and prevent side effects of restraint use. 3. eliminate factors requiring restraint use.

Excerpted from the CMS RAI Training Manual

RAPs for Activities and Social Services

Although the Activity and Social Services Departments may only be responsible for completing a few of the RAPs, it is necessary for these disciplines to review the entire MDS and all triggered RAPs prior to completing the care plan. This is usually done in care conference; but if not, each discipline must take the responsibility to complete a thorough review of the RAI.

The MDS responses, especially in Cognition, ADL, Incontinence and Nutrition, will give more in-depth assessment information and possibly more current information than was gathered on admission. Many of the RAPs require or suggest interventions by the activity and/or social services professionals in conjunction with the other interdisciplinary team members.

The following charts list the RAPs and suggested interventions to be considered by activities and social services when developing the resident care plan.

RAPs Requiring Activity Intervention

Delirium	• Caused by recent relocation: Orientation program to provide calm, gentle approach with reminders and structure to help resident settle in. • Caused by diagnosis: Activity program to help prevent further cognitive decline and improve quality of life while problem is being treated.
Cognitive Loss or Dementia	• Provide positive experiences for the resident (e.g., enjoyable activities) that do not involve overly demanding tasks and stress. • Design programs to enhance resident's quality of life. • Provide opportunities for independent activity and participating more in decisions about daily life. • Segment tasks to make them easier to accomplish. • Provide small group programs. • Create special environmental stimuli (e.g., markers, special lighting).
Communication	• Provide opportunities to communicate, e.g., availability of partners. • Provide tactile approaches to communication. • Participate in restorative communication treatment program.
ADL	• Provide a program that supports rehabilitative goals for the resident.
Psychosocial Well-Being	• Provide social relationships. • Alter environment to allow access to others or routine activities. • Provide activities to address cognitive/communication deficits that may cause a lack of interest in activities or interactions with others. • Focus on a daily schedule that resembles the resident's prior lifestyle.
Mood State	• Passive residents with distressed mood may be overlooked. • Evaluate those with no involvement in activities (alone or with others) or little initiative.
Behavior Problems	• Participate in support programs that focus on managing behaviors. • Participate in activities where coping skills, relaxation and anger management techniques are taught.
Activities	• Focus on: residents who have indicated a desire for additional activity choices; cognitively intact, distressed residents who may benefit from an enriched activity program; cognitively deficient, distressed residents whose activity levels should be evaluated; and highly involved residents whose health may be in jeopardy because of their failure to slow down.

RAPs Requiring Social Services Intervention

Delirium	Assess and intervene if caused by: • isolation, • recent loss of family/friend, • depression/sad anxious mood, • recent relocation and/or • sensory losses.
Cognitive Loss or Dementia	• Develop strategies to assist staff. • Teach staff and resident how to deal with behavioral manifestations of cognitive loss. • Develop a behavior control program. • Assess if problem could be remedied through improved staff education, referral to OT/RT for training or an innovative counseling program. • Assess if emotional, social, excess disability and/or environmental factors play a role in cognitive decline.
Visual Function	• Referral to optometrist/ophthalmologist if necessary. • Evaluate for appropriate use of visual appliances: glasses clean, labeled, reading glasses not used for walking. • Evaluate for effect of sad or anxious mood on visual dysfunction. • Provide appropriate devices for level of vision: large print calendar, clock, high wattage light, large print signs. • Refer to activities if necessary.
ADL	• Evaluate the effect of mood or behavior problems on ADL performance and motivation. • Develop a behavior control program to improve functioning.
Incontinence	• Evaluate the effect of incontinence on psychosocial well-being and social interactions and assist resident with coping with the dysfunction.
Psychosocial Well-Being	• Evaluate the effect of mood and behavior problems on feelings about self and social relationships. • Develop treatment program to focus on mood and behavior problems. • Develop corrective strategies to address distressing relationships and concern about loss of status.
Mood State	• Evaluate the need for new or altered care strategy when manifestations of mood state problem are present: sad mood; feelings of emptiness, anxiety or unease; loss of weight; tearfulness; agitation; aches and pains; bodily complaints and dysfunction.
Behavior Problem	• Develop alternate interventions and treatments to address behavior problems. • Identify the various factors involved in the manifestation of problem to identify behaviors that could be resolved and eliminate the problem.
Psychoactive Drug Use	• Develop monitors and care plan to address possible decline or impairment of cognitive and behavior status.
Physical Restraints	• Evaluate conditions associated with problem behaviors and physical restraint use: delirium impairment, cognition impairment, unmet communication needs, psychosocial needs, sad or anxious mood, resistance to treatment, medication, nourishment, motor agitation, confusion, gait disturbance. • Evaluate resident's response to restraint use. • Evaluate the philosophy, values, attitudes and wishes of the resident regarding restraint use. • Develop monitors and care plan to address possible negative outcomes from restraint use.

How to Complete or "Work" a RAP

The Interdisciplinary Team can complete RAPs as a group effort or RAPs can be assigned to certain disciplines. Usually the social services professional completes the Mood, Behavior and Psychosocial RAPs. The activities professional is usually responsible for completing the Activities RAP. A copy of each of these is provided in the appendix and should be referred to when reading this section.

The RAPs function as decision facilitators. They provide the basis for developing a problem list and formulating the resident's plan of care. After the MDS and RAPs are completed, the interdisciplinary team will be able to decide if:

- The resident has a troubling cognition that warrants intervention and addressing this problem is a necessary condition for other functional problems to be successfully addressed.
- Improvement of the resident's functioning in one or more areas is possible.
- Improvement is not likely, but the present level of functioning should be preserved as long as possible with rates of decline minimized over time.
- The resident is at risk of decline and efforts should emphasize slowing or minimizing decline and avoiding functional complications (e.g., contractures, pain).
- The central issues of care revolve around symptom relief and other palliative measures during the last months of life.

The most important requirement for RAP documentation is that the thought process in working the RAP is evident. There are no mandated formats or forms for the RAP process. A separate form can be used for RAP documentation or the RAP review can be included when completing the disciplines assessment form or the progress note. In general four areas should be addressed when completing a RAP review:

- Nature of the condition
- Complications and risk factors that affect the staff's decision to proceed to care planning
- Factors that must be considered in developing individualized care plan interventions
- Need for referrals or further evaluation by appropriate health professionals

To complete the RAP review, use the following steps: (*have the RAP found in Appendix B available for review*)

1. Determine Why the RAP Triggered by Reviewing Section II (Triggers) of the RAP

This is an essential step in working the RAP. A RAP cannot be properly reviewed unless the reason for triggering is understood. A RAP is triggered by the MDS coding. A review of Section II Triggers will show the MDS responses that could trigger each RAP. Review the list, note which questions were answered on the MDS. One response or several responses can trigger a RAP. All should be noted.

2. Review the Guidelines in Section III (Guidelines) of the RAP

The guidelines are developed to help the clinician determine whether or not a problem truly exists or was "falsely triggered." They also provide a series of probes to help identify possible causes, risk factors and complications that may affect the resident. These guidelines should be read each time a RAP is triggered until the clinician is very familiar with the content. The RAP key following each RAP provides a summary and sometimes a clarification of the information in the guidelines and can be used as a quick reference once familiarity with the text is gained.

3. Rule Out Suggested Complications and Risk Factors

Keeping in mind why the RAP was triggered, review the guidelines and determine which factors are NOT related to the problem. It is not necessary to record the factors that do not apply.

4. Determine Which Factors are Related to the Problem

After eliminating the factors that do not apply and again keeping in mind why the RAP triggered, determine if there are any remaining factors or complications that will affect the resident's functioning, whether or not they can be eliminated, reversed, prevented from causing decline or whether complications can be avoided. Address these in the RAP review note.

5. Document the Rationale for Proceeding or Not Proceeding to the Care Plan
The clinical decision-making process should be very clear in the documentation. A lengthy statement is not needed but enough information should be given to clearly identify the rationale for proceeding to the care plan. Or if the decision is made not to address the problem in the care plan, you must make it clear why you determined that the triggered condition is not a problem for the resident.

6. Determine the Need for Referral to Another Health Professional
In some cases, the resident may benefit from a consultation by a qualified specialist. This could be a psychologist, dentist, audiologist, the facility dietitian or pharmacist or other professional.

A Sample RAP Note Using the Steps Above:

Refer to the Activities RAP on the next page. For purposes of instruction, the RAP Key is being used. In practice, the full RAP guidelines would be consulted as well. Note that many of the Guidelines have been struck out. This illustrates Step #3, the elimination or "ruling out" process. Note the items marked with a ♥. This illustrates Step #4, the identification of factors that have been determined to be the causes of the resident's lack of participation. These factors are then addressed in the RAP review.

The numbers in the RAP review are included only to highlight the steps being completed. The resident being reviewed is a female admitted for rehabilitation following a fracture. She is expected to return to home when her therapy is completed.

(#1) Triggered due to <u>involved in activities little of the time</u>. (#4) Resident is <u>new to the facility</u>, with <u>reduced energy reserves</u>. Her <u>routine is much different than at home</u>, where she <u>was very involved in taking care of her frail husband</u>. She is receiving physical therapy and occupational therapy and is <u>focused on her rehab program</u> and does not want to become involved in facility life. She is too tired to read, doesn't like television. She prefers to rest when not involved with rehab. (#5) Will proceed with care planning to provide her with company to prevent complications of boredom and to support her discharge plans.

RAP Exercises

Try applying the six steps to complete the RAP in the following case studies. Photocopy the appropriate RAP Key from the RAP in Appendix B. Circle the reason for triggering and strike out the Guidelines that are not applicable. Then try and write a RAP review note addressing the remaining Guidelines. After you have practiced writing out your sample RAP review notes you are welcome to compare your notes with the samples at the end of this chapter.

Exercise #1 — Mood RAP

Mr. James is an 88-year-old with Alzheimer's disease. His memory and decision-making skills are impaired (B2, B4). He repeats continuously, "Where is my car?" "Where are my keys?" (E1i) and paces continuously up and down the hallways (E1n) looking for a way out to the parking lot to find the car. These behaviors have not improved and in fact are becoming more frequent (E3). At this time he is easily redirected from the door and no behavioral symptoms are present. He spends little time in activities (N2). He has no reversible conditions present, is on no psychotropic medication and can communicate his basic needs.

ACTIVITIES RAP KEY *(For MDS Version 2.0)*

TRIGGERS - REVISION	GUIDELINES

TRIGGERS - REVISION

ACTIVITIES TRIGGER A (Revise)

Consider revising activity plan if one or more of the following present.

♥
- Involved in activities little or none of time [N2 = 2,3]

- Prefers change in daily routine [N5a = 1,2] [N5b = 1,2]

ACTIVITIES TRIGGERS B (Review)

Review of activity plan suggested if both of following present.

Awake all or most of time in morning [N1a = checked]

Involved in activities most of time [N2 = 0]

GUIDELINES

Issues to be considered as activity plan is developed.

♥
- Time in facility [AB1]
- ~~Cognitive status [B2, B4]~~
- ~~Walking/locomotion pattern [G1c, d, e, f]~~
- ~~Unstable/acute health conditions [J5a, b]~~

♥
- Number of treatments received [P1]
- ~~Use of Psychoactive medications [O4a, b, c, d]~~

Confounding problems to be considered.

♥
- Performs tasks slowly and at different levels (reduced energy reserves) [G8c, d]
- ~~Cardiac dysrhythmias [I1e]~~
- ~~Hypertension [I1h]~~
- ~~CVA [I1t]~~
- ~~Respiratory diseases [I1hh, I1ii]~~
- ~~Pain [J2]~~

Other issues to be considered:

♥
- Customary routines [AC]
- ~~Mood [E1, E2] and Behavioral Symptoms [E4]~~
- ~~Recent loss of close family member/friend or staff [F2f, from record]~~

♥
- Whether daily routine is very different from prior pattern in the community [F3c]

Exercise #2 — Mood RAP

Mrs. Snow is a 91-year-old with dementia. Her memory and decision-making skills are impaired (B2, B4). She cries continuously, she has a sad, pained expression and repeatedly calls out, "Help me." (E1c, l and m). Her mood is not easily altered (E2) and has deteriorated (E3) from the last assessment. Her ADL ability has deteriorated (G9). She is on an antidepressant (O4). She has no reversible conditions present, no behavior or relationship problems and can communicate her basic needs.

Exercise #3 — Psychosocial RAP

Mrs. Smith is an 88-year-old with severe COPD. She is oxygen dependent. She has no mood or behavior problems, no recent losses or changes. She participates in facility life, getting along with residents and staff. She likes to set her own schedule for activities and her daily care. She is coded as F1d = establishes own goals.

Hints for Completing RAPs

The suggestions shown in this section will help you to understand the purpose and intent of the five RAPs most often completed by activity and social services professionals. Be sure you also refer to the CMS RAP guidelines.

Mood RAP

- The Mood RAP will tend to "over trigger" because all symptoms are coded regardless of assumed cause. Create a care plan entry because of this RAP only if the problem identified is a true mood problem and is causing the resident distress. Do not proceed if the symptom is a manifestation of a physical problem or if it does not cause the resident distress.

- Signs and symptoms coded in Section E1 may be manifestations of actual disease problems — pained expression due to severe pain from terminal cancer, repetitive movements due to Parkinson's, legitimate repetitive health complaints due to unresolved gastrointestinal problems, pacing due to Alzheimer's.

- Presence of actual physical problems — especially pain — should be ruled out before assuming the resident is depressed or has a mood problem.

- If a true mood problem is identified, the goal is to *resolve* the problem. The RAP suggests that an altered care strategy is required when a mood problem persists.

- The Mood RAP states, "those residents with stable behavior and no unusual confounding problems do not require care plan alterations." A resident's repetitive complaints may be a long-standing personality trait with no need for any intervention other than to accept that person for who s/he is. It would be impossible to change whom that person is, and therefore no altered care strategy is needed.

Behavior RAP

- The Behavior RAP will also "over trigger" because the coding focuses on a resident's actions and not the intent.

- The first focus of this RAP is to determine if a behavior is serious, endangering the resident and others or causing distress to the resident or others, or if it is a behavior that can be easily accommodated.

- A care plan may not be warranted for behaviors that do not present a danger or cause distress to the resident and which can be easily accommodated. Take for example a resident that is delusional and believes that she is still working in an office; her behavior could be accommodated by allowing her to sit at a desk and sort papers.

- The second focus of the Behavior RAP is to identify potential causes of the problem that could be resolved to reduce or eliminate the behavior. As in the Mood RAP, illnesses and physical conditions, as well as the other factors listed, should be ruled out as possible causes before turning to a drug to manage the behavioral symptom.

- Always rule out pain as a potential cause of the behavioral symptom if coded in Section J3 of the MDS.

- The RAP will also trigger due to an improvement in behavior. In this case the RAP suggests potential factors that could mask the problem, such as physical restraints that stop the wandering or antipsychotic medications to control physical abuse. These should be evaluated for continued need or possible reduction.

Psychosocial Well-Being RAP

- The Psychosocial Well-Being RAP identifies both problems and strengths.

- When negative symptoms are exhibited, such as problems with roommates or concern about loss of status, a mood or behavior problem is often present as well. The primary focus should be to address the mood or behavior problem with hopes of increasing the resident's feelings of well-being.

- The RAP notes for Mood, Behavior and Psychosocial can be combined when the problems overlap.

- Strengths are identified to focus on the need to maintain a resident's independence and involvement in life that may be quashed by an institutional environment. In most cases, a care plan is not warranted if the resident continues to display these positive attributes.

Activities RAP

- The Activity RAP states, "Activity planning is a universal need in the nursing home." Every resident will have some type of activity care planning. The focus of this RAP is to identify those that need a *revised* activity care plan. The question to answer is whether or not the resident's participation level is meeting his/her need to be physically and mentally challenged and whether or not the current activity plan is appropriate for the resident.

- The RAP targets residents whose inactivity "may be a major complication in their lives." The probes in the guidelines focus on questioning whether or not the resident is suitably challenged, whether his/her active involvement can be improved and whether or not the routine of nursing home life contributes to resident apathy.

- In some cases, the current plan may be appropriate for the resident and provide all of the challenges that the resident can tolerate even though participation time is low. In this case, it is not necessary to proceed with a care plan revision.

- In other cases, the resident is clearly not challenged or is apathetic and bored. Although nothing seems to work, the activity professional needs to continue to revise the care plan to strive to meet the resident's needs.

- The RAP also targets residents whose high activity involvement or failure to slow down may cause medical complications. Residents with cardiac diagnoses may need to pace their activities and take rest periods to avoid overexertion.

Cognitive Loss/Dementia RAP

According to the RAI Manual (MDS 2.0), a cognitive loss or dementia problem is suggested if one or more of the following is present:
- Short Term Memory Loss   (B2a = 1)
- Long Term Memory Loss   (B2b = 1)
- Impaired Decision Making   (B4 = 1,2, or 3)
- Problem Understanding Others   (C6 = 1,2 or 3)

The Cognitive Loss/Dementia RAP guidelines look at cognitive losses that are reversible (10% of skilled nursing residents) along with interventions. The guidelines also look at chronic cognitive losses and how we can provide the best quality of life through environment, activities and sustaining current functional capacities and strengths. These three areas should be goals for the programs that we provide. Some contributing factors to cognitive losses could be:

- Depression
- Lack of motivation
- Medications
- Diet
- Sensory impairments
- Malnutrition
- High fever
- Fluid imbalance
- Meningitis
- Anemia
- Hyperthyroidism
- Anxiety
- Traumatic brain injury

- Stroke
- Substance abuse
- Dementia due to HIV
- Neurological disorders
- Pain
- Need for task segmentation
- Communication disorders
- Lack of involvement in surroundings and ability to make decisions
- Low self-esteem and lack of self-confidence
- Excess disability (decline related to environmental stimuli that exacerbates any current deficits)

It is important for the treatment team to create cognitive challenges at all levels. Below are suggested guidelines for interventions and activities for three different levels of cognitive function. Which guidelines you choose for a particular resident depends on the resident's MDS scores. The three levels are 1. Improvement or Retaining, 2. Restoration and 3. Maintaining and Sustaining.

Improvement or Retraining

Goal: Improvement or retraining of cognitive and functional ability level.

These residents have potential for orientation and score independent to modified independence on cognitive skills for daily decision making on MDS Section B4 = 0 or 1.

Remember that according to the diagnosis and contributing factors, individuals may fluctuate from level to level and the documentation needs to substantiate these changes. An example would be working with an individual who is recovering from a CVA or a recent head injury.

In addition, many of these individuals will not want to participate in the general activity program because they think of themselves as a short term stay patient and not a "resident." Small groups designed with other individuals at this level will prove more successful. The activity professional must work very closely with the therapy staff in addressing therapy goals specific to the person's treatment plan.

With the new Electronic Data Submission (EDS) and the Prospective Payment System (PPS) being implemented as the final final rule of OBRA, the Interdisciplinary Team will want to assess and capture a resident on Medicare Part A at the lowest level of function, mood and behavior in order to assure coverage for the services needed towards rehabilitation goals. Some of the activities that are appropriate for a person at this level are

- Activities designed by the therapist and supported by activities
- Physical and movement activities
- Creative writing
- Crossword puzzles, word and board games specific to cognitive functions
- Memory aides to enhance individual strengths
- Adaptations to prepare for independent living and a lesser level of care
- Community reintegration skills: Learning the skills and resources needed to be reintroduced to living outside of the facility
- Memory book
- Independent leisure interests and supplies needed (reading, painting, crafts, letter writing, movie watching)
- Communication enhancing activities

Restoration

Goals: Restoration of cognitive and functional ability level.

These residents have potential for reality orientation and score modified independence to moderately impaired on cognitive skills for daily decision making on MDS Section B4 = 1 or 2. Some activities and ideas that are appropriate for these individuals are

- Daily reality orientation including date, weather, location and daily events
- Memory aides. Use visual aides to reinforce information
- Repetition is very important. Allow more time for responses and for individuals to be as independent as possible
- Games that promote attention and expression
- Memory book
- Reading out loud, word games, simple crossword puzzles, Scrabble
- Creative writing beginning with writing the date and individual's name
- Activities that enhance and reinforce social skills. From re-orientation, the professional works on remotivation and re-socialization skills
- Activities that require a certain level of active participation in speaking and answering questions
- Reminiscing groups
- Resident Council
- Physical movement and exercise activities
- Problem solving games. This could be as simple as reading Dear Abby and asking how each individual would resolve the problem to more advanced questions and games. This creates a clustering of skills and allows the leader to build on more advanced cognitive skills of understanding, abstract thought and communication
- Life skills such as grooming issues, money management, social skills, cooking, writing lists, sequencing events
- Card games and board games
- Geography classes including completing a USA map puzzle for visual and tactile reinforcement
- Musical activities that demand a greater level of active participation or assisting other residents in need
- Create activities that require a higher level of social interaction and perhaps require team work and cooperation
- Current events, cultural activities, newspapers, magazine review

Maintaining and Sustaining

Goal: Maintaining and sustaining cognitive and functional ability level (taking into account progression of disorders).

These residents have little or no potential for reality orientation and score moderately to severely impaired on cognitive skills for daily decision making on MDS Section B4 = 2 or 3. Activities that are appropriate for these residents include:

- Sensory stimulation
- Aroma therapy
- Pet therapy
- Sensory motor activities
- Physical movement and games
- Body awareness
- Name identification
- Object identification
- Sorting games, matching skills
- Sensory boxes
- Focus on long term memory skills (trivia, reminiscing, multi-sensory)
- Looking at and/or reading the daily paper or magazines
- Creative writing, group poems
- Singing and music making
- Cooking skills, life skills, basic money management, shopping skills
- Motor skills, range of motion
- Validation therapy
- Task segmented activities for all of the above
- Photo albums and picture albums of familiar objects and things
- Completion of familiar sayings such as "too many cooks spoil the --------."
- Humor and laughter: people remember better and respond at their potential when they feel safe and are smiling and feeling good about themselves

How to Decide to Proceed or Not Proceed

- *Proceed* when a triggered condition affects a resident's functioning or well-being. In this case, a realistic and achievable goal should be evident.

- *Do not proceed* if the triggered condition does not affect a resident's functioning or well-being. In this case there would be no problem to resolve, no goal to be met. If the resident does not want to pursue a problem, e.g. an overweight resident does not want to lose weight even though it may affect her health, a care plan is not warranted. A goal cannot be met without the resident's participation.

- *Do RAPs have to be done with each full assessment?* No. If an annual MDS or significant change MDS is completed and there have been no coding changes on the MDS and no new triggers for the RAP, a brief note can be made to indicate that the existing RAP was reviewed and continues to accurately reflect the resident's status. RAPs are not required for quarterly MDS or the PPS/MDS.

RAP Summary

The RAP summary form (on the next page) provides information on which RAPs were triggered, where the RAP review information can be found, and whether or not the team has decided to proceed with care planning. Completion is required with each comprehensive assessment MDS.

The location and date of the RAP review documentation is entered on the form in Section VA. Only the primary source of documentation need be listed. It is not necessary to list secondary sources used to assess. An entry may be:
- RAP review 3/11/00 or
- Activity progress note 3/11/00

The care planning decision column is completed after the interdisciplinary team meets and discusses the care planning focus. The required completion date is seven days after the VB2 date.

Care Planning

Purpose of the Care Plan

The goal of care planning is to aid the resident in attaining or maintaining his/her highest practicable physical, mental and psychosocial well-being. While care plans do identify problems to be managed or eliminated, they also identify strengths to be built on to help the resident achieve the highest possible quality of life. These areas are pinpointed in the MDS and brought forward for further assessment in the RAP process.

The care plan is the culmination of the assessment process. It is the final distillation of the resident problems, needs and strengths. The care plan provides a "road map" to the resident's caregivers describing conditions to be treated, expected outcome and the care to be given.

SECTION V. RESIDENT ASSESSMENT PROTOCOL SUMMARY Numeric Identifier _____

Resident's Name:	Medical Record No.:

1. Check if RAP is triggered.

2. For each triggered RAP, use the RAP guidelines to identify areas needing further assessment. Document relevant assessment information regarding the resident's status.

- Describe:
  — Nature of the condition (may include presence or lack of objective data and subjective complaints).
  — Complications and risk factors that affect your decision to proceed to care planning.
  — Factors that must be considered in developing individualized care plan interventions.
  — Need for referrals/further evaluation by appropriate health professionals.

- Documentation should support your decision-making regarding whether to proceed with a care plan for a triggered RAP and the type(s) of care plan interventions that are appropriate for a particular resident.

- Documentation may appear anywhere in the clinical record (e.g., progress notes, consults, flowsheets, etc.).

3. Indicate under the Location of RAP Assessment Documentation column where information related to the RAP assessment can be found.

4. For each triggered RAP, indicate whether a new care plan, care plan revision, or continuation of current care plan is necessary to address the problem(s) identified in your assessment. The Care Planning Decision column must be completed within 7 days of completing the RAI (MDS and RAPs).

A. RAP PROBLEM AREA	(a) Check if triggered	Location and Date of RAP Assessment Documentation	(b) Care Planning Decision—check if addressed in care plan
1. DELIRIUM			
2. COGNITIVE LOSS			
3. VISUAL FUNCTION			
4. COMMUNICATION			
5. ADL FUNCTIONAL/ REHABILITATION POTENTIAL			
6. URINARY INCONTINENCE AND INDWELLING CATHETER			
7. PSYCHOSOCIAL WELL-BEING			
8. MOOD STATE			
9. BEHAVIORAL SYMPTOMS			
10. ACTIVITIES			
11. FALLS			
12. NUTRITIONAL STATUS			
13. FEEDING TUBES			
14. DEHYDRATION/FLUID MAINTENANCE			
15. DENTAL CARE			
16. PRESSURE ULCERS			
17. PSYCHOTROPIC DRUG USE			
18. PHYSICAL RESTRAINTS			

B. _____
1. Signature of RN Coordinator for RAP Assessment Process   2. Month — Day — Year

_____
3. Signature of Person Completing Care Planning Decision   4. Month — Day — Year

MDS 2.0 September, 2000

MDS Section V

Time Frames

The comprehensive care plan is mandated to be completed seven days after completion of the MDS and RAPs (the VB2 date). It is reviewed and updated as necessary with change in resident status and at least quarterly with the MDS review.

Components of the Care Plan

There is no mandated format or language for care planning. The only required components are
- a problem or need statement,
- a goal, and
- specific staff approaches or interventions.

Care plans should be simple. Remember the purpose of the care plan is to deliver care to the resident. The entries should be written at a level that can be understood by all caregivers and the resident or his/her family.

There is no magic number of required care plan entries. The resident's functional level and medical needs will determine the number of entries.

In order to keep a care plan simple and concise, problems are often merged or blended. Very often a problem may present many manifestations. For instance, a resident that is depressed may have declined activity participation, had a weight loss, used an antidepressant and become more dependent with ADLs. If each of these problems were written up separately, there would be five problems on the care plan. It is likely that each of these problems would have similar interventions. None of these problems will resolve individually until the resident's depression is resolved. By merging or blending these problems into one entry, the interdisciplinary team can work toward a common goal.

When merging problems, there may be several goals. Each discipline will be adding interventions to meet these goals. The examples of care planning below give an idea of how a merged problem might look.

How to write a problem, need or strength statement

- Be specific in your description of the resident.
- Use words found in the MDS and RAP documents.
- Needs will be suggested by the RAPs, but do not rely on these alone. All conditions requiring intervention identified in the assessment process should be included in the care plan.

How to write a goal

- Be realistic.
- State the desired resident outcome using descriptive words so that it is obvious when the goal has been met.
- Make the goal measurable.
- Include a time frame to indicate when the goal should be reevaluated.

How to write interventions

- Be specific about how the intervention applies to the resident.
- Do not list interventions generic to all residents such as "need to escort to activities," "calendar in room" or "provide calm environment."
- Do not list one time interventions such as "psych eval."
- Include the discipline responsible for providing the care with the intervention statement.

Gathering Data for the Care Plan

Although the RAI is the major source for care planning, the team should not neglect problems or risks identified through other sources. Data gathered from the individual discipline's assessments, risk assessments and information from families should always be considered when developing the care plan. For example, if a risk assessment identifies the resident as a high risk for falls, this should be considered for care planning even though the Falls RAP was not triggered.

Using the RAPs to Create Care Plan

Completing a RAP almost writes the care plan by itself. The following RAPs will illustrate this concept. Note the underlined words— these are the beginnings of the care plan. Note that this care plan also combines the discharge planning care plan (marked in *italics*). Social services and activities have merged entries with common goals.

> Triggered due to <u>involved in activities little of the time</u>. Resident is <u>new to the facility</u>, with <u>reduced energy reserves</u>. Her routine is much different than at home, where she was very involved in taking care of her frail husband. She is <u>focused on her rehab program</u> and does not want to become involved in facility life. She is too tired to read, doesn't like television. She <u>prefers to rest when not involved with rehab</u>. Will proceed with care planning to <u>provide her with company</u> to <u>prevent complications of boredom</u> and to support her <u>discharge plans</u>.

Need Statement	Goal	Interventions
involved in activities little of the time As evidenced by: prefers to rest in bed when not involved in rehab Contributing factors: new to facility reduced energy reserves Strengths: focused on rehab program	Will not manifest complications of boredom as seen by: No apathy towards discharge or rehab plans for the next 2 weeks *Discharge to home with in home health care in the next 2 weeks*	1. Daughter to bring husband to visit 3 x wk for dinner (DSS/CNA) 2. Short daily visits from AD and SSD to provide her with company 3. Calendar in room to mark off days until return home AD to use pink highlighter with daily visits (AD) 4. Radio by bedside. Tune to easy listening station. (AD/CNA) 5. Daily visits from SSD to *review discharge plans*, and progress in rehab (SSD)

This next care plan will combine ADL, Mood, Psychoactive Drug Use and Activities RAPs in care planning.

> Triggered due to <u>calling out for help, crying and sad pained expression</u>. Her mood is <u>not easily altered</u> and has not responded to antidepressant therapy. She is in obvious distress and her mood is <u>affecting her ADLs</u> and <u>psychosocial functioning</u>. Will create a care plan to address her <u>need for relief from her symptoms</u>. Refer to psychologist and pharmacist for medication review.

Need Statement	Goal	Interventions
Decline in Mood, ADL and psychosocial functioning

As seen by:

calling out for help, crying, sad, pained expression

does not respond to attempts to alter mood

current antidepressant ineffective

decline in activity participation and socialization

more dependent with ADLs

Contributory factors: dementia memory and decision making skills impaired

Strengths: Strong family support | Will demonstrate benefit from antidepressant and relief of symptoms of distress as seen by:

No side effects from change in antidepressant in 2 weeks

Return to participation in AM coffee social and PM sensory awareness group in 4 weeks

Improvement in dressing to limited assist in 4 weeks | 1. Follow psychologist plan for mood alteration: see attached interventions (All Staff)

2. Observe for side effects of new medication: Prozac (LN)

3. Visit with resident daily for AM coffee. Bring out to group if resident expresses willingness (AD)

4. Ambulate resident to sensory group daily. Allow to watch and participate if willing (CNA/RNA)

5. Use task segmentation for dressing. Do not overwhelm with choices in daily attire. (CNA)

6. Engage family in mood alteration plan with weekly visits (SSD) |

This care plan demonstrates several points about care planning. In intervention #1 the psychologist's plans are referenced but not repeated on the care plan. If specific detailed plans for care have been outlined by a discipline, it is not necessary to repeat them. A copy can be placed behind the care plan entry, which can then be referred to by all caregivers. Also note that all of the interventions begin with an action verb and are related to the goals. This is the idea behind care planning. State specifically what needs to be done with the resident to accomplish each goal.

Revising the care plan

The care plan is a dynamic tool for resident care. It should be revised as often as the resident's needs change. At minimum the care plan is reviewed every 90 days with completion of the quarterly MDS. Changes in coding on the MDS may indicate a need to revise the care plan either due to an improvement or a decline in functional status. The process for determining if the care plan needs to be revised is as follows:

- review all sections of the MDS for coding changes from the previous assessment
- review the care plan entry specific to the MDS section with coding changes
- determine if the problem statement is accurate or needs to be revised, rewritten or discontinued
- determine if the goal is still realistic, if it has been met, if the time frame needs to be changed or if a new goal is needed
- determine if the interventions are still appropriate and in effect or if a revision is needed. As a rule of thumb, when a goal is not met it indicates that interventions were not effective. It may also mean that the goal was not realistic or achievable.

Procedures for changing the care plan vary for each facility. What needs to be evident are the changes made, the date of revision and a signature. This can be accomplished by using a highlighter pen, a red line or some other method that meets with legal documentation principles. If the care plan is reprinted, the changes made should be evident on the old copy of the care plan.

Updating the care plan for a temporary change of condition

When a resident experiences a temporary change in condition, such as the flu, urinary tract infection or pressure ulcer requiring bed rest, the activity and social services professional need to assess the resident for a risk for decline due to increased isolation or decreased activity. Most care planning systems have a short term problem care plan separate from the comprehensive care plan. If after assessing the resident for increased risks it is determined that a temporary change in interventions is needed, the activity or social services professional should add to the problems on the short term care plan.

Care Plan Examples

Getting a feel for writing a care plan can take some practice, so here are a few more examples of care plans. Each is written in a slightly different style to help you find a way of writing care plans that is comfortable for you.

Mrs. Y has triggered the Mood, Psychosocial, ADL, Activities and Nutritional RAPs. The Interdisciplinary Team has decided that her most acute need is to resolve her mood problem as this is causing most of her other problems and impeding her rehabilitation goals. The team care plan merging all of the above RAPs is shown below.

Sample Social Services Care Plan

Problem, Need, Strength	Objective	Interventions	Dsc
Alteration in Mood as evidenced by: • expresses sadness over lost status • anger at nursing home placement • spends little time in activities • leaves over 25% uneaten • lacks interest in rehab • frustration over lack of speech Contributory factors: • Recent CVA with dysphasia • Recent decline in ADLs • Recent nursing home placement Strengths: • Close family and church group support • Good rehabilitation potential	will eat 80% of breakfast & lunch QD by 1/20/01 will verbalize acceptance of disability and need to participate in rehab by 1/20/01	1. Hipro with each meal 2. DSS to provide substitutes for food refused 3. Encourage husband and friends to bring in favorite foods 4. Introduce to stroke support group 5. Visit with facility dog 6. Discuss Discharge Plan in positive terms 7. Ask yes/no questions 8. Allow time to express thoughts 9. Psych visit 1x wk 10. PT to describe interim goals to be met to achieve discharge 11. Space to be arranged for daily visits from friends	D D All SS AC DC All All Psy PT AC

Sample Activity Care Plan Entries

The *Care Planning Cookbook for Activities and Recreation* by Hall and Nolta[56] contains problem/need statements, goals and over 300 care plan approaches and interventions. A sample care plan on anxiety is shown below. Choose the entries that are appropriate for the resident and integrate them into the care plan. Tie in with existing problems/needs if possible.

Category: Emotional Issues   **Subtopic:** Anxiety

Problem Description, Concern, Need or Strength	Goal/ Objective	Approach/ Interventions
Refer to MDS Section E • Resident often appears to become anxious during activity programs evidenced by wringing hands, jumping at every sound, rigid posture, frequently yelling for help, _____. • Resident often states, "I'm not sure I should be here. I have lots of things to do in my room." • Resident needs one-on-one attention to promote participation during activity programs secondary to displaying anxious behaviors.	• Resident will not exhibit anxious behavior of _____, for ____ minutes, at _____ group activities, ____ times per week. • Residents will participate in _____ activity programs by following the group's general directions, ____ times per week.	• Invite, assist Resident to group activities of interest (i.e. _____ _____). • Explain the activity program's format to Resident prior to the start of program. • Allow Resident to choose seating placement at program. • Introduce to other alert peers. Identify similarities between Residents to promote conversation and friendships. • Ask the Resident direct questions to promote participation. • Refocus the Resident's attention to the specific activity task of _____ if anxious behavior is exhibited. • Compliment the Resident for following the activity program's directions.

---

[56] Hall, Beth A., CTRS and Michele M. Nolta, CTRS, ACC, 2000, *Care Planning Cookbook for Activities and Recreation*, p. 5-5, Recreation Therapy Consultants, San Diego, CA.

The chart below shows more possible entries in a resident care plan specific to activities. These could be combined with existing problems/needs on the care plan.

Problem/Need	Goal	Approach
Poor pathfinding skills — needs to go between room and dining room	Resident will be able to go between room and dining room without assistance within 3 months.	1. Visual cue on door. 2. Walk with Resident to and from dining room. 3. All staff to praise efforts of Resident.
Sensory deprivation — needs tactile stimulation	Resident will receive a minimum of 20 minutes of tactile stimulation a day.	1. Pet visits 2x weekly. 2. Massage hands with lotion 3x weekly. 3. 1:1 with sensory stimulation kits 2x weekly
Personal appearance sloppy, beard stubble, uncombed hair, body odor — needs to improve grooming	Resident will shave at least every two days, comb hair daily and bathe daily.	1. AC to visit with grooming items 2x weekly. 2. Grooming group 2x weekly. 3. CNAs to assist with AM care.
Hearing impairment — needs to be seated next to group leader	Resident will learn to sit next to leader where s/he can hear and respond to reminiscing questions.	1. Seat Resident next to leader in Current Events 1x weekly. 2. Reinforce advantages of sitting where s/he can hear. 3. Use visual cues.
Blindness and deafness — needs increased social contact	Resident will have at least 20 minutes of structured social contact 7x weekly.	1. AC to assist weaving hand over hand 4x weekly. 2. Resident will roll yarn ball for project. 3. Include in cooking, gardening and outdoor events for social interactions 5x weekly.
Self-stimulation — needs to keep hands busy due to dementia	Resident will fold napkins for social events by 3 months.	1. AC to set up folding station for Resident 1x daily. 2. AC/volunteer to visit Resident with tactile stimulation 2x weekly.

Other Resident Care Plan Considerations

If your facility uses hand-written resident care plans, you can leave a few lines between your entry and the ones above and below. As the resident's needs change and interventions are revised, there is room to add new entries.

Be realistic, both in your identification of a problem and the approach. Do not enter "will visit 4x weekly" on the care plan, if you realistically cannot visit more than 2 times weekly.

Be specific in your interventions. For example, do not enter "Group activities 1 x wk," but rather "Go to sing-along 1x week."

Be sure that the goal that is stated on the care plan is the same as the one discussed in the quarterly note. You must be sure that all parts of the care plan come from observations in the assessments and that every observation of problems or needs in the assessments — especially triggers in the MDS if the team decides to proceed — are addressed in the care plan. The team may choose not to proceed with a triggered RAP, but they must document why they made that decision.

There are some terms to avoid in identifying a problem on the care plan. The following chart offers some alternatives that are more descriptive and offer clearer connections between the problem and the treatment.

Don't say this	Say this to be more descriptive
social isolation or loneliness	needs to be aware of people around him/her or needs to feel useful to others
non-responsive	fear of answering inappropriately in a group setting.
confusion	needs to improve problem solving skills
short attention span	needs to follow one directive in exercise class or needs to stay on task with project for 5 minutes
disorientation	needs to locate room
too tired	needs energy conservation techniques due to COPD
boredom	needs to develop one new leisure interest
lack of awareness	needs to stimulate short term memory retention
anxious	cries easily due to CVA or has anxiety due to CVA
need for diversional activities	needs diversion to decrease agitation
needs sensory stimulation	needs to respond to _____ stimulation as seen by (blinking eyes, holding object etc.) Be specific as to what type of stimulation — tactile, visual, auditory, etc.
refuses to attend	This is the resident choice and is not a problem for the resident. Your problem is to devise activities that the resident will participate in.
needs transportation to activities	no alternative, this is your problem, not the resident's

Sample RAP Notes

The three sample RAP notes are for you to compare with the RAP notes you were asked to write earlier in the chapter.

Sample Mood RAP Note for Exercise #1

Triggered due to continuous pacing and repetitive questions. Behaviors have increased in frequency in the last several months due to advancing Alzheimer's disease. Activity participation is very limited due to his very brief attention span and continuous pacing. Will not proceed with care planning at this time, as this is not a true mood problem but a manifestation of his ongoing disease process. His behavior is stable. Current staff expectations and interventions are appropriate. Altered care strategy is not required at this time.

Sample Mood RAP Note for Exercise #2

Triggered due to calling out for help, crying and sad pained expression. Her mood is not easily altered and has not responded to antidepressant therapy. She is in obvious distress and her mood is affecting her ADLs and psychosocial functioning. Will create a care plan to address her need for relief from her symptoms. Refer to psychologist and pharmacist for medication review.

Sample Psychosocial RAP Note for Exercise #3

Triggered due to establishing own goals. Very active in directing her own care, has set plans for her daily schedule. There is no conflict with institutional routine, no impediments to her continuing to exercise her independence. Will not proceed to care plan.

Chapter 13
Monitoring the Treatment Plan

Assessing the participant and writing the care plan are not the end of the treatment process for the individual's care. There must be an ongoing process to monitor the status of each participant. You must make notes in the participant's chart whenever there is any change of condition that affects the individual's functioning or ability to participate in programming. Every quarter the care team must meet to perform a quarterly review of each participant's care plan, which includes determining if the most recent assessment of the participant's condition is still correct.

Monitoring Tools — Activities

There are several ways to make sure that your treatment plan is still appropriate for the participant. The methods include:
- Daily Activity Attendance (Participation) Records
- Bedside Log Notes for one-on-one visits
- Progress Notes

Participation Records

Records must be kept on each individual's participation in activities and treatment programs. The records must be kept seven days a week. Participation in an activity can be either positive or negative. Just documenting that an individual attended or participated in an activity is telling only part of the story. Dave Dehn developed a method of easily documenting the quality of participation during any type of activity. (This scale can be found in Chapter 6: Activities). This method not only helps the professional document an individual's status but also provides the individual with an easy way to understand what "healthy" participation looks like. The following pages show a set of forms you can use to keep a record of participation. (You may want to refer back to Chapter 6: Activities and use the five point participation scale to document the quality of the individual's participation.) We recommend that the activity professional use two different kinds of forms for documentation of participation:
1. Activity Participation Record
2. Special Programming/Bedside Log

The first form, the *Activity Participation Sheet*, shows a way to keep track of each individual's participation in group activities. You don't have to use this exact form, but it includes the set of information that you do need to keep. (You, of course, need to have the activities from your facility listed.) The important components to include are participant name, type of activity, date and length of time. You also want to use a code that shows the level of participation (active or passive, positive or negative). When an individual refuses an invitation to an activity or room visit, be sure to mark "R" for refuse. This will document that you attempted to include her/him and that it is her/his right to refuse.

For individuals who are restricted to their beds or who do not attend activities 2–3 times per week, you need to keep additional documentation to show their involvement in activities. One way to do this is with a bedside log shown in the second form. Whatever type of log you decide to use, it must describe the type of visit (what you did), length of the visit, date and the individual's response.

Activity Participation Sheet

Participant Name _____

Room # _____

Active = A
Refused = R

Observed = O

Month _____

	1	2	3	4	5	6	7	8	9	10	11	12	13	14	15	16	17	18	19	20	21	22	23	24	25	26	27	28	29	30	31

Special Programming Bedside Log

The activity professional must provide specialized and individualized programs for participants unable and/or uninterested in attending group activities at least 2 - 3 times per week.

Each participant who needs in-room activities will have a Bedside Log Form. The form is used and kept by the month and the year.

Activity Code: These are the types of activities that you may be providing. They need to be the same as on the care plan "approaches." Numbers 17 and 18 are there in case you wish to add any activity not listed on the form.

Activities should be at least fifteen minutes in duration and two to three times per week in frequency. After the visit you record onto the log.

Example:

Date	Length of Visit	Code	Participant Response
1/16/99	20 minutes	2 & 4	Mrs. Idder held and petted the kitten and afterwards we wrote a letter to her son. She expressed thanks and enjoyment for the visit.
OR			
1/16/99	15 minutes	15 a, c	Mr. Miller opened his eyes when I turned on relaxation tape. He visually followed my movement around his bed and seemed to be intent on listening to the sound of my voice while I was talking to him.

These records can be kept either behind the individual's attendance participation records or in a separate binder. If the bedside logs are not in the attendance participation records, you should note in the participation records where the bedside logs can be found.

Special Programming: Bedside Log

Name _____

Month/Year _____ / _____

Activity Code:

1. Reality orientation
   a: oral
   b: written
   c: picture book/board
2. Pet visits
3. Art projects
4. Creative expression
5. Exercise
6. Music
7. Religion
8. Games
9. Reading material
10. Grooming
11. Participant volunteer
12. Community involvement
13. Work type activities/project oriented
14. Discussion, conversation
15. Sensory stimulation
    a: scent
    b: tactile
    c: sound
    d: visual
16. Rehab Goal Support
17.
18.

Date	Length of Visit	Activity Code	Initials	Participant Response

Monitoring Tools — Social Services

Keeping up with a participant's needs (psychosocial and concrete) and changing conditions (health and behavior) is an ongoing challenge. It is only partly done if you know what the need/concern/problem is. To complete the cycle you must reflect your knowledge and your plan in writing in the participant's record.

Although this is not a regulation and will not even appear in any of the surveyors' guidelines, it is a good social services practice to make an entry in the participant's chart every week for at least the first two months. You can start it with each new participant and use it as a form of tracking his/her adjustment to the facility. Chart each week on some significant clue to the adjustment (or lack thereof) by indicating such things as knowledge of the facility: various rooms; recognition of faces, if not names, of staff and roommates; and familiarity with the approximate routine within the facility.

This charting will help you track the participant's moods, find behavior patterns which might escalate into problems or begin to work toward appropriate discharge planning. Very importantly, you can determine if your current entry on the participant care plan is still a reflection of the participant's need. Use a standard social services progress note form. A narrative style of documentation seems to work best for most social services entries.

If you find that weekly charting is not necessary because the participant's overall independence and adjustment or, at the other extreme, very poor orientation and inability to respond to standard reality orientation, you can record this observation in the chart by making a note to that effect and change the frequency of the tracking.

Another way to document social services interventions is to keep a Social Services Log for each participant. This log is a record documenting services and counseling provided to the participant by the social services professional. The form could be a narrative or it might be similar to the Bedside Log used by the activity professional. Be sure to identify date, nature of service, participant's response and the follow-through that is required.

Quarterly Review

Care conferences are held quarterly for each participant to discuss his/her current status and care plan. The formal part of this process is the requirement to update the MDS for the resident. It is a chance for care team to meet together and check each participant's care plan. The team needs to be sure that the information about the participant's condition is up to date and that the care plan reflects the participant's current condition.

Your responsibilities are to write a quarterly progress note, complete your part of the MDS and then carefully read the MDS and notes for the other disciplines before you attend the care plan meeting. (Activity professionals are required to write quarterly notes. Social services professionals are only required to write annual notes, but we strongly recommend that they write quarterly notes, too. Both have portions of the MDS to complete.)

Quarterly Progress Notes

When you write your quarterly progress notes and complete the MDS, realize that you are reflecting on three months of a participant's life. It is essential, therefore, that you take the time to do a comprehensive review of all of the most recent entries in the medical chart: from the doctor's progress notes to nursing summaries, to dietary and therapy entries and your own interventions. Also check the participant care plan for any changes, the medication book for new drugs or discontinued ones and, when indicated, behavioral monitors that reflect a participant's mood or behavior. Review your last quarterly note to ensure that you have addressed unfinished issues from the last quarter.

Both activity and social services professionals should end the note with a goal for the quarter. This goal will be the same as on the care plan.

Quarterly Progress Notes — Activity Professional

Below you will find a checklist for a comprehensive activity quarterly progress note. Follow these guidelines for a note that identifies all of the important areas of an individual. If there are areas not needing attention such as special diets, skip them in the note.

Directions: When writing your quarterly note, review the necessary areas of information on this checklist form. Include as many of these areas as possible in order to document in a *comprehensive* manner.

Content Areas

	Cognitive Status
	Communication Deficits and Needs
	Behavioral Issues and Interventions
	Mood and Behavior, Depression
	Family Involvement & Relationship with Roommate and Staff
	Previous Leisure and Lifestyle Interests
	Specific Involvement in Activity Program
	Level of Responsiveness in Group Activities
	Strengths and Abilities
	Necessary Information About Vision, Hearing and Speech
	Psychoactive Medications
	Restraint Use
	Special Notes About Diet
	Therapy
	All Areas on Care Plan with Activity Approaches
	RAP Information
	Activity Treatment Plan & Quarterly Goal

Quarterly Progress Notes — Social Services

Your responsibilities at the time of the quarterly update are to complete your section(s) on the MDS, review your prior progress note and review the existing care plan. In the case of a participant for whom behaviors are being monitored (with or without chemical intervention), you will need to review the audit record to assure that the MDS is filled out accurately.

This being completed, proceed with a quarterly note and necessary care plan revisions. The social services professional looks at different parts of the individual's life. View your note as a summary of events; recap important occurrences in the quarter and note any changes. Consider the following:

1. Is the participant alert? Oriented? Has there been a change in his/her cognitive status?
2. What is the participant's involvement with family or other participants?
3. What is the participant's daily pattern? Where does s/he spend most of his/her time (in his/her room; in activities)?

4. Have there been any changes in the types of activities that the participant has chosen to participate in?
5. Have there been any changes in the level of participation?
6. Does s/he socialize with other participants or does s/he seek out staff?
7. Does s/he have visitors? Who? How often? Has this changed since your last quarterly note (e.g., a family death or illness)?
8. Who tends to his/her concrete needs (family, social services professional)?
9. In general, what has changed over the last three months? Has s/he become agitated? Calmer? Why?
10. What comments do you have about personality, characteristics and special individual traits seen now versus previous reported lifestyle?
11. Has any special consultation been received (psych, etc.)?
12. Have there been any changes related to dentures, glasses, hearing aids, funding, and durable equipment?

Reflect, where appropriate, the components of these elements of a participant's record:
*   Review all physician's notes for the quarter.
*   Check to see if there have been any medication changes (especially regarding medications that modify behavior).
*   Assess the behaviors that are being monitored in the medication/treatment book. Is the monitor sheet a true description of behavior? Are there any patterns emerging that can be analyzed?
*   Assess restraint use and whether it has had any effect on psychosocial functioning.
*   Check for any consults and results during the quarter (e.g., psych. or dental).
*   Check for changes in function (see nursing and therapy notes).
*   Reread your own interventions to refresh your memory.

At the end of your note, it is advisable to address:
*   The issue of placement (Is it appropriate to consider discharge to a lesser level of care or are needs still best met in the current setting?)
*   Are the individual's Advance Directives in place or has s/he at least been offered the opportunity to express his/her wishes?
*   Do the care plan and the accompanying goal and approaches remain adequate to address the individual's need (s)?
*   Is the goal reasonable and obtainable?

The Care Plan

Now it is time to reflect on the care plan entry.
*   Does any change in the MDS require a change in the care plan?
*   How closely did the problem/need/concern actually reflect the individual's need(s) during the quarter?
*   How close is the participant to the goal you established for him/her?
*   Have the planned approaches been successful/adequate?
*   Does the problem, need or concern still reflect your assessment of the participant?
*   Have things changed enough so that you need to start again or add to the care plan?

Your quarterly entry is the place to answer these questions. It is okay to change; in fact, it is essential to change any part or even all of the individual care plan entry if it is no longer a reflection of the individual. If the goal will never be accomplished, change it; then alter the approaches to support the goal. Remember that all changes in the care plan require input from the individual and/or guardian.

When you have done this, support your changes in the progress note. If you have been honest in your updated assessment of the individual, you will know whether the care plan needs changing. Remember — the individual care plan goal must be reflected in your progress notes. If your entry does not help to paint an accurate picture of the individual, it needs to be changed.

A few sample quarterly progress notes for activity and social services professionals are shown below:

Activity Quarterly Progress Notes

6/10/01 Activity Quarterly Progress Note

Mary is alert and aware of people and things around her. She has occasional periods of confusion, which seem to occur in the late afternoon. When in a group setting, she is hesitant to speak up due to an embarrassment about her word retrieval skills.

She spends most of her day in her room, feeding birds on the patio and waiting for her daughter to visit.

During one-on-one visits 2x weekly, she converses and expresses interest in our conversation.

Mary has a wonderful sense of humor and a strong sense of curiosity. She is receiving speech therapy 1x weekly for language deficits 2° to a mild left CVA. The speech therapy goals for her will be reinforced in one-on-one conversation and word/memory games. She will also be encouraged to join in the small morning discussion group for social interaction and communication building skills.

E. Best CTRS, ACC

9/10/01 Activity Quarterly Progress Note

Mary is alert with periods of confusion reported about 1x per day, usually in the early afternoon. Some progress is being made in conjunction with the speech therapist to solve problems pronouncing words, but she still has significant difficulty being understood at times.

Most of the day, she can be seen looking out of her window, waiting for her daughter or feeding the birds out on the patio. Her daughter visits weekly and she receives mail monthly from a distant relative in Iowa.

She seems to enjoy our visits 2x weekly and has enjoyed participating in the small morning discussion group. She has contributed a lot of insight to our discussions and is much appreciated. I have had to interpret what she said to the other members about 20% of the time (down from almost 50% when she first joined the group), but this has not been a problem for the group. We have worked with the speech therapist on the continuing areas of difficulty.

One thing that I have continued to appreciate is Mary's strong sense of curiosity and a wonderful sense of humor.

GOALS:

Res. will continue to practice communication techniques (see speech therapy goal for revised plan) during the small discussion group 2x per week for the next three months. Activity professional will assist participant to practice new communication skills learned in speech therapy during the small discussion group.

Check more carefully to try to pinpoint time of confusion. Nursing is considering the possibility that it may be related to medication.

E. Best CTRS, ACC

Quarterly Progress Notes

6/08/01 Social Services Quarterly Progress Note

Lydia has been here for three months now and has worked very hard to make an adjustment to this environment. She came here from a loving home environment which could no longer support her, given the escalation in her personal care needs related to a compression fracture in her spine which compounds the existing circumstance related to a CVA she suffered in 1999. She very appropriately mourned the loss of her life as she had known it and SSD spent at least an hour a week with her reminiscing, dissecting the pros and cons of her present situation and gradually looking to a future (something she had verbalized to me after about six weeks into her admission that she had no sense of).

Lydia has rejected the idea of an antidepressant (which her physician had asked her to consider) feeling instead that she would rather "feel her emotions and deal with the issues now — not prolong the pain of separation." There have been no observed indications of depression; Lydia has maintained as excellent appetite (gaining eight pounds over the quarter), sleeps well at night and says she has "nice dreams," all counter indications of the usual signs and symptoms of depression. Her weight gain of eight pounds keeps her well within range of her normal body weight. (For further clarification, see dietary note.)

Lydia's family, husband and one of two daughters who lives nearby, visit several times a week and have made her room homey, reflecting Lydia's love of clowns and flowers.

Lydia remains oriented, interested in her care and gradually has entered into an activity of her choosing.

Her placement remains appropriate at this level of care because of her dependence for care, her incontinence and her non-ambulatory status. Lydia's advance directives are in the chart: she has expressed clear end-of-life wishes.

There are no apparent unmet concrete needs at present: she has new glasses, her dentures fit well and she is not hard of hearing.

SSD goal of visiting at least once a week to allow her to verbalize her feelings related to adjustment, with the additional intention of establishing a trusting relationship with at least one staff member, has been met thus far. Because she is becoming more independent, emotionally and physically, within the facility, this goal will be revised to biweekly visitation for the next quarter.

M. A. Weeks, SSD

6/08/01 SS Quarterly Progress Note

John is a very stable participant of three months duration in the facility. He has a diagnosis of Alzheimer's disease (probable). His signs and symptoms are consistent with that as he is no longer able to identify himself, find his room or ask for what he needs. He is alert, however, and seems interested in his surroundings; he is a passive observer in most activities, responds to his name by making eye contact and appears to recognize his wife when she visits (daily at lunch) because he will smile and reach for her.

John had been receiving Ativan for agitation and anxiety BID [two times a day]. He had been placed on this medication at home because of his behavior and the physician chose not to discontinue it upon admission, choosing instead to monitor and assess his behavior on the drug in this new setting.

At first John would become very restless, moving himself in his chair, reaching out to passersby and pulling at his clothes. This was noted especially in the evening, beginning at about 7 pm. After several weeks of a trial with the medication, the staff was not noticing a major change in his behavior pattern and it was decided to attempt behavioral interventions to address John's anxiety. The goal of reducing his episodes of nightly anxiety was addressed by removing John from the main activity room and putting him in the room where there was quiet music being played and there were never more than five other participants in attendance. Staff would speak very calmly and softly and if John began to show any signs of motor restlessness, he would be calmed with a gentle and reassuring touch to his hand. These approaches have been successful to the extent that the physician discontinued the Ativan at his last monthly visit.

All concrete needs have been addressed at the present time: John has a new upper denture; he used to use glasses only for reading but no longer reads, thus is not in any way dependent on glasses. He has a hearing aid in his right ear, which he tends to remove. It can usually be found in his pocket. His family is aware of the risk of loss and feel that, at this point in his diagnosis, he wears the aid out of habit, not for "hearing." The hearing aid is kept in the medication cart at night.

John's care needs require the supervision necessary at this level of placement. He has a Durable Power of Attorney in the medical chart.

SSD goal has been revised; John is visited at least monthly and during those visits, the goal is for him to respond in conversation by making eye contact when his name is used; he is also assessed for any personal care or clothing needs. If there are any, contact is made with his wife.

M. A. Weeks, SSD

The best advice we can give you on actually getting these done is to stay organized and try not to let progress notes pile up. The requirements of the PPS (the facility doesn't get paid unless the MDS is completed) make it likely that you will have a great deal more support from your facility management in getting your quarterly reports done than you did before the PPS was instituted. Doing them each week before the MDS review and participant care conference is the regulation. It is your responsibility to do your reports and provide other members of the interdisciplinary team with your unique perspective as they, too, comply with quarterly entry requirements.

Updates in the Progress Notes for a New RAI

Not only must you comment on the reason for the new Resident Assessment Instrument (RAI) when an individual's health status changes, but you must also discuss any impact that this may have had on the psychosocial well-being of the participant. For example, if the participant has had a stroke, s/he may have lost some of his/her ability to socialize. Clearly this can have an effect on his/her ongoing orientation and a new plan must be developed to address this.

Remember, because the MDS starts the clock anew, this update note will in essence be a quarterly progress note. If it has been a while since you have written a comprehensive note, now is the time to write one.

Annual Review

Once a year you will participate in an annual review of each individual. The purpose of the annual review, unlike the quarterly review, is to completely reassess the individual. The team does a new MDS and any RAPs that are triggered. New, rather than revised, care plans are written.

Your participation is the same as it was in the initial assessment of the individual: supplying information for your section of the MDS, assisting with RAPs, reading through information from all the other disciplines and participating in the care plan conference.

Social services professionals are responsible for an annual update in the progress notes. This note is an overall summary that reflects change over the entire year. The annual date is determined by the date of the previous, full, validated MDS.

Sample activity and social services annual progress notes are shown below:

Social Services Annual Progress Note

9/6/01 Social Services Annual Progress Note

Lydia has continued to make progress with an adjustment that started out with difficulties related to her mourning her previous life at home. She has been consistently verbal and able to express her feelings and has maintained an ongoing relationship with me, which has included at least biweekly "check-in" visits after the first quarter of weekly visits.

Her health has remained stable with no further fractures or indications of new problems related to her original CVA. Her mood is optimistic and she has reached out to other alert individuals and they have formed a dining group that meets every day at lunch. This group is also the nucleus of the Resident Council and Lydia seems delighted to use her organizational skills as the elected secretary.

Her daughters offer love and support to her; her husband has himself suffered some major health problems during the year and his pattern of visiting four times per week has been reduced to two times per week. Lydia has been able to accept this new pattern without evidence of a setback in her mood, probably, she says, because she realizes that her husband, after so many years of focusing on her, must allow others to tend him now. She misses him but is always so happy to see him when he does visit that they spend their time catching up on events in their separate lives.

There have been no new medications needed; the MD's progress notes regularly reflect Lydia's stability and good humor.

SSD goal of biweekly visits has been revised to quarterly visits, which is a reflection of a well-integrated individual.

M. A. Weeks, SSD

9/8/01 Social Services Annual Progress Note

John has had an expected decline due to his diagnosis of probable Alzheimer's disease. He is no longer alert as evidenced by his keeping his eyes closed much of the time and he does not seem to respond to his wife any longer, not even opening his eyes when she speaks to him. He spends much of the day out of his room with the possibility that he will receive some form of stimulation. John seems calm with no restlessness or aimless body movements noted. He is nonverbal and all of his needs must now be anticipated. Additionally, John has had a weight loss over the year representing about 10% of his body weight. He remains well within range of his ideal body weight but with his diagnosis a gradual weight loss is not inconsistent, even though he is fed all of his meals, consumes 75–90% of each and receives protein drinks between each meal and at bedtime.

John signed a Durable Power of Attorney for Health Care when he was well and his wife is able to make decisions regarding his care. She has asked that all possible comfort measures be provided, including relief of pain if necessary; he will remain with us, even if he develops further health care problems. She does not wish him transferred out to the acute care hospital.

John's physician has noted the obvious decline during the past five monthly visits to him; there is no medication indicated.

The SSD goal has been revised to reflect these changes: during monthly visits with John, his concrete needs are assessed, he is monitored for any obvious change which should then be discussed with his wife.

M. A. Weeks, SSD

Scheduling Updates

As important as documenting your service is the design of a documentation update system. This is a means of having your own documentation audit system. Remember that you are on the same schedule for updates as all other departments. This is a backup system for your internal departmental needs.

An easy system is a 3x5 card file. Each individual has a 3x5 card with his/her name, date of care plan entry and quarterly progress note date. You may find it helpful to include specific information related to interests, likes, dislikes, care plan problem and need, therapy goals, etc. The box is organized with monthly dividers from January to December.

If an individual has his/her first care plan entry on August 8, 2001, his/her card will be filed behind November. This will be the month that the review is due. Many facilities have due dates set up according to the individual care conference schedule. If this is the case in your facility, you will keep in sync with their calendar.

When the first quarterly update is due, be sure that this review date is the same date as for the care plan review. If both dates are the same, you will always have these two items due on the same day — a good time management technique.

Sample card:

MYRTLE SMITH
8–8–01
Loves music, dislikes large groups. Responds well to pets
Speech therapy for improving communication by pronouncing
words

Chapter 14
Councils

The people we serve have the right to form and run a self-governing council. This council usually takes one of two forms: a Resident Council run for and by the residents of a facility and a Family Council run for and by the family members of residents who live in a facility. The idea is that residents (and their families) should be involved in policy decisions that affect resident life. These councils provide the residents (and their families) with opportunities to participate in decision making through voicing their views and helping resolve issues and concerns.

Resident Council

According to OBRA, every long term care facility is required to have a Resident Council. Other facilities, including adult day programs, assisted living centers and hospitals may also have some type of council. The activity or social services professional is usually the chairperson for the council and is responsible for assuring that this very important meeting occurs each month and that minutes are kept and issues resolved.

What is the Resident Council?

The Resident Council is the political voice of the individuals who use or reside in your facility. Many of the residents are *unable* to voice their opinions and/or concerns and need to rely on residents who are capable and interested in facility events to speak for them.

A president, vice president and secretary/treasurer should be elected from the group. Because the Resident Council is so important, during the annual survey process, the survey team will ask to meet the president and/or vice president of this council. The surveyors will also lead a Resident Council meeting with only residents involved to determine whether there are issues that residents wish to confide in them without staff present.

The regular monthly meeting consists of all interested residents, representatives from the Ombudsman program, any guests that the residents invite and/or request to speak and the chairperson (the staff person responsible for assisting the resident council). The resident council members need to approve any staff member or visitor to these meetings. They can also request to have time alone without any staff present in order to discuss issues confidentially.

Many residents will be hesitant to take on the responsibility and leadership of a council position, as it may be a new and intimidating experience. Because of this, be sure to explain how the meetings work, what the responsibilities are and encourage members to share a position if they are interested. The president is the spokesperson for the council. This resident sits at the head of the group along with the chairperson and other officers. Each council has its own personality. Create the positions to meet the needs of the current group along with the stated responsibilities of the council.

The Resident Council is required to take place *one time per month*. In large facilities, additional meetings may be called as the need occurs. The chairperson keeps the minutes of these meetings. A copy of the minutes always goes to the administrator for review so that s/he is always current on issues, concerns and resolutions.

How Should a Meeting Be Organized?

Each meeting should begin with attendance and recognition of each member. The chairperson usually opens the meeting unless the president wishes to open. Because this is an official meeting, there should be an agenda to follow. An example of an agenda would be:
- Attendance.
- Review of last month's minutes including resolutions to each issue addressed.
- Department heads speak on any issues that may have come up. Residents need to know that when an issue is addressed, the responsible discipline follows through with the concern and speaks to the group in regards to policy, changes and educational information.
- Review of one or more specific resident rights.
- Review of one or more quality of life issues.
- Reminder of the right to review the past year's survey results and where they are located. These should be both available and accessible for review.
- Discussion of activity planning so that the residents have a voice in future events and evaluation of the program.
- Voting issues should always be mentioned so that all members know that they can register to vote, can request assistance with absentee forms and change of address forms. A current list should always be kept of residents who are registered to vote.
- Open forum for any and all residents in the council to voice an opinion and add additional information and recommendations for group projects.

New discussions: every six months or so, review with the resident council all of the concerns/grievances that have arisen during those six months. Are they still concerns or has the facility addressed them to the satisfaction of the residents. If not, keep trying. The surveyors will certainly want to know that there are ongoing attempts to address concerns and it is the facility's responsibility to correct any problems.

As with any group, if complaints and concerns are the only agenda, members will become disinterested in attending. Find worthwhile projects for the council to become involved in. Some examples could be welcome cards and visits to new residents, Employee of the Month award voted by council members, inservice training, invitations to outside speakers, congratulation letters to community groups and individuals recognized for special efforts, recognition projects for staff and other residents in the facility, a council newsletter, inspirational announcements each morning and the list goes on and on.

What if Only a Few Residents Attend the Meetings?

In relationship to the census in a facility, the number of council members is always on the low end. Some very alert and independent individuals may be found in their rooms because they are not interested in attending these meetings. Others may not attend because the effort required is too great. Sometimes it is appropriate to bring the meeting to them. After the official meeting is adjourned, go individually to the rooms of residents so they can review issues and address concerns with you on a one-on-one basis. Keep a record of these council room visits attached to the council minutes. If there are issues addressed, be sure to document these and have the responsible department head write up the resolutions. These should be signed and dated also.

How Do You Document Tough Issues in the Minutes?

As the legally responsible chairperson, your duty is to document the facts and issues verbalized by the council members. There must be an atmosphere of trust and responsibility in these meetings. If a resident requests to remain anonymous, this is his/her right and you must respect this right. If there are individuals who are "chronic complainers" even when the issue has been resolved, discuss the resolution during the meeting and add this to the minutes. This documentation will substantiate both the resolution and the fact that this resident needs to vent each meeting regardless of past resolutions. Be sure that this resident does not have the opportunity to take over the meeting. The chairperson may have to designate a five-minute period near the end of the meeting for this member's voice to be heard.

When documenting tough issues in the minutes, be specific but not narrative. The minutes are not the place to write the story, but to record the information so that the responsible department head can address and help find resolution to the issues and concerns. Ask your administrator for assistance in writing these minutes when the issues get complex.

What Exactly Are the Chairperson's Responsibilities?

The chairperson is responsible for scheduling the monthly meeting, announcing the meeting and posting an invitation to family members, creating the agenda, facilitating the meeting, recording the minutes and typing them up and, most importantly, taking the issues and concerns to the responsible department head for review and resolution. This is not *your* meeting. This is a legal requirement of the facility and you are the designated chairperson.

All grievances and concerns need to be resolved by identified departments. You must get these staff members to write a plan of action, date it and sign it on the council forms. These minutes are kept on file and are always to be made available for surveyor review, corporate review, administrative review and ombudsman review. They are never thrown away as they are legal documents for the facility.

Policy and Procedure — Resident Council

Purpose:

To provide residents with an opportunity to meet and discuss issues that affect their daily lives and quality of life as residents in skilled nursing facilities.

Policy:

It is the policy of this facility to provide a regularly scheduled resident council meeting as required by federal and state regulations.

Procedures:

1. Resident Council meetings will be held at least one time per month.

2. Additional meetings can be scheduled per special request or need.

3. The activity coordinator or social services coordinator will chair the monthly meetings.

4. All residents are invited and encouraged to attend the monthly meetings.

5. The council members can request and recommend specific visitors, guests, staff or speakers to attend the next month's meeting if approved by the members.

6. The council members can request to meet privately without staff or visitors present during each meeting. The chair will add this to the minutes.

7. Attendance records and minutes of the resident council shall be written or compiled by the activity coordinator and secretary of the council.

8. Two resident rights are reviewed, discussed and documented in each month's minutes. The right to vote and the right to review previous survey results should be addressed at each meeting as a reminder.

9. Resident Council members will review the activity program and give input to programs, special events and requests at each meeting.

10. The original copy of the council minutes will be kept on file in the activity office. The original copy should include the plan of action.

11. A copy of meeting minutes will be given to the administrator for review and comment.

12. All issues addressed by the council need to be documented with a plan of action written, signed and dated by the responsible discipline. This plan needs to be written only by the department representative responsible for follow through.

13. The past month's issues will be reviewed with a discussion of resolution as old business at the next meeting.

14. The agenda for each meeting should include the following:
    a. Welcome
    b. Attendance
    c. Review of past month's minutes
    d. Review of past month's resolutions to issues
    e. Review of specific departments such as nursing, dietary, social services, activities, maintenance, therapy and administration
    f. New business and issues
    g. Request for visitors for the next month's meeting

Use of the Resident Council Forms

The Resident Council form on the next page has an area for attendance, old business, review of resident rights, activity review and new issues. The new issues area is very important. Write the issue and then have the responsible discipline write the plan of action. Attach the plan of action to the minutes. Add the title of the plan of action to the new issues section of the minutes and have the person who wrote the plan of action date and sign the appropriate box. You can also use the Department Response to Issues form shown after the one-on-one form. Your signature is on the bottom of the form along with the date. The one-on-one form needs to be completed by the chairperson also. Any issues that come from the one-on-one form should be addressed the same way as issues from the Resident Council meeting.

This form is meant to show you what areas need to be addressed. Depending on your facility, you may need to add more space for different parts of the form. Having the form as a template in your word processing program and typing the information after the heading is probably the most efficient way to use the form.

Resident Council Meeting Minutes

Attendance: _____ _____ _____

_____ _____ _____

_____ _____ _____

_____ _____ _____

_____ _____ _____

_____ _____ _____

_____ _____ _____

_____ _____ _____

Business:

1. **Review of Past Month's Issues/Resolutions:**

_____

_____

_____

_____

2. **Review of Resident Rights: Review at least two specific rights per meeting**

_____

_____

3. **Review of Quality of Life Issues: Review at least two specific quality of life issues per meeting**

_____

_____

_____

_____

_____

4. **Activities: Review of Calendar/Input by Residents:**

_____

_____

_____

_____

5. **New Issues**

Issue	Responsible Department	Plan Completed Signature and Date

Resident Council Chair _____ Date _____

Resident Council Meeting
In-Room Form

Resident Name	Comments/Concerns

_____
Resident Council Chair   Date

Department Response to Issues

Department: _____

Date of Meeting Referring to: _____

Issue(s) Identified by   ☐ Resident Council   ☐ Family Council   ☐ Resident

_____

_____

_____

_____

_____

_____

_____

_____

Department Response

_____

_____

_____

_____

_____

_____

_____

_____

_____

_____

_____

_____

_____

_____

Department Supervisor _____ Date _____

Administrator _____ Date _____

Family Council

Organizationally, the Family Council is wide open and its success is dependent upon the available family population and their energy level and interest. Theoretically, it is a self-governing body, which serves in an advisory capacity to the administration. Underlying its motivations is the support that can only be given and received by people sharing situations in common. Because each council sets its own standards and determines its own needs, each is unique.

Family Council provides a wonderful opportunity for personal support within the group and also forms a ready and willing audience for giving information about the facility, the staff and the long term care system in general. The ideas generated by those most directly affected by facility policies can make a difference in the overall atmosphere. When the group is part of the decision making process (from remodeling to laundry problems), everyone — the people we serve, families and staff — benefits.

The presence of staff should be occasional and limited to 1 to 2 people who have been invited or have a direct purpose for being in attendance (e.g., explanation of a program or policy). The social services professional is the appropriate resource person and his/her presence will be monitored by those in charge of the Family Council.

It can be very difficult to convene an entirely autonomous Family Council. For some, any leadership commitment is an additional drain on an already taxed spirit and some feel the transitory nature of their involvement in the facility. The size of the group doesn't matter. Whether it is five or fifteen members, regard the council as the body that speaks for all of the families. As the members begin to become involved in the facility through the family council, they will be the best advertisement for new members.

Family Councils are not mandatory but facilities must allow such organizations to exist. The support required by the facility is space for meetings, privacy and, by invitation only, staff. The other obligation is to follow-up on grievances and recommendations, which are directly, related to the person we serve and his/her quality of life.

The meeting can be announced by direct mail, e-mail, newsletter and/or posters within the facility. Vary the time, the day and the topics in order to appeal to the schedules and interests of a number of family members. Coming together for a meal will frequently create the informal, relaxed atmosphere desired in the early stages of a Family Council. Speak with your dietary manager, plan a meal or a snack, choose a program (the Ombudsman, Medicare, your rehabilitation program, etc.), announce the meeting and see what happens.

Once convened, families will soon realize what a relief it is to share with others. Long-lasting friendships are often made through these meetings because most find that their concerns, complaints, recommendations and emotional highs and lows are remarkably similar. Proceed from this point of sharing; encourage varying agendas, projects (e.g., a facility garden), a newsletter or legislative activity. Be creative.

Even if no one agrees to take on the leadership roles, you do not need to abandon the Family Council concept. You must simply assume more responsibility yourself, at least temporarily, especially if it appears that there are very interested families and very real concerns. Be mindful always of not imposing on the families' right to privacy.

The Family Council may be one of your most frustrating ventures as a social services professional; not because it isn't worthwhile, but because of the turnover of families and the frequent lack of interest in being in charge. We find that families really enjoy coming together and they like receiving new information. When the time is right and someone feels that s/he would like to do more, step aside. Until then, continue to provide a welcoming environment yourself.

Someone once told us to expect it to take 18 months for a Family Council to get organized. We think that's an underestimate, but keep at it and it will get done.

The form on the next page can be used to record the minutes of a Family Council meeting. You can use the same Department Response to Issues form, shown in the Resident Council section, to record responses to issues raised by the Family Council.

Family Council Meeting

Meeting Date: _____

Attendance: _____ _____ _____

_____ _____ _____

_____ _____ _____

_____ _____ _____

_____ _____ _____

_____ _____ _____

Agenda: _____

_____

_____

_____

Minutes: _____

_____

_____

_____

Action Items:

Concern: _____

Department: _____

Response (including Plan of Correction): _____

_____

Concern: _____

Department: _____

Response (including Plan of Correction): _____

_____

Recommendations:

_____

_____

_____

Chapter 15
Volunteers

"Volunteers" is the first word that you will hear from the administrator after you accept the position of an activity or social services professional. Not only do you need volunteers as part of your departmental team, the people you serve need a variety of personalities and a collection of talents to enhance the quality of their interactions. It is important however to inject a word of caution. Do not begin recruiting volunteers until there is a structure to your program. In terms of priorities, the department needs to be well organized and structured and you need to know both the resident needs and the volunteer needs. If you encourage volunteers without a vision for how the experience will benefit them and the people you serve, it will be disappointing to all involved. And most importantly, the volunteer will not stay long.

Both federal and state regulations identify the need for volunteers and address this as a function of the Activity Department. Social services also has a need for volunteers working more on a one-on-one basis. LITA, which is a good example of a one-on-one volunteer program, is discussed at the end of this chapter.

Activity Department Volunteers

There are many excellent resources on designing and developing a volunteer program. Contact the local volunteer center in your community and request brochures and job descriptions. Arrange to go to training sessions that they offer. Go to facilities and organizations that have a strong and successful program in place. Although the settings and needs are different, the basic development of a volunteer program is similar.

Priority steps in developing a volunteer program:
- Identify what needs the department has for volunteers.
- Write volunteer policies and procedures.
- Design a job description with specific responsibilities, qualifications and time needed.
- Have a choice of possible work and responsibilities for volunteers to choose from.
- Identify volunteer skills, talents and strengths for the growth of both volunteer and program.
- Create forms for applications, orientation to facility, work, attendance records and evaluation.
- Recruit and select volunteers. This process should be as structured as it was for you to be interviewed and selected.
- Train and orient all volunteers well. The more information that a volunteer has, the better able s/he is to meet the demands of the work, the people you serve and the setting.

- Supervise. By working with a volunteer on site you continue his/her training and assure follow through with the responsibilities of the work.
- Evaluate. It's easiest to evaluate volunteers according to the duties and outline of the specific work. Everyone needs feedback on how s/he is doing and this is one of your responsibilities as the volunteer coordinator. Evaluation should be on a regularly scheduled basis.
- Recognize. Individuals who volunteer are doing so for personal reasons. There is a personal goal that they have identified as being important in their lives. For most it is the opportunity to help others in need or to build work skills that can be transferred to employment. There are other volunteers who are completing hours either for school or to work off minor violations through a community service program. These volunteers also need feedback and recognition for their work. The ways to recognize volunteers are many. What are more important than "prizes," are recognition and individual honors. Volunteers need to know that they are making a difference to the organization and lives of the people you serve. Having the people you serve involved in this recognition is very meaningful.

If you have ever volunteered, you know how important it is to manage this time into your already busy schedule. Be clear on how much time is needed per day or week or month. If a volunteer feels that there is not enough organization or direction, s/he will seek out another agency that is better prepared.

Another important area to consider is how you identify needs to determine what volunteer jobs should be created. Think beyond the needs of group activity and individual visits. These both are very important and demand assistance from volunteers. However, there are many other ways that individuals and groups can be involved. Some ideas are

- writing and typing the newsletter,
- decorating the facility,
- shopping,
- letter writing,
- sewing and mending,
- caring for facility pets,
- sharing talents in performances,
- creating visual aids and cards for residents who are sensory impaired,
- making the new month's calendar of activities,
- monitoring residents who are confused and disoriented in structured parallel sensory activities,
- filing and organizing the office,
- reaching out to the community with presentations and flyers,
- developing an intergenerational exchange program with a local school or agency, and
- having a business or agency adopt your facility one time monthly.

The list is endless so the best way to begin is with a wish list. Volunteers help create a quality activity program! It takes work to recruit and supervise a good set of volunteers, but all staff, residents and families feel the benefits.

> "Sometimes our light goes out, but is blown again into flame by an encounter with another human being. Each of us owes the deepest thanks to those who have rekindled this inner light." — Albert Schweitzer

Social Services Volunteers

The social services volunteer differs significantly in function from the volunteer in the activity program mainly because emphasis is on one-on-one contact as opposed to group involvement. This means that a volunteer who wishes to interact directly with an individual must maintain contact with the social services professional to stay abreast of changes in the emotional or physical status of the individual s/he visits.

In our experience, however, it can be difficult to recruit and train the true social services volunteer — the person who is not threatened or intimidated by the ongoing contact with one person at a potentially intimate emotional level. There is a high turnover rate with one-on-one volunteers as they begin to feel that they are not qualified or are not prepared to interact with an individual so intensely. Often a volunteer will come to the facility with some time to share but with no idea of how emotional this experience can be. Also, some volunteers begin to relate too personally in this setting because they themselves are elderly or have an aging relative. These factors also contribute to the high turnover rate among volunteers.

When we are fortunate enough to find individuals who are willing and able to take on the role of social services volunteers, they act as a direct adjunct to the social services program and extend the contact that the social services professional is able to have with the person.

The social services volunteer may be a Friendly Visitor (some begin in this rather casual role and stay for years), a support to someone in the adjustment crisis, a source of support for someone in the terminal state or one of several variations on these themes. The key to success in terms of individual needs is a solid mix of warmth, compassion, consistency and a true interest.

The social services professional has the responsibility of providing ongoing support for the volunteer, beginning with a well-rounded orientation to the facility and a definition of role expectations. An introduction to Resident Rights, especially confidentiality, is essential. After that, a weekly check-in is vital. The volunteer can offer "untrained" insights and ask questions which will assist in a better overall psychosocial plan for the individual; the social services professional can share information from a professional perspective and elicit feelings and concerns from the volunteer.

Your support may be what makes the difference in keeping a volunteer in your facility — for the benefit of all concerned.

One to One Volunteer Friendship Programs

A Volunteer Program That Every Facility Needs

One of the most important gifts that you can give to an individual is the gift of ageless friendship. A volunteer not only adds to the services provided by activity and social services departments, s/he also adds to the quality of life of the individual. The losses associated with being in a care setting are profound, and depression is prevalent in every setting. One way to lessen the loneliness is to bring in volunteers of all ages to visit on a one-on-one basis and match them with an individual who has no family or visitors close by.

Such a volunteer program has existed in California under the name of **LITA**, *Love is the Answer* for the past twenty-five years. The mission statement of this non-profit organization is to lessen loneliness in long term care settings by providing one-on-one friends for isolated residents. The concept is a simple one, to be a friend. The commitment for the volunteer is a weekly visit of at least 15–30 minutes with the matched resident friend. Matches are made with only one resident at a time as developing relationships takes time and attention.

LITA has recently joined with other volunteer friendship agencies and programs to establish a network for volunteer friendship programs. The goal of this new organization is to strengthen existing volunteer friendship programs in the San Francisco Bay Area in order to reach more isolated elders and help them maintain vital connections to their communities. Another goal is to encourage the formation of new programs that will work together to keep pace with the burgeoning number of elderly people.

We encourage you to look within your geographic area and identify agencies and programs that offer volunteer services to the elderly. This may be a volunteer organization, church affiliated program, or a service provided through your community's area agency on aging. Find ways in which to link onto an already existing program if possible. Also, contact other skilled nursing facilities and assisted living settings to see if they would be interested in organizing a program similar to LITA. It makes such as difference.

For more information, or to share your successful friendship stories, call 415-453-6130.

Volunteer Resources:

Activity Policy and Procedure Manual, Recreation Therapy Consultants, 6115 Syracuse Lane, San Diego, CA 92122. (858) 546-9003. (This publication has excellent forms for volunteer programs.)

Elements of a Successful Volunteer Program. Nancy E. Hughes, 210 Sylvia Way, San Rafael, CA 94903. (415) 479-9316.

Job Descriptions for Volunteers. Jacquelyn L. Vaughan. Available from idyll Arbor, PO Box 720, Ravensdale, WA 98051.

101 Ideas for Volunteer Programs, Steve McCurley and Sue Vineyard. Heritage Arts/VN Systems, 1807 Prairie Avenue, Downers Grove, IL 60515.

Volunteer Blueprint for Success! Kennie Benner. Available from Idyll Arbor, PO Box 720, Ravensdale, WA 98051.

Chapter 16
Quality Assurance, Infection Control and Risk Management

This chapter covers three important aspects of working in any health care setting: quality assurance, infection control and risk management. *Quality assurance* looks at the ability to provide the highest quality services and treatment, *infection control* is concerned with the ability to eliminate the spread of infection from one individual to another and *risk management* discusses the ongoing process of making the environment safer.

Providing the individual with quality services — meeting his/her needs — does not happen by accident. It takes knowledge, thoughtfulness and some old fashioned self-evaluation to do good work. And, it does not matter how good your services are or how successful your treatment is if you cannot guarantee the person you serve a basic level of safety while s/he is in your facility. Each individual has the absolute right to be free from bodily harm or psychological damage while receiving care. It is up to each staff person to act in a manner that ensures that each of the people we serve is safe. A solid quality assurance program, knowledge of the basic principles of infection control and a solid understanding of risk management are required to ensure a good program. These issues are discussed in this chapter.

Quality Assurance

Quality assurance is a process of continually self-evaluating the services you provide and then improving the service based on problems you have identified and corrected. In order to continually evaluate your department, you must have a Quality Assurance Program in place.

Quality Assurance is not a new term but is much more frequently used in nursing homes now that OBRA regulations (Tags F520 and F521) have mandated that each nursing facility have a quality assurance program. Almost every type of facility will have some kind of quality assurance program. A quality assurance program must include policies and procedures for quality assurance and a committee that meets at least quarterly to review current studies and issues.

A long term care facility must maintain an ongoing assessment of the quality of services provided and have a quality assurance committee to monitor the overall effectiveness of the facility's quality assurance program. The quality assurance committee consists of:

1.   the director of nursing services,
2.   a physician designated by the facility and
3.   at least three other members of the facility staff.

The quality assurance committee must meet at least quarterly to identify areas that could and should be improved and to develop and implement appropriate plans to correct identified quality deficiencies.

What is Quality Assurance?

Quality assurance (QA) is the process of internally monitoring your own work. It is an on-going program that looks at the quality of the services provided as well as the cost effectiveness of those services. It is not enough to find out at survey time that there are problems. We should always know, during the entire year, what are our weak areas. And we should always be working on improving our services by taking a systematic approach to problem solving. Just as we have written out care plans identifying ways to meet resident needs (with measurable objectives), we have a written out quality assurance program which identifies ways to meet our quality improvement needs.

How Can a Facility Assure that the QA Process Will Be Successful?

The best way to begin the process is by educating all staff on the importance of monitoring their performance. Stress that they are not only a part of the process but also accountable for the end results.

Quality assurance has been a part of the long term care setting for many years but it became all the more important when OBRA added it to the regulations. The Final Rule (OBRA 1995) included quality assurance as a part of the survey process and plan of corrections guidelines.

How Do I Start a Quality Assurance Program or Study?

Your facility already has a quality assurance program, policy and procedure manual and quality assurance committee. If you are not a member of the committee, ask to sit in on these meetings to better understand the process. Each professional should be a strong element of this committee because of his/her involvement in the area of *Quality of Life*, *Resident Behavior and Practices* and *Quality of Care.*

The quality assurance process is, by definition, an interdisciplinary process. When the committee has identified an area needing attention, all departments will work to solve the problem. But in addition to working on identified problems, each department should be on the lookout for potential problems and issues specific to its service.

What Type of Studies Would Activity or Social Services Departments Address?

There are many areas to study. Some of these might include:
•   Does the current program meet the needs of the current population?
•   Are some individuals having difficulty getting to activity groups of interest? If the individual is not getting to the activity, this is an issue to address in QA.
•   Is the role of activity or social services professionals in the behavior management programs to decrease the use of psychoactive medications clearly defined?
•   Is the role of activity or social services professionals in the physical restraint reduction programs for use in groups or one-on-one activities clearly defined?
•   Are the people we serve satisfied with their rooms, food, opportunities, interactions with staff or any other quality of life issues?

- Is the space where activities are held large enough? Is the lighting at the proper level for individuals who have visual impairments?
- Are all levels of cognitive and functional needs being met in group or individual settings?
- According to the percentage of men or younger residents in the facility, are there appropriate and available leisure activities for their interests?

There are specific steps involved in the design of a quality assurance study. The chart on the following page shows the five steps you need to take for a successful quality assurance program. For more information about quality assurance programs see Cunninghis and Best Martini's book, *Quality Assurance for Activity Programs, Second Edition* (1996) from Idyll Arbor, Inc.

The following forms can be used as quality assurance review forms for survey preparedness. The first two forms (one for activities and one for social services) provide a review of what you should be doing that will help you prepare for survey. The next two department checklist forms can be used to review your activities. They can be used as time management tools and for orienting new employees to their duties. The last form can be used to make sure that you meet all of the requirements for admitting a new individual.

Steps of Quality Assurance Programs[57]

Step 1	*Identifying Issues and Selecting Study Topics*	Obviously it is essential to begin with a determination of what service needs to be improved to provide quality service. This first step has you look closely at the problem to specifically identify what is not right. Unfortunately, many quality assurance programs concern themselves with issues that are not important or with procedural items that can be easily remedied, rather than those that justify being part of long-range planning.
Step 2a	*Establishing Indicators*	Identifying elements that can be monitored to measure changes made. The elements or characteristics of the service you select to measure should be a general statement about what the service would look like if there were not a problem.
Step 2b	*Developing Criteria*	Developing criteria for each indicator. Writing a plan that spells out exactly what should be found and ideally in what quantity and in what time frame.
Step 3a	*Determining Methodology*	Establishing the exact method to be used to collect information: from which sources, by whom, how often, how long and how the results are going to be used.
Step 3b	*Collecting Data*	Implementing the chosen methods of data collection.
Step 4a	*Understanding the Problem*	Reviewing and assessing collected data to see what, where and how serious the problems are. Deciding which problem areas should be the focus of further study.
Step 4b	*Setting Standards*	Standards are set to describe the desired outcomes in a measurable way.
Step 4c	*Finding Solutions*	Searching for possible ways to reach the standards set.
Step 4d	*Writing an Action Plan*	The methodology for implementing a change is determined along with decisions about who is to have the responsibility and what the time frames will be.
Step 4e	*Implementing the Plan*	Putting into action the strategies that have been developed.
Step 5a	*Assessing the Outcomes*	Did the plan work? Do the problems still remain? Has there been some improvement? This procedure often entails a repeat of steps 3 and 4: going back and re-collecting the data and then analyzing the results to see if the standards have been reached.
Step 5b	*Identifying New Issues or Continuing to Work on the Old*	If the problems are not solved, new strategies must be planned. If, however, the process has been successful, a new plan should be developed for the next area of focus. As stated earlier, quality assurance is an ongoing process and does not stop once a particular problem is corrected. It is also necessary to periodically go back and monitor earlier plans and see if the goals are continuing to be met. Two or three past issues may be chosen at random for an on-going audit in addition to the main topic of study. These could be changed periodically on a rotating basis to assure that new problems have not arisen in any of these areas.

---

[57] Cunninghis, R. N. and E. Best Martini, 1996, *Quality Assurance for Activity Programs, Second Edition*, pp. 18-19, Idyll Arbor, Inc., Ravensdale, WA.

Quality Assurance Checklist for Activities

Reviewed by: _____ Date: _____

Review this list to determine the level of compliance for your department.

Staff: **Yes/No**
1. proof of training/qualifications .... _____
2. consultation reports & qualifications .... _____
3. job descriptions .... _____
4. weekend coverage .... _____
5. evening coverage .... _____
6. professional involvement .... _____
7. inservice training .... _____

Documentation:
1. initial activity assessment form .... _____
2. MDS form, activity portion (LTC) .... _____
3. input to RAP summary sheet (LTC) .... _____
4. care plan entry .... _____
5. 30-day re-evaluation .... _____
6. daily attendance (7 days per week) .... _____
   Did you include level of participation and refusals? .... _____
7. bedside log .... _____
   Did you include type, frequency and response to visit? .... _____
8. individual included in assessment and care plan process .... _____
9. quarterly activity progress note .... _____
   Did it end with a goal? .... _____
   Is this the same as on the care plan? .... _____
10. change of condition note .... _____
11. physician's orders for activities, outings, and work related activities .... _____

Physical Environment
1. large calendar posted and legible to visually impaired .... _____
2. individual calendars in each room .... _____

Program Evaluation
1. Activity Analysis Form completed for all activities offered ..... _____
2. Activity Program Review completed .... _____
3. programs offered that meet the diversity of resident needs and abilities .... _____

Resident Rights
1. Resident Council minutes .... _____
   proof of resolution to issues .... _____
   posted invitation to monthly meetings. .... _____
2. review of resident rights .... _____
3. review of last survey results .... _____
4. accessibility of survey results to interested residents .... _____
5. opportunity to register to vote .... _____

Quality Assurance Checklist for Social Services

Reviewed by: _____ Date: _____

Review this list to determine the level of compliance for your department.

Staff: Yes/No
1. proof of qualifications ...._____
2. job description ...._____
3. consultant reports & qualifications..._____
4. professional improvement ...._____
5. inservice training ...._____

Documentation
1. social history..._____
2. initial psychosocial assessment ...._____
3. initial discharge plan..._____
4. MDS form, psychosocial aspects (LTC)..._____
5. RAP summary sheet input (LTC) ...._____
6. care plan entry ...._____
7. quarterly social services progress note.._____
8. annual social services progress note.._____
9. annual discharge plan update.._____
10. MDS update (change of condition) (LTC) ...._____
11. care conference attendance sign in ...._____
12. durable power of attorney for health care, living will directive to physicians
    and/or conservator papers..._____
13. advance directives signed (such as no CPR) ...._____
14. surrogate decision maker listed ...._____
15. room change notification; introductions made ...._____

Optional Recommendations:
1. community resource file..._____
2. family council minutes ...._____
3. theft and loss log..._____
4. social services groups..._____
5. social services newsletter ...._____
6. social services log..._____
7. social services volunteers ...._____
8. grievance log ...._____
9. log for marked dentures, glasses, and hearing aids ...._____
10. client follow up after discharge ...._____
Notes:

Activity Department Checklist

Activity Professional _____ Starting Date _____

Daily — Areas To Be Completed	Mon	Tue	Wed	Thu	Fri	Sat	Sun
Attendance							
MDS — RAP Summary							
Initial Interviews & Assessments Completed							
Schedule Changes & Revisions							
Quarterly Progress Notes							
Volunteer Sign-in & Supervision							
Room Visits/Bedside Log							
Office/Department Readied for Next Day							
Other							
Weekly							√
Shopping & Inventory							
Community Contacts							
Care Conference							
Completion of Special Planning							
Interdepartmental Meetings							
Calendars/Decorations/Newsletter							
Department Head Meetings							
Monthly							√
In-service Training							
Resident Council Minutes							

Notes:

Social Services Department Checklist

Starting Date _____

Social Services Professional _____

Daily — Areas to be completed	Mon	Tue	Wed	Thu	Fri	Sat	Sun
Department Head Meetings							
Complete Assessments on New Admission							
Complete Multidisciplinary Discharge Summary							
Paperwork Related to Room Changes							
Introduce Residents to New Roommates							
Fix Up Room Changes with Visit about Move							
Chart Room Changes and Adjustments							
Document Significant Behavior Changes							
Document Significant Changes in Condition							
Record Lost Dentures, Glasses and Hearing Aids							
Clothing and Personal Care Needs							
Transportation Needs							
Family and Resident Counseling							
Deaths							
Other							

Weekly	√
Quarterly, Annual Progress Note Updates (Including MDS)	
Attend Resident Care Conferences	
Attend Rehabilitation Meetings	
Organize Rehabilitation Meetings with Resident and Family	
New Resident Adjustment Issues	
In-Service Training	
Staff Meetings	

Monthly	√
Send Out Notices for Next Month's Resident Care Conferences	

Notes:

New Admissions Checklist — LTC

Name of Resident _____

Date of Admission _____

Date Assessments to be Completed _____

Date MDS to be Completed _____

Social Services Professional _____

Activity Professional_____

Therapists _____

Item	Act	SS	RT
Social history			
Capacity statement completed by physician and in chart			
Psychosocial assessment, activity assessment			
Discharge plan			
MDS and RAPs			
Care plan entry			
Letter inviting new person or responsible person to care conference			
Review care plan with the individual and/or responsible person if not in attendance at care conference			
Add individual's name to voting status form, birthday list, alcohol list, outing list			
Mark glasses, dentures and hearing aid(s)			
Weekly charting by social services for the first two months			

Notes:

Quality Indicators

The Quality Indicators (QIs) are a MDS based quality monitoring system for evaluating care in nursing homes. They are used to focus quality monitoring and quality improvement activities by Federal and State regulatory agencies.

The QIs are flags to draw attention to potential problem areas that need further review and investigation. QIs can help facilities identify areas or systems in the facility that may be improved and can be used with the facility's Quality Assurance program. A QI report can be downloaded from the MDS submission site and should be reviewed at least quarterly, if not more frequently, to identify potential problem areas in the facility. The QI reports are also available to state and federal survey agencies. They are used to focus onsite surveys to potential problem areas and also to monitor for quality of care issues between surveys.

At present, the monitoring system has 24 quality indicators organized into eleven care domains. It is expected that this system will continued to be revised to more accurately identify potential problem areas. The domains are: 1. Accidents, 2. Behavioral/Emotional Patterns, 3. Clinical Management, 4. Cognitive Patterns, 5. Elimination/Incontinence, 6. Infection Control, 7. Nutrition/Eating, 8. Physical Functioning, 9. Psychotropic Drug Use, 10. Quality of Life, and 11. Skin Care. The domains that are of particular interest to the activities and social services professional are: Behavioral/Emotional Patterns, Cognitive Patterns, Psychotropic Drug Use, and Quality of Life. Table 16.1 defines the quality indicators for these domains.

Prevalence of the indicators listed on the table in an individual facility will be compared to prevalence in facilities in the state, the region, and the nation. Because the indicators point to potential problem areas, a facility with a higher than average prevalence may be subject to a focused review by Federal or State regulatory agencies. A high prevalence of quality indicators does not necessarily mean that there is a problem in the facility. It does mean that facilities should be prepared with documentation of investigation to determine whether the prevalence of the QI is really identifying a quality of care problem.

If a resident's most recent MDS reflects any of the indicators listed above, documentation in the social services or activities progress notes should address the significance of the indicator and reflect the interventions taken to manage the problem, if needed. For example: if a resident has used a hypnotic for more than two days of the week, the cause of the resident's sleeplessness should be assessed and corrective interventions should be documented. This could include both social services and activities interventions such as the teaching of relaxation techniques, a change of room, or an increase in physical activity. The care plan must be updated to reflect the problem and the corrective interventions. An example of the Quality Indicators that activities, therapy, or social services can impact is shown on the next page.

Quality Indicators Impacting Activities, Therapy, and Social Services

Domain	Description / Definition	MDS Component
II: Behavioral/Emotional		
3. Prevalence of behavioral symptoms affecting others	Residents with behavioral symptoms affecting others on most recent assessment	Behavioral symptoms: E4b,c,d = > 0 verbally or physically abusive, socially inappropriate behavior
4. Prevalence of depression	Residents with symptoms of depression on most recent assessment	Sad mood: E2 = 1,2 AND 2 or more symptoms of functional depression: Symptom 1 - E1a = 1,2 Symptom 2 - E1n = 1,2 E4e = 1-3 E1o = 1,2 E1p = 1,2 Symptom 3 - E1j = 1,2 N1d = checked or awake 1 period and not comatose Symptom 4 - E1g = 1,2 Symptom 5 - K3a = 1 OR I1ee or I1ff is checked and E2=1,2 OR I1ee or I1ff is checked AND at least 1 symptom of functional depression
5. Prevalence of depression without antidepressant therapy	Residents with symptoms of depression and no antidepressant therapy	Depression AND O4c = 0 AND No psychotherapy (P1b&e)
IV. Cognitive Patterns		
7. Incidence of cognitive impairment	Residents who were newly cognitively impaired on most recent assessment vs. residents who were not cognitively impaired on previous assessment	Cognitive impairment: B4 = 1,2 and B2a = 1 Severe cognitive impairment: B4 = 3 and B2a = 1
IX. Psychotropic drug use		
21,23 Prevalence of antipsychotic and antianxiety/hypnotic use	Residents who used antipsychotics, antianxiety or hypnotics on most recent assessment	O4a,b,d = > 0
24 Prevalence of hypnotic use more than two times in last week	Residents who received hypnotics more than 2 times in last week on most recent assessment	O4d = > 2
X. Quality of Life		
27. Prevalence of little or no activity	Residents with little or no activity on most recent assessment	N2 = 2,3 (Excludes comatose residents)

Infection Control

The spread of infection requires three elements: 1. a source of infectious material, 2. a resident who is susceptible to the infectious material and 3. a means of transmitting that infectious material to the susceptible resident. Just by the nature of health care facilities it is not possible to exclude infectious material (people come in sick), nor is it possible to exclude individuals who might be susceptible to infection. The only way to truly control the spread of infection in facilities is to control the transmission.

There are four main routes of spreading infections:

1. Contact transmission
   a. Direct contact (staff to resident or resident to resident)
   b. Indirect contact (germs transmitted by touching an object, e.g. a tape recorder passed from one resident to another)
   c. Droplet contact (transmission of germs from a person sneezing, coughing or talking within a distance of three feet)
2. Vehicle Route Transmission Through Contaminated Items (food, water, drugs, blood)
3. Airborne Transmission (infectious materials which adhere to moisture or dust in the air and are suspended for long periods of time)
4. Vectorborne Transmission (infection spread through an insect or animal as in mosquito-transmitted malaria)

Handwashing is the best way to control the spread of infections. Staff will need to wash their hands after coming into physical contact with any resident, using the restroom or coming into contact with activity supplies which may have contaminated surfaces. It would not be unusual for activity professionals to wash their hands over 30 times a day — activity assistants even more.

Using good handwashing technique is important. First, get the hands wet. Place soap in the hands and lather up the soap. Once the soap is lathered, scrub all parts of the hands while slowly counting to ten. The hands should be rinsed under running water while continually rubbing the hands, again counting to ten slowly. Dry the hand using disposable towels or air-dry them. Turn off the water using the paper towels, not the newly cleaned hands, to turn the handles.

Many of the supplies used by activity professionals are considered to be "reusable equipment" versus "disposable equipment." Nursing and other health care professionals have turned to using disposable equipment to help significantly reduce the spread of microorganisms but this would prove too costly for activity departments. It is therefore important that the activity professional learn the basics of good disinfecting techniques.

When cleaning items that can tolerate getting wet, use the following technique:
- The staff or volunteer doing the cleaning should wear waterproof gloves while cleaning all items.
- When using equipment that has moving parts or comes apart to be cleaned and has body secretions on it, take apart the item immediately after it is used. This allows cleaning to take place later without the pieces becoming stuck together after the secretions dry.
- When rinsing the item to be washed, always use cold water first. Body secretions are more likely to coagulate (to thicken and become glue-like) when placed in hot water versus cold water.
- Soap and sudsy water work well for loosening up dirt. Let items soak if possible.
- When doing the actual cleaning, use water as hot as your hands will tolerate. Hot water and soap help break the dirt into tiny particles, making them easier to rinse off.
- Use a cloth or sponge if you need to clean using friction (scrubbing). This friction, combined with hot water and soap, breaks down the dirt and microorganisms into even smaller pieces, allowing for easy rinsing.

- Use a stiff bristled brush to remove dirt and microorganisms from grooves in the equipment, being careful not to allow any of the dirt to fly up into your face. Wear a face shield or a mask and goggles for extra precautions.
- Use abrasive cleaners to remove stains that soaking doesn't remove. Use alcohol or ether to remove oily stains that don't come out with just soap and water. Remember to rinse items cleaned this way thoroughly.
- Rinse all items under hot, running water to detach any remaining dirt and microorganisms.
- Thoroughly dry all supplies prior to putting them away.
- Clean all of your cleaning supplies and then wash your hands, even though you wore gloves.

For items that cannot be washed using water and soap, follow your agency's disinfecting or sterilization techniques. When using disposable equipment, dispose of the equipment immediately after use to reduce the chance of further contamination of other equipment.

Risk Management

Risk management is the act of identifying situations in the workplace that may harm the person we serve, the staff or the facility. Most facilities will have many policies and procedures related to making the workplace safe. This section will talk about how the staff controls for risks.

Controlling risk is like placing a safety net under the person we serve. It requires around-the-clock management by each staff person — on duty as well as off duty. Krames Communications, in the booklet "Risk Management: Your Role in Providing Quality Care" (1989) lists the eight areas of around-the-clock management. Specific questions for the professionals have been added to Krames Communications' categories.

Around-the-Clock Risk Management

On the Job

Safe Environment
- Are the activity supplies appropriate for the individual's abilities?
- Are all the fire exits unblocked?
- Is the water temperature below 110°F?

Ongoing Monitoring
- Do individual assessments represent the individual's actual abilities and needs?
- Are staff diligent in changing the individual's care plan as the individual's abilities change?
- Are staff continuing to be careful about individual safety and infection control?

Off the Job

Continuing Education
- Have you kept your knowledge and skills up-to-date by continually seeking out new information?
- Are you seeking continuing education in the areas where you have the weakest knowledge and skill, not just the areas that are convenient or interesting to you?

Journals
- Do you regularly (e.g., at least monthly) spend an hour or more reading up on new information and developments in your professional journals?
- Do you support the body of knowledge by writing up important information or developments and submitting them for publication?

Clear Communication

- Do staff communicate important information to each other concerning an individual's status and workplace concerns?
- Do staff communicate with the people we serve and their families in a timely and appropriate manner?

Handling Incidents

- Do all staff know the facility's policies and procedures well enough to implement them all of the time?
- Have staff had the proper training to be able to carry out the administration's intent for handling the different types of incidents?

Professional Groups

- Are you an active member in at least one national and state/local organization?
- Do you find time to discuss issues with other professionals outside of your facility, especially if you are a one-person department?

Healthy Lifestyle

- Are you responsible enough to make sure that you get enough sleep prior to going to work to reduce the chance of mistakes being made?
- Do you eat food that is good for your physical health and exercise on a regular basis to be able to perform your job well?
- Do you balance your work life with your play life to be able to be refreshed?

How do you ensure that each individual is safe while s/he is in your environment and receiving your services? One of the most successful ways of ensuring that the individual is receiving quality care and services is to make sure that your department is adhering to professional standards of practice. Standards of practice usually outline minimum standards for management of the service, minimum standards for delivery of the service and minimum qualifications for staff. (You will find the Standards of Practice for the National Association of Activity Professionals in Appendix C.) However, even when you seem to be following standards of practice completely, you may still run into problems. Risk management and quality assurance are similar — only on different ends of the continuum. Quality assurance is the process of improving good services to make them better. Risk management is the process of reducing or eliminating harmful or dangerous situations.

The ability to identify and control harmful or dangerous situations in the environment and in the delivery of service is called Risk Management. Risk Management has six steps:
1. To recognize that there is a problem.
2. To be able to identify what in the system is causing the problem.
3. To be able to identify who is impacted by the problem.
4. To be able to identify if the problem is changeable (or if other systems need to be changed to accommodate for what cannot be changed — a long term care facility cannot decide to exclude all individuals who are HIV positive — they need to change their systems of infection control to accommodate those individuals).
5. To develop a method of correcting the problem.
6. To develop a means to measure if the problem was corrected.

joan burlingame, CTRS, ABDA, studied the worst breakdowns in resident safety in her 1992 study of Immediate Jeopardy citations. She was able to identify ten basic principles of reducing risks to resident safety. By being aware of these risks, the activity professional can help manage harmful or dangerous situations within his/her own facility. These basic principles are:
1. Water temperature at the taps should never be over 110 degrees Fahrenheit.
2. Fire doors and fire routes must always be free of clutter. Fire safety standards must always be followed.
3. Floors should be free of objects that may cause the individual to slip or to trip.
4. Walkways (including hallways) must be free of protruding objects — many individuals have poor vision and may walk into a protruding object and injure themselves. (Protruding objects may stick out only 4 inches from the wall between the height of 27" to 80" from the floor.

Exceptions are made for drinking fountains or telephones that are mounted on posts. They may stick out 12 inches.)

5. The building must be maintained in a manner that ensures it is always structurally safe.
6. Staff must always talk to and treat each individual respectfully.
7. Only life threatening events should get in the way of any staff helping an individual resident move/turn who is at risk for pressure sores and is in need of movement/turning.
8. Staff should always practice good infection control principles.
9. Staff should always ensure the physical safety of each individual — including protecting him/her from self-inflected injuries.
10. Food and fluid should always be treated as if they were a prescription item — never given to an individual unless in a manner which follows the medical orders.

The most important thing for staff to remember is — if something doesn't seem right, it probably isn't. Even if your supervisor assures you that the way a resident is being treated is all right because the treatment team agreed to the treatment, if you feel that it may be abusive or neglectful treatment, *act!* Approach your facility administrator. If that doesn't work, each state has a law that says a staff person must report a potential case of abuse or neglect (usually in 24 hours or less). It is not up to that staff person to obtain proof that the treatment is abusive or neglectful. If the staff person suspects abuse or neglect, s/he is to leave it up to the state investigators. When you call, you do not need to give your name. Remember, you may be the best advocate that the resident has!

Immediate Jeopardy[58]

When a survey is conducted, the surveyors determine whether or not a facility meets the Conditions of Participation (the federal regulations) for receiving Medicare and Medicaid funding by assessing whether the facility meets all of the requirements in the federal regulations. Usually, a deficiency means that the provider must submit a plan of correction to be acted upon within 30 days.

However, sometimes the surveyors discover situations that are so severe that stronger sanctions are required. In these cases, the guidelines for determining "immediate jeopardy" (also known as "fast track") are applied. The provider must correct a condition of "immediate jeopardy" immediately or "immediate termination action" will be taken; i.e., the residents will be removed and the facility closed.

To assist surveyors in determining when circumstances pose an "immediate jeopardy" to an individual's health and safety, a set of criteria has been developed. This guide is intended to provide greater consistency among surveyors when reviewing specific situations and assessing provider failures.

The standards for the funding for health care services (and therefore, the standards of health care practice) in the United States depends heavily on the actions of the Congress of the United States. For administration purposes, health care is divided into two separate entities, the Centers for Medicare and Medicaid Services and the Public Health Service. Almost every activity or social services professional who works in a clinical setting is under the auspices of the Centers for Medicare and Medicaid Services or CMS. (In 1991 CMS was responsible for oversight on 54,586 facilities.)

Specific minimum standards are set for each type of facility, e.g., hospitals, home health care, long term care (nursing homes), etc. All changes and new health care laws are released on October 1st

---

[58] This section is by joan burlingame, CTRS. Used with permission.

of each year in the government publication called the **Code of Federal Regulations** or **CFR**. While most regulations are facility-type specific, there are two federal health care regulations that apply to all health care under the jurisdiction of CMS. The first regulation is the Civil Rights Act (Title Six). The second regulation, the most stringent, is called *Immediate Jeopardy*, also known as Appendix "Q". (Prior to October 1, 1992 it was called "Immediate and Serious Threat.")

With just a few exceptions, every facility that is surveyed by either the Joint Commission or by CARF: the Rehabilitation Accreditation Commission fall under the jurisdiction of CMS. The loss of CMS certification is actually more severe than the loss of accreditation by either the Joint Commission or by CARF. A facility may maintain its business license without Joint Commission or CARF Accreditation. Without CMS certification, it is not likely that a facility can maintain its business license. In such a case, it often requires legislation on the state level to maintain the facility.

Definitions from Appendix Q and Appendix J

Immediate and Serious Threat An immediate and serious threat is defined as having a high probability that serious harm or injury to residents could occur at any time or already has occurred and may well occur again if residents are not protected effectively from the harm or the threat is not removed.

Patients Includes all persons receiving treatment, care or services from the provider.

Physical Abuse Refers to any physical motion or action (e.g., hitting, slapping, punching, kicking, pinching, etc.) by which bodily harm or trauma occurs. It includes use of corporal punishment as well as the use of any restrictive, intrusive procedure to control inappropriate behavior for purpose of punishment.

Provider/Facility Means all Medicare providers and suppliers and Medicaid only facilities (intermediate care facilities for the mentally retarded — ICF-MR).

Psychological Abuse Includes, but is not limited to, humiliation, harassment and threats of punishment or deprivation, sexual coercion, intimidation, whereby individuals suffer psychological harm or trauma.

Verbal Abuse Refers to any use of oral, written or gestured language by which abuse occurs. This includes pejorative and derogatory terms to describe persons with disabilities.

Guiding Principles (taken directly from Appendix Q)

1. An immediate and serious threat need not result in **actual** harm to the resident. The threat of probable harm is perceived as being as serious or significant.
2. The threat could be perceived as something which will result in potentially severe temporary or permanent injury, disability or death and must be perceived as something which is likely to occur in the very near future.
3. Mental abuse can be as damaging as physical abuse and may constitute an immediate and serious threat.
4. Only one resident needs to be jeopardized; the entire or large percentage of resident population **does not have** to be threatened or injured.
5. The absence of adequate staff training does not, in and of itself, pose the threat. However, if the staff lacks the skill or knowledge necessary to properly care for the residents, this may present the same serious problems as when there are insufficient numbers of staff and will make it more difficult for the provider to correct or eliminate the problems.
6. The situation is severe enough that it outweighs potential concerns of resident transfer to another facility.

7. The situation may or may not be a threat considering such factors as season of the year and geographic location.
8. The deficiency cannot be corrected quickly to prevent a resident from being severely harmed.
9. Immediate and serious threat termination is the only response to the problem.

Immediate Jeopardy may be "called" without having to close a facility. By citing Immediate Jeopardy the survey team is stating that there exists an unacceptable threat to a resident, which must be corrected within hours or days, or else termination action will begin. Termination action usually does not officially occur (with public notification) until the fifth day after Immediate Jeopardy has been called.

Sentinel Event

A sentinel event is the term used by the Joint Commission on Accreditation of Healthcare Organizations (JCAHO) that is similar to Immediate Jeopardy. A sentinel event is

> An unexpected occurrence involving death or serious physical or psychological injury, or the risk thereof. Serious injury specifically includes loss of limb or function. The phrase, "or the risk thereof" includes any process variation for which a recurrence would carry a significant chance of a serious adverse outcome. Such events are called "sentinel" because they signal the need for immediate investigation and response.

JCAHO Web Site

The Joint Commission of Accreditation of Healthcare Organizations publishes a *Sentinel Event Alert*. Since January 1995 Joint Commission has reviewed 798 Events. This organization has reported 34 Sentinel Events in the long term care industry for 4.3% (as cited in *Sentinel Event Statistics*, 11 March 2000). Examples of Sentinel Events that are voluntarily reportable under the Joint Commission's Sentinel Event policy (as cited in *Sentinel Event Alert*, 11 May 1998):

- Any patient death, paralysis, coma or other major permanent loss of function associated with a medication error.
- Any suicide of a patient in a setting where the patient is housed around-the-clock, including suicides following elopement from such a setting.
- Any elopement, i.e., unauthorized departure, of a patient from an around-the-clock care setting resulting in temporally related death (suicide or homicide) or major permanent loss of function.
- Any procedure on the wrong patient, wrong side of the body or wrong organ.
- Any intrapartum (related to the birth process) maternal death.
- Any perinatal death unrelated to a congenital condition in an infant having a birth weight greater than 2500 grams.
- Assault, homicide or other crime resulting in patient death or major permanent loss of function.
- A patient fall that results in death or major permanent loss of function as a direct result of the injuries sustained in the fall.
- Hemolytic transfusion reaction involving major blood group incompatibilities.

JCAHO expects a facility to identify possible conditions within the facility that may lead to a sentinel event. An example might be a situation where activity assistants are moving radios, which are probable sources of serious infections, between residents without cleaning them appropriately, thereby posing a risk for the residents who are getting the radios. The activity director would work with the nursing department to identify what is known as a "root cause," or the basic reason(s) that there is a failure to follow the facility's infection control policy. A "root cause analysis" would be done to help identify the basic factors that would cause some staff to follow the infection control policy and for others not to follow the policy. The activity director and nursing staff would look for both "errors of omission" and "errors of commission." An error of omission is a problem that is caused by action not being taken and an error of commission is a problem that is caused by an action being taken that should not have been taken. A sample of developing a root cause analysis of potentially infected radios being taken out of isolation rooms (a potential sentinel event) can be found below.

Sentinel Event and Root Cause Analysis		
Possible Sentinel Event		Radios are said to be removed from rooms of residents who are in wound isolation because of resistant organisms present in two residents' bedsores.
Root Cause Analysis	**Error of Omissions**	• Staff have not had the inservice on infection control. • Staff are not aware that the resistant organism can live on radios. • Staff are not able to read and/or understand the words on the infection control notice. • Staff "wipe down" the radio with the residents' blankets before taking the radio to another resident, thinking that it should be "good enough."
	Error of Commissions	• Staff do not pay attention to infection notices outside of rooms. • Staff decide to ignore infection control policy.
Action Plan		• Ensure that all staff have current infection control inservices. • Ensure that all staff can demonstrate appropriate infection control/cleaning techniques. • Determine which staff have basic competencies in reading and understanding key written communication. Limit job tasks of all staff to areas where they can demonstrate competency. • Counsel staff who are not meeting minimum standards of infection control. Document all infractions in personnel record. Provide inservice training as appropriate.

Chapter 17
Management

This chapter discusses some of the important management issues not covered in the rest of the book. The issues include resident rights, restraints, behavior management, time management, budgets, writing policies and procedures, OBRA regulations, surveys and medications for the elderly.

Resident's Rights

Residents in both assisted living centers and nursing facilities have specific rights outlined in federal and state laws. This section discusses some of the most important rights. The primary right of a resident is to make decisions. This right is never taken away, just modified. If the resident is no longer competent to make decisions, another individual is named to represent the resident's wishes. Other resident rights include the right to informed consent, the right to participate in his/her care plan and the right to be free of unreasonable restraint.

Determining Capacity

Capacity is defined as "the ability to make choices that reflect an understanding and appreciation of the nature and consequences of one's actions." If the resident is unable to make decision for himself/herself, these rights are granted to his/her legal representative. Many states have provision for representation of the resident who has no legal representative or who may not have any interested family member and is not capable of making decisions. The capacity of the resident may be established in several ways. A court may determine that the resident is unable to make his/her own health care decisions and formally declare him/her incompetent. In this case a conservator of person will be appointed. If an individual is not available to act as conservator, a public guardian may be appointed. It is important when reviewing conservatorship papers to determine whether the conservatorship is for person or property or both. Only a conservator of person can make health care decisions for the resident.

In the absence of a court order, the physician may make the determination of capacity. On admission it should be assumed that the resident has capacity unless there is documentation to prove otherwise. If the staff are not aware of any court ruling concerning the resident's ability to make decisions and if the staff question the resident's capacity, the nursing staff or the social services professional should contact the physician for a determination. The physician should get feedback from family and close friends when evaluating the resident's capacity. The determination of decision-making capacity should then be documented in the health record.

If the resident has executed a durable power of attorney, the durable power of attorney for health care (DPAHC) agent has authority only when the resident loses decision-making capacity. Depending on the laws of the state, the physician may appoint a surrogate in the absence of conservatorship or a DPAHC.

Often when making changes in the treatment plan or obtaining informed consent, the staff will defer to an involved family member and neglect to discuss the changes with the resident with decision-making capacity. It is very important for the professional to be sure that the resident is allowed to exercise his or her right to free choice.

Informed Consent

The overriding principle governing informed consent is that residents have the right to control what happens to their bodies. Informed consent is a legal term which means that the resident or surrogate has the right to understand both the positive reasons for making a decision and also the possible negative consequences of any decision made. This includes informed consent for psychoactive medications and physical restraints. To meet the legal test of informed consent, the resident must have been presented five types of information. The first type of information is a clear description of the problem presented in a language and manner that the resident can understand. The second is a description of the suggested solution presented in a language and manner that the resident can understand. The third is an explanation of the possible negative consequences (or possible side effects) of going along with the proposed solution. The fourth piece of information is the possible negative consequences of not going along with the proposed solution. The fifth type of information is other, possible treatment options. When the resident is given these five different types of information, s/he should be able to make a decision about the proposed solution.

The professional is required to document in the health record that informed consent has been obtained. Except in a few situations outside the scope of practice of activity professionals, social services professionals and recreational therapists, when informed consent is required, the staff cannot initiate treatment until the consent is documented in the record. As in all circumstances of resident's rights, the staff must be sure that the resident is being afforded the right to exercise free choice.

Advance Directives

The Patient Self-Determination Act (PSDA) 1991 requires that all skilled nursing facilities accepting Medicare or Medicaid funding inform residents of their rights to accept or refuse treatment and to formulate advance directives.

Definition

An advance directive is a written instruction relating to the provision of health care when an individual is incapacitated. It can be a living will, a durable power of attorney for health care or other instrument recognized under State law. Simply put, an advance directive makes your wishes for health care known when you are not able to express them.

With a durable power of attorney for health care, an agent is appointed to make decisions. Alternates may be designated in the event that the primary agent cannot fulfill the obligation. With a living will choices about treatment are stated in advance of an incapacitating illness. The two functions can also be combined in a single document.

Documentation

There are two requirements that the social services professional must address on admission:

- First, s/he must determine if the resident has executed an advance directive. The answer must be documented in the health record. If s/he has, a copy must be obtained and filed in the record.
- Second, the resident must be informed of the right to formulate an advance directive. If the resident is incapacitated on admission, the provider may give advance directive information to the legal representative or the family. A PSDA pamphlet explaining advance directives is available from most medical societies or local hospitals.

Honoring an Advance Directive

Providers are not required to provide care that conflicts with an advance directive. Life sustaining treatments such as feeding tubes and antibiotics may be withheld if stipulated in the advance directive.

The provider can conscientiously object to implementing the advance directive if state law allows. In this event, the resident may be transferred to another facility or to another physician's care. The notice of transfer regulations would apply.

When there is a disagreement between the surrogate decision maker and other interested parties, every effort should be made to reach consensus. The parties may need to consult an institutional or regional bioethics committee.

Conservatorship vs. Durable Power of Attorney

The agent appointed by a resident in the DPAHC take precedence over all others, including the court appointed conservator, family and close friends. The only person who can overrule the DPAHC is the resident who possesses current decision-making capacity. The DPAHC agent only has authority in the event that the resident loses decision-making capacity.

Right to Participate in Care Planning

An important right the resident has is the right to participate in the plan of care *including the right to refuse a treatment or a service* (Tags F154, F155, F157 and F280). In other words, the resident must give consent before any treatment or service is initiated. In some cases, informed consent is required (e.g. for a restraint program). The regulations specify that even if the resident's ability to make decisions is impaired or the resident is formally declared incompetent by a court, the resident should still be informed of changes in his/her plan of care and consulted about preferences. OBRA requires that a resident be fully informed in advance about care and treatment and of any changes in that care or treatment that may affect the his/her well-being (483.10 (d) (2)). The resident must receive information necessary to make health care decisions, including those involving activity and social services. When planning an activity program for a resident or when developing social services interventions, be sure to include the resident or the surrogate decision maker in the planning.

Residents (or their legal representative) have the right to refuse any and all treatments or services. When a resident refuses medication, treatments, food, fluids, socialization or activities, the social services professional must assess the cause of the refusal and discuss with the resident or surrogate decision maker the risks and consequences of refusal. The counseling of the resident must be clearly documented. The refusal must be shown to be consistent and persistent. Alternative treatments must be offered and all attempted interventions should be documented in the progress notes and on the care plan. Every effort should be made to safeguard the resident's health and safety while also respecting his/her right to refuse treatment.

Right to be Restraint Free

The resident has the right to be free from any physical or chemical restraint not used to treat medical symptoms (Tags F221 and F222). In fact, the resident is guaranteed the right to make an informed choice about the use of restraints. Except for a few situations (e.g., medical crisis), informed consent must be obtained before restraints can be used. Posy vests and lap belts are easily recognized restraints, but bed rails, geri-chairs and seizure medications may also be used to modify a resident's behavior. Any piece of equipment, furniture or medication that is used to control any aspect of the resident's behavior is considered to be a restraint and requires specific consent.

Before using restraints, the facility must show that reasonable attempts were made to determine the cause of the problem and that non-restraint interventions were exhausted. It must be determined if the resident's behavior is due to a lack of a meaningful activity program or the need to manipulate his/her environment. Is the resident's behavior due to environmental factors — e.g., too hot, too cold, too noisy, too crowded — or is it related to a recent loss, such as the loss of a family member or a roommate? Perhaps individual needs are not met or customary routines are not being followed. Activity, social services and recreational therapy professionals, because of their expertise in these areas, should participate in these assessments and interventions. See the section on restraints in this chapter for more information on when and how restraints can be used.

Visitation Rights

The resident must be given immediate access to his/her immediate family or relatives, his/her physician, the state ombudsman or other individuals of his/her choosing. *Visiting hours are not legal!*

Transfer and Discharge Rights

Resident rights safeguard the resident from discharge at the facility's discretion. This is an area that is scrutinized very closely by survey agencies.

The local Ombudsman is often asked if there are any problems surrounding transfers or with residents being allowed to return to the facility. Family members of former residents may be interviewed as well to determine if the discharges met legal guidelines and facility policy.

During closed record review, surveyors are instructed to look for appropriate notices for residents transferred to the hospital or absent on a therapeutic leave. The notices must meet the requirements specified in federal regulation 483.12.

The social services professional is the lead person in assuring that a transfer follows facility policy and does not violate the resident's rights. This includes discussion of facility policies on admission with the resident and family and follow up with the family on transfer of the resident to another room or to another setting.

Room Transfers

The resident's preferences must be taken into account when a change in room or roommate is proposed. Federal regulations require that the resident be notified in advance of any changes. Frequent room transfers can be very disorienting to residents. Surveyors review these closely to determine if the changes are being made for the facility's benefit or to accommodate resident needs. In certain cases the resident has the right to refuse the transfer. Facility policies should be consulted for transfers from a Medicare section to a Medicaid section of the hospital.

Documentation of room change should show that the notice was given in advance of the transfer, that the resident or legal representative agreed to the transfer and that family was notified. The reason for the transfer should be clearly documented. The social services professional should assess the resident for adjustment to the new room a few days after the transfer and document the findings.

Notification of family is very important. It can be very awkward when a family member comes in to visit and the resident's bed is empty and his/her belongings are no longer in the room.

When a change in roommate occurs, the documentation should show that introductions were made. A follow up note is needed to assess the adjustment of all parties to the new arrangement.

Bed-Hold Notice

A bed-hold is the period the resident has to return and resume residence in the nursing facility after leaving for the hospital or other therapy. State law defines the number of days the bed will be held. If the resident does not exceed the duration of the bed-hold s/he must be allowed to return to the same bed as soon as s/he is discharged from the hospital or returns from therapy.

Residents who exceed the duration of the bed-hold must be readmitted to the facility when the next empty bed is available. They must require skilled nursing care and be Medicaid eligible.

Federal regulations require that the nursing facility notify the resident and a family member or legal representative of the facility's bed-hold policies. This notice must be provided twice — on admission and when a facility transfers a resident to a hospital or allows the resident to go on a therapeutic leave.

The notices must be in writing and a copy kept either in the financial file or in the health record. The second notice must document whether or not the resident or legal representative wishes to pay for the bed if the absence exceeds the bed-hold duration. For non-Medicaid residents, the resident or legal representative is asked if s/he wishes to pay for all days of the bed-hold.

The social services professional needs to explain the facility's bed-hold policy to all residents and their families. The explanation should include how the resident is afforded the right to return if the bed-hold duration is exceeded.

Notice of Transfer and Right to Appeal

Federal regulations specify when the resident may be discharged. These regulations exist to prevent the facility from discharging a resident for reasons such as difficulty of care, expensive treatments, abrasive personality or refusing treatment. The resident or legal representative may appeal any discharge.

Criteria for Discharge

A transfer or discharge is allowed when:
1. *The resident's needs cannot be adequately met in the facility.* The resident needs emergency treatment and is transferred to the hospital.
2. *The resident's health has improved so that the resident no longer needs the services provided by the facility.* The resident no longer needs skilled nursing and can return to a lesser level of care.
3. *The safety of individuals in the facility is endangered.* The resident is assaulting other residents. Documentation shows that all attempts to manage the behavior have failed.
4. *The health of individuals in the facility is endangered.* The resident has an infectious disease that cannot be managed in the facility.

5. *The resident has failed to pay for a stay at the facility.* Documentation supports that payment has not been made after reasonable and appropriate notice.
6. *The facility ceases to operate.*

When the facility initiates a discharge or transfer of a resident they must:
- Record the reason for the discharge or transfer in the resident's clinical record and include a copy of the notice sent to the resident, family or legal representative.
- Provide 30 days advance notice or, as soon as practicable, if it is an emergency transfer or the resident has not resided in the facility for 30 days.
- Include in the notice: the effective date of transfer or discharge; the location of discharge; the right of appeal; the name, address and phone number of the Ombudsman and appropriate protective and advocacy agencies.
- Notify a family member or legal representative of the proposed transfer or discharge.

Facility initiated discharges are usually for reasons 1, 3, 4, 5 and 6 listed above. Note that a transfer within the facility from the part that handles Medicare residents to another part of the nursing home is considered a discharge and requires the above notification.

Resident/Family Initiated Discharges

When the resident or family initiates a transfer or discharge and the facility anticipates the discharge they must:
- Provide adequate counseling and referrals.
- Provide a recapitulation of the stay that summarizes the resident's status and provides for continuity of care (commercial forms are available to meet this requirement).
- Provide a post-discharge plan of care.
- Resident/family initiated discharges are usually for reason 2 listed above. Their preferences for discharge are usually clear on admission. Initial and subsequent discharge planning notes should clearly indicate that it is the resident's or family's desire to return to a lesser level of care.
- Although not required, in some cases where the success of discharge may be questionable, the social services professional may want to provide the Notice of Discharge to the resident or family.
- The recapitulation of stay and discharge summary is required for all discharges to home, board and care or to another nursing home.

If the resident/family-initiated discharge is considered inadvisable, documentation should reflect the alternatives offered and notification of appropriate advocacy and protective services. The physician may choose to document that the resident left against medical advice (AMA).

Protection of Resident Funds

The long term care facility may not require that the resident deposit his/her personal funds with the facility.

If the resident does choose to deposit his/her funds with the facility, there are strict guidelines for the handling of the resident's funds. If the resident's funds are in excess of $50, they must be deposited in a separate account and the resident must receive all interest earned on the deposited money. If a resident's deposited funds stay under $50 at all times, they may be deposited in a non-interest bearing account or in a petty cash fund as long as full accounting is kept.

The facility has five legal responsibilities for the funds deposited:
1. to assure a full and complete, separate accounting of each resident's personal funds,
2. to maintain a written record of all financial transactions involving each resident's personal funds deposited with the facility,

3.   to provide the resident or his/her legal representative with reasonable access to the record of deposits, withdrawals and interest,

4.   to convey promptly the resident's personal funds and final accounting record to the administrator of the resident's estate upon the resident's death or transfer and

5.   to purchase a surety bond to provide assurance that the resident's funds are protected from staff theft.

Theft/Loss: An Issue of Identity

Theft and loss occur in facilities. The way to handle situations of theft and loss are part of both federal and state law. It serves a facility well to explain its philosophy about theft and loss very early in the admission process to prepare individuals and families for the reality of the situation. It also behooves all of us in the facility to take very seriously any claims concerning missing items and to use the quality assurance process to reduce the number of incidents of theft and loss by eliminating situations that allow theft and loss to occur.

The prevailing philosophy is that everything, from a misplaced robe to a lost radio, is assumed stolen until it is found again. It is our experience, however, that episodes of theft are less frequent than episodes of loss. The number of items that are lost far outweighs the number of items that are stolen. Additionally, it is assumed that anything that is not found has been taken by a staff member when in fact individuals are known to wander into rooms and "rearrange" other peoples' radios, clocks, glasses, dentures, watches, etc. This is especially true in facilities that have individuals who are able to walk freely but, due to dementia, lack judgment. In any case, before accusations of any kind are made, a thorough search of the facility is in order.

Another common occurrence is misplaced laundry. Our advice: In the short run, be patient. In the long run, fix the system. Laundry has a way of finding its way back to one's closet although the route can be circuitous, taking several days, even weeks. When that happens, the facility needs to put procedures in place to prevent it from happening again. It can be very difficult to keep track of laundry, but the facility is expected to do it, even the socks and underwear.

Never negate the impact on a family of seeing their mother's clothes on someone else — or vice versa. This is a terrible shock and a very emotional experience when this happens (and all too frequently, it does). Try to prepare both the person you serve and family about this in advance; it may ease the trauma.

If everything fails after an item has been reported missing, time spent in room searches and laundry area forages, families and the people you serve may be entitled to some compensation. The circumstances governing this must be very clearly defined in the facility theft and loss policy using federal and state mandates as guidelines.

Never forget that inherent in all of this is the fact that everything, including items of clothing, has an intrinsic value. We must treat all possessions as prized items because the fewer "treasures" left to us, the greater the trauma associated with any loss.

Voting

Every individual has the right as both a citizen of the United States and (as a resident) within the Resident Bill of Rights to continue his/her responsibilities through voting in local and national elections. The information regarding whether an individual is interested and registered is gathered upon admission by either the admissions clerk or through the activity and social services assessment process.

The activity assessment form in *Chapter 2: The People We Serve* has a space on the upper right side for this information.

The activity professional needs to know the following information regarding voting:
- Is the individual interested in being registered to vote?
- Is s/he currently registered to vote and if so at what address?
- Would s/he like to vote by absentee ballot?
- Is s/he capable of making this decision or does s/he have a power of attorney?
- Does s/he need any special devices or assistance in order to use voting equipment?
- How many individuals in the facility are registered?
- Where do you keep this information and how do you update it?
- Do you know whom to contact in the community to assist the individuals with current issues and initiatives? (League of Women Voters, Registrar of Voters)
- Would you like the facility to be a polling place for the community? If so, contact the Registrar of Voters and request information on this and the guidelines necessary.

Voting Policy and Procedure

Policy:

It is the policy of this facility that each resident, according to federal and state regulations, has the right and the opportunity to vote as a citizen of the United States.

Procedures:

1. Upon admission, the resident will be asked about voting status. Are they registered to vote and would they like to be registered to vote.

2. The activity coordinator will document this information on the activity assessment form.

3. This name will be added to the current list of voters.

4. The activity coordinator or social services coordinator will send in a change of address notification for all interested residents.

5. The activity coordinator or social services coordinator and other staff members will assist residents with completing their absentee ballots.

6. The staff will assist in encouraging and informing residents of issues and the importance of their vote.

As you can see, there are many important issues to address regarding voting. The form on the next page will assist you in keeping this information up to date. Add every resident's name onto the form and identify his/her current voting status.

Voting Status Form

Record each resident's name on form. Check off appropriate column and date the last column when completed. List also if they need assistance with voting forms.

Resident Name	Interested Yes/No	Registered Yes/No	Absentee Form Yes/No

Restraints

Federal law requires that the least invasive approach be tried first before more invasive approaches to modifying an individual's behavior are tried. This is especially true when one considers restraints. Restraints can be either physical (like geri-chairs or lap belts) or chemical (like Ativan or other psychoactive medications).

While it is usually the physician, in consultation with the nursing staff, who decides if an individual is to be restrained in any manner, *it is not the staff's right to make that decision independent of the person and his/her guardians*. Any time a restraint is needed, there should be clear documentation as to the path taken to achieve consent from the person or his/her legal guardian. This documentation should also show a progression of the least restrictive restraints being tried first, before more restrictive ones.

The physician and the nursing staff may be the primary individuals initiating the use of restraint, but all professional staff are expected to be advocates for the individual and notify the treatment care team that a violation of the person's rights may have occurred. This violation is a very serious violation. Each department head is responsible to ensure that all of his/her staff are aware of the importance of person's rights and to notify the administrator immediately if there is a potential violation. In some states this may be considered a case of resident abuse and, by law, needs to be called into the appropriate state agency within 24 hours.

Restraint Reduction

The interdisciplinary team (IDT) needs to look for ways to reduce restraints and find alternatives to guarantee the highest possible quality of life. Modification of behavior works best when the entire team and environment are working together, in a unified and integrated approach. As a member if the interdisciplinary team, the activity professional plays an integral role in providing the best possible quality of life to the people we serve. Because an individual will be in the activity program for some portion of the day, the IDT works together to determine the specific role that the activity professional will be playing as part of this program.

A facility should have a set of procedures in place to initiate a restraint program for individuals who would benefit from a restraint program and another set of procedures that allow the frequent review of possible reductions in the use of restraints for every individual who currently is involved in a restraint program. This may include having a specific group of staff (including the activity professional, recreational therapist and the social services professional) to help identify strategies for restraint reduction. This restraint reduction committee should be well versed in ways to reduce the use of restraints based on each person's abilities and strengths.

After the IDT or restraint reduction committee has tentatively identified a resident as needing a reduction of restraint, six steps are taken. The steps are
1. assessment to determine if the individual would benefit from a restraint reduction program,
2. approval from the individual's physician for a restraint reduction program,
3. identification of the possible levels of reduction,
4. identification of responsibilities,
5. approval from the individual (or surrogate) and
6. inservice for the staff on the specific aspects of the program.

The first step is to assess if the person is a good candidate for a reduction in his/her restraint program or if alternatives to the current program are indicated. "Good candidates" usually come from people who are doing exceptionally well or exceptionally poorly on their current program. If a person is doing exceptionally well on his/her restraint program, it may mean that s/he could tolerate and even thrive with a less restrictive program. If an individual is not doing well on his/her current program (e.g., the desired results are not being achieved), then a change in the restraint program is definitely called for. A checklist for behaviors that make an individual a "good candidate" can be used or other types of assessment forms can be created by staff. The "scoring" or data placed on the assessment tool should include input from all other disciplines.

The second step involves the individual's physician. The physician needs to give approval and orders for any reduction. The orders need to be signed and in the medical chart.

The third step is to identify possible levels of physical restraint reduction or alternative strategies. There will be different levels of reduction within any restraint reduction program. These include the removal of the restraint (least restrictive), alternatives to provide maximum freedom within safety margins (moderately restrictive) or the identification that a restraint is required (most restrictive). If the team (and the individual/surrogate) recognizes that some kind of restraint is required, effort can be made to minimize the type and time of the restraint being used.

The fourth step is to identify who is responsible for implementing the various parts of the individual's restraint/restraint reduction program. It should be clearly defined which staff member is responsible for each duty. Communication is crucial for the security of the person and success of the program. When the individual participates in an activity, it is important to identify who is responsible to release the restraints and who will re-secure them at the end of the group.

Informed consent is step five. In the ideal situation, the person and/or his/her surrogate will have helped define the restraint reduction process. Sometimes this is not possible, but at this point, once the restraint reduction program has been formally defined, s/he must give informed consent.

The sixth and last step of a restraint reduction program is to let all the staff know what they will be expected to do. Each restraint reduction or alternative program will likely follow similar guidelines but vary according to the individual's needs, teamwork goals and individual goals. All staff need to be educated about the goals of the program, the program structure and expectations of staff involved.

In addition to the specifics of each person's restraint reduction program, the training of all staff needs to include gait belt use; restraint options, use and techniques; positioning; and transfer techniques (when included in the policy).

You will need to determine which activities are appropriate for this reduction. You will supervise and observe responses while the person is restraint-free in a structured activity. Small groups are better than large groups for evaluating the effect of any restraint reduction on individual's performance and affect.

The names of each participant, information regarding his/her restraint reduction needs or goals and seating position should be available for any staff who are assisting in the room in which the activity is held. This could be a diagram posted behind the door or on a clipboard for reference. All of the professionals working with the individual will want to be evaluating, assessing and documenting behavior, mood, safety issues and functional levels.

In terms of chemical restraint reduction or alternatives, a Behavior Management Program is often the most successful approach.

Behavior Management[59]

With the implementation of OBRA and MDS version 2.0, staff are called upon to deal with unwanted behaviors through behavioral interventions first, before using any psychoactive medications. If behavioral interventions fail, then the use of medication to modify behavior may be tried. Gone are the days when we saw an unwanted behavior and called the attending physician for a psychoactive medication to control the behavior. This change is a good thing. It asks us to pay attention to the specific behavior and to be creative and professional in dealing with it. On the MDS we are asked if a behavioral plan has been implemented. This section will provide some ways to deal with managing behavior instead of using psychoactive medications, prior to using psychoactive medications or in conjunction with them.

A behavior is an observable action. Many behaviors are a result of experience, values or beliefs. Others are caused by organic changes within the individual's own body (e.g., psychosis). There are three primary ways we can effect behavioral change: help the individual change his/her own behavior, change the environment that the individual is in or use psychoactive medications (medications that change a person's behavior by changing his/her body chemistry).

Often when we look at behaviors, it is the environment that has created the behavior. For example, an individual who has moved into a facility learns that s/he gets his/her needs met quicker when s/he yells out. After a time s/he begins to yell out just to get attention. By modifying the environment (having staff respond quicker to his/her call bell) and by re-training the individual, we can decrease the yelling.

The first place to begin modifying unwanted individual behaviors is to make sure that the environment within the facility promotes positive, cooperative behaviors. It is also important to train all staff in appropriate behavioral interventions. These interventions are not necessarily part of a formal behavioral management program, but are consistent behaviors used by all staff to encourage appropriate individual behaviors. When the facility is able to offer a positive environment with appropriate staff behaviors, the need for formal behavioral modification programs will drop significantly. This is a win-win situation. The individuals have a better, more social place to live and the staff spend less time with the paperwork required of a formal behavioral management plan.

Environmental Management

Environmental management means changing the environment to affect the behavior. This may be as small a change as playing classical music versus rock and roll in the activity room to painting the double door that leads off the unit to look like a bookshelf. (Painting a mural of a bookshelf across the door that leads off the unit confuses individuals with dementia who wander, making it less likely that they will leave the unit.) By using environmental management we may be able to deal with unwanted behaviors without using psychoactive medications. It could mean changing rooms, roommates, the showering schedule or meal times. Be creative and listen to what the individual is telling us through his/her words and actions.

This is an example that happened during one of my consultations. A long time resident of a nursing home became a little more agitated than normal. She had a long history of psychiatric problems. The behaviors associated with her psychiatric diagnosis were generally not disruptive but included episodes of hallucinations. While I was there, the nurse received a phone call from the individual's physician with an order for Haldol 1 mg BID for three days for agitation with delusions. This order was unexpected, as the individual's behavior did not seem significantly different than her normal baseline — a baseline that seemed well within the facility's ability to

---

[59] This section is by Kay Garrick, LCSW. Used with permission.

accommodate without the use of psychoactive medications. As the nurse did some detective work, she found that the individual had called her daughter and told her the nursing home was making her stay in a room with a dead person. Because of the individual's psychiatric history, the daughter assumed the individual was becoming psychotic and called the physician. The nurse came to me with the dilemma of whether to implement the physician's orders or to call the physician back to discuss the situation. The nurse was concerned because she felt the individual was not hallucinating as the individual's roommate was in the process of dying. I suggested we check with the individual to see if she wanted to move to another room. The individual gladly accepted the move. We called the daughter, explained the situation and then called the physician who canceled the medication order. The individual was moved to another room. By being sensitive to the individual's concerns and what was happening in her environment, we were able to solve the problem without using medications.

Behavioral Intervention

Behavioral intervention is just another term for providing the person with gentle, normal consequences for inappropriate behavior. Staff frequently create unrealistic "community" standards for social skills within the facility. Instead of ignoring grabbing behavior, the staff should be taught how to respectfully ask the person not to grab them and, just as important, figure out why the individual felt the need to grab. Behavioral interventions can be used when the behavior is seen in limited situations — when the behavior is not pervasive. An example would be an individual who yells when s/he is in an activity and not at other times. Talk to the individual about the behavior when the behavior is not happening. If an individual calls out in group, talk to him/her before the group. Tell him/her what behavior you have noticed and then ask what s/he thinks is causing the behavior. (This is for individuals who have the mental ability to understand.) Let him/her know that it is affecting other people and how it is affecting others. Ask the person if s/he has any suggestions to solve the problem. Perhaps his/her hearing is bad and if s/he sits in the front of the group, s/he would not yell out. If s/he has no suitable ways to solve the problem, let the person know what you will do. If s/he disrupts the group again, you will need to remove him/her from the group.

Remember to maintain the person's dignity as much as possible. If the situation arises where you must remove an individual from an activity, do not discipline him/her in front of the group. Simply go to the person and take him/her out of the activity. Outside of the group remind him/her that his/her behavior was disruptive to others. Use a consistent simple phrase that describes the behavior and use it every time the behavior happens. Do not touch, smile sweetly or show anger. In our guilt at taking this kind of action, our behaviors can reinforce the wrong behavior. Keep your facial expression blank. Later, visit privately with the person to see how s/he responded to the intervention.

Make a plan to meet the needs of the individual. If you have a person who consistently yells out in group and not when s/he is in his/her room, why do you continue to bring him/her to group? Perhaps one-on-one visits would be more effective. Often individuals with dementia get over-stimulated in large groups. Try smaller, quieter activities. Physical activities may be successful also.

In one facility a newly admitted resident with a diagnosis of dementia called out constantly, "Nurse, nurse, nurse." It was her first admission to a nursing facility and the Director of Nurses was ready to discharge her on her date of admission because of her calling out. The resident loved to receive hugs. I pulled the clock at the nurses' station off the wall and went to the resident and put the clock in her lap. I used simple phrases but told her she needed to be quiet for five minutes and that if she was quiet she would get a big hug. I showed her the clock and where the hands of the clock would be when she would get a hug. Her face lit up. I left her in her wheelchair across from the nursing station and sat nearby but out of her range of vision. When she called out, I got her attention and made a quiet signal and verbally cued her to three more minutes until her hug. I kept my face blank and did not touch her. At the end of five minutes she had called out three times and I went to hug her and praised her for the good job she did being quiet. Then I increased the time to ten minutes with the "hug" reward at the end and continued increasing the time in increments of five minutes up to an hour. When the resident was up to an hour, she called out only once.

The Director of Nurses was sold on behavior management along with the rest of the staff. The Maintenance Director found a large kitchen timer that rang after the appropriate amount of time. The certified nurses' aides took the resident to her room, set the timer and when the bell rang they would go to her and give her a big hug and reward her behavior. Initially it took me all morning to work this through with the resident and staff. We were able to eliminate the yelling out behavior so that the resident felt safe and her quality of life was improved. The staff bonded with the resident and gave her attention and praise for appropriate behavior. She was able to be maintained at the facility instead of being placed elsewhere.

Behavior Management Programs

When a negative behavior is serious and frequent enough to require a systematic change, the team will need to develop a behavior management plan. Behavior management plans should be implemented when the behavior is affecting most aspects of care and the quality of life for others is impacted. It is a more complex system that involves all disciplines and the person and/or family in an organized, planned approach to eliminate the behavior.

The reason that this situation is complex is that it has reached the point where the unwanted behavior is ingrained. Instead of having just isolated occurrences, this behavior has been established as a coping pattern. To break this pattern, all staff have to work together in a systematic way. Each staff person needs to know how to discourage the behavior as well as promote healthy ways of coping.

We can change a behavior *if* there is something an individual *likes*. I prefer to use positive reinforcements rather than negative. Positive reinforcements are more successful. It is often easier for staff to use positive rewards.

Many folks believe that if a person has a diagnosis of dementia, behavioral management is not effective. That is not my experience. Individuals with dementia *can* benefit from behavioral plans. Does the person really like hugs, candy, to sit outside, time with family/staff? We then use what the individual likes as a reward for the appropriate behavior and behavior can be changed.

Behavioral programs take time initially but, when they are effective, they take less time than responding to the inappropriate behavior. This may be difficult for staff to understand. Just have the staff add up the amount of time they spend answering a person who uses the call light frequently. Changing the behavior will eventually save time. To change a behavior, we must act like a detective and find out the reason for the behavior. The best way to find out the causes is usually at a special care planning conference where all disciplines are represented and can give input related to the behavior. It is very helpful to have the certified nurses' aides who work with the person present at this meeting. Has something changed in the person's life that triggered the behavior — a new room, a new roommate, a new nurses' aide, family out of town? What is the individual's diagnosis? What are the medications the person is taking? What happens before the behavior occurs? These are called the "antecedents." Is it change of shift? Does the nurses' aide try to provide care? Does the family leave? What exactly is the behavior? We need to be very specific. Is the individual verbally abusive or did s/he raise his/her voice and yell at the staff? We cannot change the behavior if we do not know exactly what it is.

What does the person get by behaving this way — space, distance, control, power, maintaining dignity? This is often called the "consequence." Has anyone told the person that the behavior is causing a problem for others? Who on the interdisciplinary team has the best relationship with the person? Would it be better to have a male staff talk to the resident? This often works best with males who are physically, verbally or sexually acting out. Could the family help us deal with the behavior? Do they have information about the behavior prior to admission? Can they come in and help at difficult times? Is there anything we can change in the environment to help change the behavior?

Consistency is crucial for a behavioral plan to work. That means all staff must behave the same way — all shifts need to be told of the plan and follow through with it. If we use a verbal phrase, all staff should repeat the same phrase to the resident. Keep your behavioral plan as simple as possible. Only work on one behavior at a time and choose the behavior that causes the most problems for the other people we serve and staff.

Behavioral plans are more difficult for individuals with a diagnosis of "borderline personality disorder." These are often the people who like to stir up tension among staff or family members. They usually do not have anything that is as rewarding to them as the tension they cause, so finding something else they like that will cause them to change can be very difficult.

When behavioral management plans are started, the person's behavior will often get worse for approximately two weeks. The individual is trying to hold on to what s/he knows, even old coping mechanisms and behaviors that are causing problems. Expect the first two weeks to be difficult, encourage staff to remain consistent, and only change the program during the first two weeks if it is completely clear that the program is going to fail or make matters worse.

Difficult Behavior

Every facility tends to have at least one person who exhibits difficult behavior. This part talks about three difficult behaviors that I am often asked to work with: inappropriate sexual behavior, suicidal thoughts and violent behaviors. These behaviors are not often discussed in behavior guides. Use a team approach, define the problem and decide your approach using some of the ideas discussed above.

Sexual Behavior

One of the most difficult behaviors to deal with is sexually inappropriate behavior. With younger individuals being admitted more frequently to facilities, sexually inappropriate behavior is becoming more of an issue for staff to deal with. Remember that this behavior can be exhibited by young and old, as well as male and female.

Sexual behavior is NORMAL. Often what comes up around the behavior are our own judgments, values and religious beliefs. We all have sexual needs and expressing them is part of life for both old and young. It is important for us to define what is "inappropriate" sexual behavior. Staff walking into an individual's room where the curtain is closed to find the person masturbating is not considered inappropriate behavior on the resident's part. It could be viewed as inappropriate on behalf of the staff. Did you allow the individual the privacy s/he wanted? Did you knock? Did the individual give the staff person permission to enter the room? Married couples have the right to share a room and are entitled to privacy.

It is crucial to know the diagnosis, as the approaches will vary depending on whether the person has mental capacity. Whether the person has capacity to make health care decisions is determined by the attending physician and can be found in the Advance Directives or in the Physician's Orders.

If an individual becomes sexually aggressive or active with another resident, determine if both individuals have capacity. If they do, they can make their own choices and consent as long as privacy is maintained. If the residents have capacity, we are not allowed to discuss this with their families unless the residents give us permission. To discuss this with the family without the resident's permission is a violation of resident rights. If the resident does not have capacity, the responsible party or agent must be informed and decide if the behavior is acceptable. Cases of sexually aggressive behavior must be reported to the appropriate reporting agency (Ombudsman, Adult Protective Services, Police). Report all episodes of sexually inappropriate behavior to your supervisor.

When a resident without capacity is demonstrating sexually inappropriate behavior, you can use the following guidelines. Remember to maintain the resident's dignity. If s/he is exposed, make sure s/he is covered or dressed appropriately. If the resident is in a public place and cannot be distracted, take him/her to his/her room and pull the curtain. Make the nursing staff aware so that they respect the resident's privacy. For a resident who exposes himself or urinates in public places, consider ordering the resident a back closure jumpsuit. They are difficult for the residents to remove. A back closure jumpsuit is considered to be a restraint. Before dressing the resident in one, the facility would have to follow the standard procedure for placing a resident in a restraint, including informed consent.

Do not talk down to the resident by saying anything that makes you want to shake your finger at the resident. The resident may not understand what you are saying but s/he may understand that you are trying to make him/her feel ashamed of the behavior. You need to look at your values about sexual behavior. Remember that you are the professional and do not personalize the behavior.

Are you doing anything to contribute to the behavior? Watch the "sweetie, honey, baby" phrases. Are you touching the resident or kissing him/her? If a resident displays inappropriate sexual behavior, do not call him/her "sweetie," or kiss him/her. Sometimes residents with this behavior ask for kisses. State professionally, "Mr. Smith I'm the Social Services Director and I will not kiss you but I will shake you hand." Remind the resident of your professional role. "Mr. Jones you must have confused me with someone else. I am the Activity Coordinator and I want to invite you to the piano recital today." Keep your face blank. Do not show shock, displeasure, laughter, smiles or anger. Remember any facial expression could encourage the behavior. If you cannot control your facial expression, turn your face away from the resident.

Do not run to you peers and giggle about the behavior. Someone will always overhear conversations. Again, this means you need to look at your own values around sexuality. Do report the behavior to the charge nurse. Is this new behavior? Is it covered in the care plan? If so, what are our interventions to deal with the behavior?

When a resident with capacity is demonstrating sexually inappropriate behavior, you can use the following guidelines. Refer the resident to the Social Services Director who will talk to the resident about the behavior. Why is it being displayed? Does the resident need more control, power or privacy? What is the resident's solution to the problem? One younger resident consistently exposed himself to older female visitors. When asked why he did this, he said that he had been in prison and that he had more freedom there than in the nursing home. He did this in hopes of being arrested and put back in prison. We were able to give the resident more control over his life and he stopped the behavior. Referral to a therapist, psychologist, social worker or psychiatrist for counseling related to the problem may be helpful. Involve the Ombudsman. Sometimes someone from outside the facility can have more impact on the resident's behavior. And remember, when the resident has been determined to be capable, s/he will need to be involved in the decision-making process.

Suicidal Behavior

Suicidal behavior is another difficult behavior to deal with. If a resident is displaying suicidal behavior, it must be determined if the facility can provide for the resident's safety. If not, the resident may need to be transferred to an acute psychiatric hospital for appropriate treatment. Suicidal statements are often a cry for help and *must* be taken seriously. Report any suicidal comments to the charge nurse *and* the Social Services Director.

If a resident threatens suicide, states a desire to commit suicide or is known to have been suicidal in the recent past, an assessment to determine whether the resident is currently suicidal will be made by the Social Services Department, possibly in conjunction with any of the following: the Nursing Department, the attending physician, a consulting psychiatrist, consulting psychologist, the Social Work Consultant, the county's mental health specialist or the family. Observe the resident for warning signs of suicide: prolonged depression, marked changes of behavior or personality, a sudden lifting of the mood (e.g., the resident who is depressed suddenly seems happy), making final arrangements as though for a final departure and/or suicide threats or similar statements.

Question resident as to motivation, method and means. If there exists a desire to commit suicide, a plan devised and a viable way to kill oneself, the risk is greater. If a risk exists, the facility interdisciplinary team will formulate an intervention to ensure the safety of the resident. However, if the resident seems to have a clear plan as to how s/he will end her/his life, the staff should question whether they could keep the resident in the facility. Determine whether there is a need for a temporary transfer. A transfer to a psychiatric unit used to handling this crisis situation is usually a reasonable choice. Check with your county's mental health specialist.

If you decide that the resident can stay in the facility, enlist all staff in monitoring actions of resident, but have one specific staff per shift who is responsible for checking the resident on a regular basis. Institute regular check-ins, usually every 15 minutes. This may require moving the resident closer to the nursing station for observation. To ensure that the frequent checks are done, a sign-off sheet should be available at the nursing station for the staff to document the resident's activity and affect every 15 minutes and then to sign-off, indicating who observed the resident during those last 15 minutes and what the resident was doing.

As much as possible, reduce environmental hazards. Remove sharp objects from resident's room and reach (e.g., matches, razors, scissors). Remove the call light cord and replace it with a tap bell. Remove any belts, cords, etc. from resident's access. Replace silverware with plastic. The nursing staff should be sure that the resident swallows his/her pills and does not hoard or cheek them.

Most residents who feel like taking their own life have mixed feelings about taking action. They frequently feel like life is out of control and want to be able to "grab" onto some strength and stability provided by someone else. Knowing that someone will be there to help gives them a sense of security. Consider using a written contract with the resident (verbal would be fine but written is more powerful). This way the resident knows that someone will be there if s/he feels the need for support. Write a contract that states "I, _____ (resident's name), agree that if I feel like harming myself in any way, I will not take any action to do myself harm. I agree to contact the Social Services Director _____ (name) or the charge nurse _____ (name)." Have a place for the resident to sign and for a staff signature. Give a copy to the resident and put a copy in the chart. Be sure to include this service/intervention in the care plan. Remember to designate staff to cover on the weekends, holidays and during staff illness and be sure the resident knows who the staff are.

Encourage the resident to talk about feelings. Often staff avoid stating the obvious, "Do you feel like killing yourself?" It will not encourage the resident to take this action but may be seen as a relief by the resident that someone will talk about it — that someone understands. Make sure you visit the resident regularly. Often staff avoid seeing the resident because they do not know what to do. All you need to do is let the resident know that you care about him/her and sit with him/her for a few minutes. Offer touch when appropriate.

Violent Behavior

Violent behavior exhibited by one or more residents can be difficult to deal with, can endanger the other residents and staff and can cause a facility to lose its license. Violent behaviors cannot be tolerated and need to be addressed immediately.

This behavior can be a result of inability to control one's impulses or feeling powerless over one's environment. Anger can be directed at others or the environment. The resident may be combative with staff, peers, and family or throw things such as food or furniture. This anger can be a result of a feeling of a lack of control, neurological damage or inadequate coping skills. It may also be a result of impulse control problems, which arise after a head injury or stroke. Staff's first responsibility is to assure that residents involved in a violent situation are safe. Do others need to be protected, moved or other staff called to assist?

Staff need to be safe, and you need to insure the safety of other residents. If someone is being violent, stay an arm's length away. Give the person space to calm down. Take him or her to a quiet place. If there is no mental decline, let the resident know that the violent behavior will not be tolerated and that staff need to keep others safe. The resident needs to know that staff will protect and set boundaries since the resident feels out of control. The behavior could lead to eviction if the resident cannot control the violent outbursts. (Although, this may not be the most prudent thing to say during the middle of a resident's violent outburst.)

Staff should avoid areas or topics that cause conflict. Avoid power struggles. Instead of "It's time for your shower." try asking, "When would you like to shower?" This gives the person more control over his/her life.

When interacting with a resident who seems on the edge of losing control, keep a neutral manner. Do not show fear, anger or laughter. Keep your face blank and present a calm professional demeanor. Do not try to shame the resident.

Controlling one's anger requires good coping skills and socially appropriate ways to express one's feelings. The resident may be justified in his/her feeling of anger although his/her way to express it is not appropriate. How would you feel if the same thing happened to you? It is good to identify the feeling and offer acceptance. "I can understand why you felt angry after what happened." Referral to a counselor, psychologist, therapist, psychiatrist or social worker may help the resident explore his/her anger and ways to express it appropriately.

Violence may be a way for the resident to release energy. Offer the resident alternatives and appropriate ways to release his/her anger thereby increasing his/her coping skills. Consider trying workouts with weights; give the resident a pillow to pound on or regular exercise such as walks around the facility.

When the violence is severe and cannot be stopped, staff may have to call 911 to have the police assist the resident. Remember, assault, no matter where it happens, is against the law. If the law is being broken, the facility may need to have professionals who are used to dealing with violent behavior take over the situation.

The following page has a sample form for a behavior management meeting.

Behavior Management Meeting

Name: _____ Date: _____

What is the individual's problem? (Do not describe the staff's problem with the individual, e.g., person is frustrated and fearful so s/he becomes combative): _____

_____

_____

How is this a problem within the facility? _____

_____

Identify the individual's strengths (e.g. is physically strong, good motor skills, maintains social etiquette, etc.): _____

_____

_____

Environmental stimulus to consider (identify environmental factors — light, noise, temperature, space, other people who are present when behavior occurs): _____

_____

_____

Medications

Antipsychotic Medication: _____

   Target Behavior: _____

   Episodes: Increased   Decreased

Antianxiety Medication: _____

   Target Behavior: _____

   Episodes: Increased   Decreased

Antidepressant Medication: _____

   Target Behavior: _____

   Episodes: Increased   Decreased

Successful non-drug approaches: _____

_____

Unsuccessful non-drug approaches: _____

_____

Last Psychiatry Evaluation: _____

Plan: _____

_____

_____

_____

Time Management

Time management is the process by which we manage our time to the extent that we feel accomplishment, completion and a personal sense of well-being. Managing our lives — being on time — is something we're always going to do … tomorrow. As a result, we tend to engage in a lot of "knee-jerk" activity; we react instead of act.

Staying on a schedule seems an especially daunting objective in a profession that deals with people and their problems. In effect, a day is never linear as we are continuously diverted to mend and fix. At the end of the day, even though we have been busy, sometimes it seems that we haven't really done any work! It is only an illusion that we can never really get it all done. In fact, we have a responsibility, an obligation to do just that: to address everything our job description says we must do.

Time management is not a skill that most people are born with; it is an acquired skill that needs attention and practice. Managing time also means that the manager needs systems designed which work for him/her. All people organize their thoughts and schedules in a unique style. For this reason, each person needs to organize in the way that best suits his/her style, type of work and personality.

Have a Schedule

We have attempted to give you a bird's eye view of the work in the sections entitled "Life of A…" For an activity professional, the schedule has some clear responsibilities at set times so this discussion will help you with the less structured times. The social services professional has more schedule freedom so what we say here applies to most of your schedule.

What you need to do is derived directly from your job description. Within those obligations, you need to develop a plan for when you work and decide on your own cues for completion. For example, you might try to do your computer work each morning before 9 a.m.; or do your quarterly notes between 4–5 p.m. after you have had time in the day to see each of the individuals you need to report on, jotting notes as you proceed throughout the day.

Set goals for the week. You can do this on Monday morning for the ensuing week or Friday afternoon in anticipation of the week ahead. Revise these goals each morning before you begin. Of course, no one working with people will ever get from A to B every time but with an idea of your task load, you can do it much of the time.

Keys To Success

- Prioritize each day's responsibilities.
- Complete the least appealing work first.
- Complete one task at a time. Too much time and energy are spent trying to complete two to three things within the same amount of time. Some people are able to do this but most find that it does not work for them.
- Discourage interruptions by scheduling calls and appointments at a good time for you. Advise staff of this schedule also. When you are leading a group, you should not be answering calls. This leaves the unspoken message to the group participants that your calls are more important than they are.
- Schedule enough time each day to complete all required documentation.
- Schedule enough time each day to visit on a one-on-one basis and record this in the bedside log.

- Keep your desk organized so that you can sort through stacks of papers according to priorities.
- Write a list of all the work responsibilities that you have. By referring to this list, you can better identify a plan and way of organizing all of the different types of duties.

Make Choices

There will always be more demands than you can possibly respond to. Be realistic as to personal goals and abilities. If the frustration becomes too great because of lack of organization, stress mounts, anxiety occurs and there is a general feeling of loss of control. Break the cycle before this happens. There are four D's in time management: *Drop it, Delay, Delegate, Do it.*

If you are a department head, you will have greater demands and expectations. Not only are you required to provide the services expected of *you,* but you are also responsible for all the other mandated responsibilities of the department, other staff members and volunteers.

When you go about trying to meet all of these demands, the most important thing you can do is to set priorities (act — don't react). Decide what needs to be done first, second and so on. Then write down your decisions so you will remember what you have to do and how soon you plan to do it.

Try to find a balance between never varying your plan and having the plan disrupted by everyone who asks you to do something. A good rule of thumb is if you already have something on your list of things to do, you should do it when you planned to even if someone just asked you how soon it would be done. The only time to change your priorities is when something new comes up. Then you need to decide where it goes in your list of priorities.

When human need arises (and that's why we do what we do), get involved up to your elbows. If you have to decide between addressing a need and writing a quarterly report, the choice is obviously to attend to the need. In fact, addressing a need as it arises is really the action position; ignoring/avoiding creates the need for reaction. However, do not allow diversion to derail you. Act, but return to your schedule of work as soon as possible. Work on your documentation skills so that you say what you need to say in a clear concise manner. Don't waste time writing too much.[60]

Chip away at your schedule and list of goals in order to keep going forward. As you finish one project for the day/week, immediately focus on your next task. There will always be something waiting for your attention; it's the nature of work like ours where we are not only dealing with people but also with paper — lots of it.

TGIF

Before you leave work for your well-deserved weekend, check the list of goals you started with on Monday (this includes the must do's from your job description, e.g. assessments and quarterlies). Is everything complete? If not, why not? Can it wait until Monday? What will be the consequence if a task remains incomplete?

If you can safely answer that everything is done that needs doing with no ill effect from a job that might be left, then you can leave!! However, you might feel better prepared to face Monday morning if you write a sketch for the coming week; that way, you will not have to dread that day or face decisions first thing in the morning after a relaxing weekend.

---

[60] For more information on documentation see Ann Uniak, *Documentation in a SNAP for Activity Programs (with MDS Version 2.0)*, 1996, available from Idyll Arbor, Inc.

Time Management Calendar

One way to determine how well you are managing your time is to complete a Time Management Calendar for one month and then analyze the results. This has been a helpful tool for many professionals. Read the codes below. These represent your responsibilities. Be sure to add duties specific to your facility.

FM (Facility Management) Any responsibility directly associated with office and departmental functions. In other words, everything related to keeping the department in order. This may also include resident shopping.

DRC (Direct Resident Care) Direct leadership and time spent with the people we serve. This would be either in a group setting or on a one-on-one basis. If you are arranging an activity for adult education teachers or a volunteer, this is listed under coordination and not direct care.

D (Documentation)

T (Transportation) Time bringing individual to and from groups.

PR (Public Relations) Time spent explaining your work to the public, press or other agencies.

TMC (Time Management Calendar) The time spent in completing this form each day for a month needs to be added on. It will be approximately 15 minutes daily.

CC (Care Conferences) The time spent preparing for and attending care conferences.

C (Coordination) This includes calendars, newsletters, interdepartmental functions, fundraising, etc.

PD (Personal Development) This is the time spent reviewing program ideas, going to workshops, reading and reviewing guidelines. You should have some of this each week.

M (Meetings) These could be staff meetings, MDS meetings, QA meetings. You should note what kind of meeting it was.

S (Supervision) Time when you are supervising volunteers and staff in the department.

CV (Consultant Visits) Add the time spent with the consultant for the department.

FC (Family Concerns) The time spent working with the family and friends of the people we serve.

G (Grievances) The time spent learning about and resolving grievances.

CL (Clothing) Making sure participants have appropriate clothing.

LA (Lost Articles) Checking on lost clothing and other articles.

DC (Discharge Planning)

L (Lunch)

O (Other) Explain how the time was spent.

How to Complete the Calendar

At the end of each day for one month, record where your time went on any standard wall or notebook calendar. Each entry must be in an increment of no less than 15 minutes. If you find that you are doing two things at one time, you must divide the time and show each one separately. Use the codes shown above. These represent the various functions of the work. If you work more than eight hours, this must be reflected on the calendar also. In order for this to be accurate, the calendar needs to be completed each day at the end of the day.

Example of how an average day will appear on the calendar when completed:

DRC	2 hours	S	1 hour	RCC	1 hour
D	1 1/2 hours	L	1 hour	PD	15 minutes
T	45 minutes	C	1 hour		

Total time: 8 1/2 hours.

By reviewing an average day over a period of one month, you will be able to see what takes the longest amount of time to complete, how much direct time is spent with the people you serve in programming, what needs more time and what may be an area of weakness.

Budgets

Every department has a budget to which it must adhere. This budget is created by the administrator and/or corporate office and is an integral part of the total facility budget. If you do not have previous experience with budgets and accounting, ask for some advice or reading materials to better educate yourself about protocols and requirements.

When you are looking at budgets, it is important to understand the difference between a supply item and a capital item. The capital items are large items that the department needs to provide a basic service. (In accounting terms, these items are depreciated rather than expensed.) Some of these items may include slide projectors, VCR and monitors, head sets with tape decks and/or radios, large bingo games, reality orientation boards, eraser boards, monthly calendars, typewriters and computers. The money for capital items may not come from the budget you use to get supplies, but you need to check this out with your administrator to be sure how your facility budgets its capital funds.

In some facilities, the activity or social services budget contains *all* costs that are incurred through this department. Some examples could be coffee supplies, paper supplies, consultant costs, entertainment and many more. Other facilities budget some of these things separately. It is important to understand how your individual facility budget works so that you can not only plan ahead but also negotiate when you know the budget will not meet the current resident needs.

As with any business, accountability is extremely important. Accountability in this instance refers to the ability of the department head to identify where every penny has gone, with receipts to back up the expenses. Without the paper backup, there is no record to substantiate purchases and payments.

At least once a year, your facility will plan the budget for the next year. You need to be part of this process. The best way to figure out what you need is to go through your records for the last year (another reason to keep these records) and add up your expenses for each category of expenditure. Make rough schedules for the next year, noting especially differences between the past year and the coming year. (Some important differences are changes in the number of participants, changes in the diagnoses, changes in requirements for consulting or needs for capital items.) Be prepared to defend your proposed budget by showing exactly where the money will go and exactly what kind of programs you will be running. Tie the programs to assessments and to regulations to demonstrate that they need to be run.

Each state varies in its rules about budgets. Some may make no reference to the activity budget. You need to understand facility and state regulations about activity budgets.

Many of the items and supplies you buy should be ordered with a purchase order. Get in the habit of using purchase orders when sending in orders and requesting supplies. If your facility does not already have a purchasing system, you can purchase your own at any office supply store. If there is a delay or question about an order, you can refer back to this transaction by the purchase order number, the date and the items listed.

Each department needs to keep an inventory of all supplies and equipment. The activity department should have an up-to-date inventory identifying all current supply items in the facility. For any of you who have taken a position in an unorganized facility, you know what it is like to try to figure out what you have, where it is, what you need to order and whether you will have enough money to last the year.

Being organized in this way is like leaving a legacy in the facility for those department heads to come. Always keep things in the manner that you would like to find them.

Policies and Procedures

Policies and procedures are the framework of any organization and any department. Each department head needs to review the current policy and procedure manual in use for the facility and specific departments. Review the policies specific to your department and determine if they are up to date with federal, state, corporate and facility requirements. If not, the department head is responsible for making sure that these policies are written. After policies and procedures are written, they need to be reviewed and approved by the policy review committee in the facility. After approval, committee members sign and date the front page of the manual.

There should be a policy for each aspect of the service provided through the department. When you write policies and procedures, keep in mind the following definitions:

POLICY: A policy identifies and defines an administrative decision about *what* needs to be done.

PROCEDURE: A procedure describes *how* the policy will be implemented.

Both the policy and procedure need to be written *clearly* enough to define the need while at the same time they need to be *general* enough to encompass a variety of situations. Be sure that the descriptions are realistic as the facility can be cited during a federal or state survey for not following through with their own policies.

Many policies are designed from federal and state regulations. An example would be an individual's right to vote in elections. This is a federal law protecting the rights of the resident as a citizen and as a resident. By writing a policy and procedure, the facility is not only complying with the law, but also clearly defining how this regulation will be adhered to and implemented in the facility. An example policy and procedure statement for outings is shown below.

Outings

Policy:

It is the policy of this facility to plan and offer resident outings away from the facility. This meets OBRA Regulations.

Procedures:
- Each resident participating in an outing needs a doctor's order to leave the facility.
- A list of participants needs to be reviewed and approved by the Director of Nursing or Charge Nurse to determine if they are physically, cognitively and emotionally able to leave the facility.
- The activity professional will contact the families to update them as to the date and time that their family member will be away from the facility.
- The activity professional will arrange for appropriate numbers of staff and volunteers. The ideal ratio is one staff member to one resident.
- All medications will be administered before the departure or after the resident returns. *No medications will be transported unless an RN or LPN goes on the outing to administer them to the residents.*

> - Residents who have approval for self-administration will be addressed on a case-by-case basis.
> - All residents need to be signed back into the nursing station upon return to the facility. The activity professional will also share any information felt to be pertinent in regards to behavior, interaction and/or condition changes, which may have occurred during the outing.

There are other special policies that will need attention. An example would be a policy and procedure for a facility pet. Although this is not a required area, the philosophy of many facilities is to encourage a homelike environment that includes a facility pet. A sample policy and procedure might look like this:

Facility Pets

Policy:
It is the policy of this facility to provide and care for a facility pet.

Procedures:
- All veterinary records and vaccination records will be kept on file in the facility.
- A designated staff member will be responsible for the feeding, grooming and general care of the pet.
- The pet will not be in the halls, resident rooms or dining areas during meal times for infection control purposes.
- The activity and social services departments will arrange a schedule for in-room pet visits.

Notice how the procedures are broadly written. For instance, the designated staff member who will be responsible for the grooming and care of the pet. Obviously this individual will have a schedule designed for when and where and how often this will occur. This may be a page attached to the original policy and procedure as additional information.

There is no mystery to writing policies and procedures. Look at your department and see if there is an area that needs a policy. Write the policy to meet either the regulations or current need. Write the procedures to describe how the policy will be implemented. After completion, have the policy and procedure reviewed and approved by the administrator and committee. *The Professional Activity Manager and Consultant*[61] has a full chapter on how to write policies and procedures. It describes each step in the process in an easy-to-follow way.

OBRA Regulations

The OBRA law contains over 180 sections concerning requirements for nursing homes. These sections are called "Tags" and each tag has a number. While there are only two tags dealing directly with activities (Tags F248 and F249) and another two tags dealing directly with social services (Tags F250 and F251), there are over 80 other tags that deal indirectly with activities, social services and recreational therapy. These other tags cover the general environment and livability of the nursing home and apply to all professionals.

Because the survey process depends largely on the Federal regulations, it is important that the professional understands how to use and interpret the regulations. The regulations are divided into 15 requirements. They are

---

[61] D'Antonio-Nocera, A., N. DeBolt, and N. Touhey, Eds., 1996, *The Professional Activity Manager and Consultant*, Idyll Arbor, Inc., Ravensdale, WA.

1. Resident's Rights
2. Admission, Transfer and Discharge Rights
3. Resident Behavior and Facility Practices
4. Quality of Life
5. Resident Assessment
6. Quality of Care
7. Nursing Services
8. Dietary Services
9. Physician Services
10. Specialized Rehabilitative Services
11. Dental Services
12. Pharmacy Services
13. Infection Control
14. Physical Environment
15. Administration

As shown in the boxes under Tags F248 and F250, each section describes the regulation and also contains a set of interpretive guidelines. The guidelines give the surveyor additional information about the meaning of the regulation and provide accepted survey procedures and probes. If you read the regulations, you will have a good idea of how the surveyor will look at this section of the regulations. It will help you prepare for a survey.

It is important to note that the interpretive guidelines are guides only and not requirements. The regulations themselves are used as the basis for survey activities.

When a problem is found during a survey, the problem is written up under the tag number that corresponds to problem. The primary tag numbers that could be used to measure how well the activity and social services staff were meeting the needs of residents are listed below along with a summary of the regulations and surveyor guidelines.

Each resident has the absolute right to be treated with dignity and to exercise his/her rights of citizenship. Just because the resident is no longer in "his/her own home" does not mean that s/he looses the rights associated with being an adult citizen. The resident is guaranteed 10 basic rights: 1. privacy and respect, 2. medical care and treatment, 3. freedom from abuse and restraint, 4. freedom of association and communication in privacy, 5. activities, 6. work, 7. personal possessions, 8. grievances and complaints, 9. financial affairs and 10. transfer and discharge. These rights include services (and recreation programs of their choice) both inside and outside of the facility.

Tag F151 The resident has the right to exercise his/her rights to make choices concerning the manner and way s/he lives subject to reasonable rules outlined by the facility and by local, state and federal law. The resident also has the right to be free from negative actions or undue pressure from the facility and facility staff when exercising his/her rights in a reasonable manner. This right includes freedom from the reduction of the group activity time of a resident trying to organize a resident group or singling out residents for prejudicial treatment such as isolating residents in activities.

Tag F152 The federal and state government has set up specific guidelines to follow if the treatment team feel that a resident is no longer cognitively able to make thoughtful, informed choices about his/her care. This part of the OBRA law provides a check and balance for residents who are at risk of well meaning staff "making choices for him/her." The system is meant to be set up so that a guardian can place the resident's needs first when making choices about care (not just what is convenient for the facility). This tag requires the surveyors to make sure that all consents (*including photo release and outing release*) are signed by the legally appointed guardian.

Tag F153 The resident and/or his/her legal representative have the right to review all of the resident's records within 24 hours of the request. This request may be either verbal or in writing;

the facility cannot insist that only written requests be accepted. This requirement is for the resident's medical chart as well as trust fund ledgers, contracts with the facility, facility incident reports and any other record that may have been made on behalf of or about the resident. The facility may charge the resident for any copies of the records that s/he may request, however, the amount of that charge may not exceed what is normally charged at places like the public library, the post office or low cost copy shops.

Tag F154 The staff and consultants at the facility must make sure that the resident is fully informed about his/her health and status in a manner that s/he can easily understand. Total health status includes functional status, activities potential, cognitive status, psychosocial status and sensorial and physical impairments. The resident should be involved in the assessment and care planning process, including the discussion of diagnoses, treatment, options, risks and prognoses. The information must be presented in advance of the treatment and must let the resident know if the treatment will affect the resident's well-being. Unless the resident has been previously determined (legally) to be incompetent or otherwise found to be incapacitated, the resident has the right to participate in planning care and treatment or changes in care and treatment.

Tag F155 The resident has the absolute right to refuse to participate in any treatment (unless it is court ordered). The resident also has the right to sign an Advance Directive and have the facility honor that Directive. This tag leads to a philosophical discussion about whether the treatment team — especially the activity or social services professional — can write up any treatment objective based on participation. If the activity professional has the care plan objective that the resident will participate in three activities a week, then the treatment being provided is *participation*. The resident always has the absolute right to refuse all treatment and the right to refuse to participate in facility sponsored activities. When most residents decline the invitation to go to any specific activity, they are not usually refusing treatment in their mind; they just are not interested in going to the activity. If the care plan objective is to participate in activities, the resident says "no thank you" and yet the staff person still tries to persuade the resident to go — that staff person is violating the resident's right to refuse treatment and is trying to coerce the resident to abandon (even if for a short while) his/her rights. This leads to potential violation of both Tag F155 and Tag F151. The prudent professional will always separate the treatment plan (therapeutic intervention) from the normal leisure pastime of going to activities. Leave participation in the domain of a normalizing activity. When you feel that the resident needs a treatment, the care plan should be based on treating the identified need (e.g., increase frequency of initiation of social communications, increase use of fine motor skills, decrease percentage of time spent alone) and not on going to activities or talking to the social services professional.

Tag F156 It is hard for a resident to exercise his/her rights if s/he does not know what they are. For this reason, the Federal Government has required that the resident receive a copy of his/her rights written in a language and manner that s/he can read (avoid small print) and understand (native language if necessary). The resident must also be verbally told of his/her rights. This notice of his/her rights (both verbally and in writing) must happen: 1. right before and/or at the time of admission, 2. immediately upon any changes in those rights, 3. upon request and 4. periodically throughout admission. The surveyors are instructed to interview some of the staff to determine if the staff know the rights and rules well enough to help implement them. This tag also covers specific information that the facility must make available to the resident.

Tag F157 Communication from the facility with the resident, the resident's legal guardian or interested family member and the resident's physician is important. In situations that the resident: 1. has been involved in an accident, 2. has experienced a significant change in health status, 3. has a need to have a change in treatment, 4. is to be discharged, 5. is scheduled to have a change of roommate and/or 6. has a change is his/her rights, the listed parties are to be notified *immediately*. A subsection of this tag requires that the facility must periodically check to make sure that all of the phone numbers and addresses that they have for legal guardians, interested family members and the resident's physician are current.

Tags F158 – F161 The resident has the right to continue managing his/her finances after s/he is admitted to the long term care facility according to Tag F158. The facility may not require that the resident deposit his/her money with the facility or at a bank of the facility's choosing. Tags F159-F161 specify the manner in which the facility may handle the resident's money if the resident chooses to allow the facility to do so.

Tag F164 The resident has the right to maintain his/her personal privacy and to have all of his/her records maintained in a confidential manner.

Tags F165 – F166 The resident has the right to complain (voice grievances) about treatment received or not received or about other things that dissatisfy him/her about the facility. The facility must take these grievances seriously by: 1. listening to the grievances, 2. investigating the complaint, 3. promptly trying to address the cause of the grievance (resolve the grievance if possible) and 4. monitoring to ensure that the cause does not lead to the same situation again. This includes addressing the resident's complaints about the behaviors of other residents and of staff.

Tag F167 The resident and the public in general have the right to see a copy of the facility's most current survey along with the plan of correction written up by the facility. This copy must be easily available and either the actually survey document or a notice of its availability must be posted in a prominent place for all to see.

Tag F168 The resident has the right to contact agencies acting as client advocates.

Tag F169 The resident has the right to be free from the requirement to work for the facility. If the resident elects to work for the facility (e.g., folding clothes, running activity groups, etc.) the facility must have in writing whether the resident is working for a wage or as a volunteer (as well as documentation that the resident is knowledgeable about his/her pay status). If the resident is getting paid for the work being done, s/he must be paid the prevailing wage for the job being done.

Tags F170 – F171 The resident has the right to receive mail and packages without them first being opened by facility staff. The laws that apply to the individual's right to privacy of mail received apply to residents of the facility just as it would if they were in their own homes. Because many of the residents are not able to go shopping for stationery, writing implements and postage stamps, the facility is expected to provide them for the residents but may attach a reasonable charge to these supplies. These tags also specify that residents must receive their mail in less than 24 hours of it being delivered to the facility and that the residents' outgoing mail must be to the post office in less than 24 hours after being given to a staff person.

Tag F172 The facility may not have visiting hours that apply to any individual whom the resident wishes to visit. Visitors must be admitted 24 hours a day if the resident wishes it to be that way. Certain state and federal officials must be allowed immediate access to any resident at any time.

Tag F173 The facility must allow the State Appointed Ombudsman access to the resident's records if the resident or his/her legal guardian gives permission.

Tag F174 The resident has the right to have reasonable access to a telephone to receive and place calls in a private manner. This phone must meet ADA (Americans with Disabilities Act) standards for height and volume control.

Tag F175 Residents who are married to each other have the right to share a room in the facility as long as both partners want to share a room.

Tags F201 – F206 To help protect the rights of each resident, the Federal government has outlined the acceptable reasons for transfer or discharge and the procedures and required steps to take before, during and after a resident is either discharged or transferred.

Tag F221 – F222 The resident has the right to be free from any physical restraints imposed; or chemical restraints imposed for purposes of discipline or convenience, not required to treat the resident's medical symptoms. **Physical restraints** are any manual method or physical or mechanical device, material or equipment attached to or adjacent to the resident's body that the individual cannot remove easily which restricts freedom of movement or normal access to one's body. Leg restraints, arm restraints, hand mitts, soft ties or vest, wheelchair safety bars, geri-chairs and bed rails are physical restraints. **Chemical restraints** are psycho-pharmacological drugs used for discipline or convenience and not required to treat medical symptoms. **Discipline** is any action taken by the facility for the purpose of punishing or penalizing the resident. **Convenience** is any action taken by the facility to control resident behavior or maintain residents with a lesser amount of effort by the facility and not in the residents' best interest. Before using restraints, a facility must demonstrate the presence of a specific medical symptom that would require the use of restraints and how the restraint would treat the cause of the symptom and assist the resident in reaching his/her highest level of physical and psychosocial well-being. Often appropriate exercise and therapeutic interventions such as orthotic devices, pillows, pads or lap trays will be sufficient. These less restrictive, supportive devices must be considered prior to using physical restraints. If after a trial of less restrictive measures, the facility decides that a physical restraint would enable and promote greater functional independence, then the use of the restraining device must first be explained to the resident, family member or legal representative and if the resident, family member or legal representative agrees to this treatment alternative, then the restraining device may be used for specific periods for which the restraint has been determined to be an enabler. Any resident who requires a restraint must have a **specific intervention in the care plan to ensure maintenance** of his/her physical, mental, psychosocial and functional status. To determine maintenance, the treatment team should administer the appropriate assessments to establish a **baseline**.

Tag F223 The resident has the right to be free from verbal, sexual, physical or mental abuse, corporal punishment and involuntary seclusion.

Tags F224 – F225 These two tags say that the facility must have policies and procedures in place to prevent abuse and specify the kind of actions the facility must take to ensure that the resident is not verbally or physically abused, including being free from the risk of being taken care of by individuals known to mistreat residents and the required actions to take if neglect or abuse is suspected.

Tag F240 The facility must care for its residents in a manner and in an environment that promotes maintenance or enhancement of each resident's quality of life.

Tag F241 The facility must promote care for residents in a manner and in an environment that maintains or enhances each **resident's dignity and respect** in full recognition of his or her individuality.

Tag F242 The resident has the right to chose activities, schedules and health care consistent with his or her interests, assessments and plans of care; interact with members of the community both inside and outside of the facility; and make choices about aspects of his or her life in the facility that are significant to the resident.

Tags F243 – F244 These two tags outline the residents' right to hold meetings in the facility, with adequate space for the meeting provided by the facility. The residents and their families have the right to meet in private and to present a written request to the facility to address grievances and/or recommendations. The facility is then required to address the grievances and/or recommendations presented in a timely manner.

Tag F245 A resident has the right to participate in social, religious and community activities that do not interfere with the rights of other residents in the facility. The facility, to the extent possible, should accommodate an individual's needs and choices for how s/he spends time, both inside and outside of the facility.

Tags F246 – F247 These two tags further define the resident's rights to receive the services that s/he wants and to have some control over who his/her roommate is. Residents have the right to refuse to have a specific aide give them a bath if they do not feel comfortable with that aide. They have the right to hire outside services (e.g., their own nursing aide or companion) without interference from the facility unless his/her action places the other residents at risk. Other issues covered under this tag include the requirement that the environment of the facility be set up for the residents, not the staff, and that measures are in place to enable residents with dementia to walk freely, to promote reorientation and remotivation, to encourage conversation and socialization and to increase mobility and independence for disabled residents.

Tag F248 This tag (provided in its complete form below) outlines the content and scope of activity services the facility is required to provided for the resident. For non-interviewable residents, the surveyors try to determine if the activities agree with assessed interests and functional level including whether cues/prompts and adapted equipment are provided as needed and according to care plan. The surveyors ask the families to describe the activities before and after becoming a resident of the facility. For interviewable residents and groups of residents, the surveyors are to ask:

- Activities programs are supposed to meet your interests and needs. Do you feels the activities here do that?
- How do you find out about activities that are going on?
- Are there activities available on the weekends?
- Do you participate in activities?
- (If yes) What kind of activities do you participate in?
- (If resident participates) Do you enjoy these activities?
- (If resident does not participate, probe to find out why not.)
- Is there some activity that you would like to do that is not available here?
- (If yes) Which activity would you like to attend? Have you talked to anybody about this? What was the response?
- Are there enough help and supplies available so that everyone who wants to can participate?
- Do you as a group have input into the selection of activities that are offered?
- How does the facility respond to your suggestions?
- Is there anything about the activities program that you would like to talk about?
- Outside of the formal activities programs, are there opportunities for you to socialize with other residents?
- Are there places you can go when you want to be with other residents?
- (If the answers are negative) Why do you think that occurs?

Tag F248 [Activities]

§483.15(f)(1) The facility must provide for an ongoing program of activities designed to meet, in accordance with the comprehensive assessment, the interests and the physical, mental and psychosocial well-being of each resident.

Guidelines: §483.15(f)(1)

Because the activities program should occur within the context of each resident's comprehensive assessment and care plan, it should be multi-faceted and reflect each individual resident's needs. Therefore, the activities program should provide stimulation or solace; promote physical, cognitive and/or emotional health; enhance, to the extent practicable, each resident's physical and mental status; and promote each resident's self-respect by providing, for example, activities that support self-expression and choice.

Activities can occur at any time and are not limited to formal activities provided by the activity staff. Others involved may be any facility staff, volunteers and visitors.

Probes: §483.15(f)(1)

Observe individual, group and bedside activities.
1. Are residents who are confined or choose to remain in their rooms provided with in-room activities in keeping with life-long interests (e.g., music, reading, visits with individuals who share their interests or reasonable attempts to connect the resident with such individuals) and in-room projects they can work on independently? Do any facility staff members assist the resident with activities he or she can pursue independently?
2. If the residents sit for long periods of time with no apparently meaningful activities, is the cause:
   a. Resident choice;
   b. Failure of any staff or volunteers either to inform residents when activities are occurring or to encourage resident involvement in activities;
   c. Lack of assistance with ambulation;
   d. Lack of sufficient supplies and/or staff to facilitate attendance and participation in the activity programs;
   e. Program design that fails to reflect the interests or ability levels of residents, such as activities that are too complex?

For residents selected for a comprehensive review, or a focused review, as appropriate, determine to what extent the activities reflect the individual resident's assessment. (See especially MDS III.1 and Sections B, C, D and I; MDS version 2.0 sections AC, B, C, D and N.)

Review the activity calendar for the month prior to the survey to determine if the formal activity program:
• Reflects the schedules, choices and rights of the residents;
• Offers activities at hours convenient to the residents (e.g., morning, afternoon, some evenings and weekends);
• Reflects the cultural and religious interests of the resident population; and
• Would appeal to both men and women and all age groups living in the facility.

Review clinical records and activity attendance records of residents receiving a comprehensive review, or a focused review, as appropriate, to determine if:
• Activities reflect individual resident history indicated by the comprehensive assessment;
• Care plans address activities that are appropriate for each resident based on the comprehensive assessment;
• Activities occur as planned; and
• Outcomes/responses to activities interventions are identified in the progress notes of each resident.

Tag F249 This tag outlines the types of credentials required of any person who is employed as the Activity Director.

Tag F250 This tag outlines the scope of social services to be provided by the facility. The entire text of Tag F250 is shown in the box below.

Tag F250 [Social Services]

§483.15(g)(1) The facility must provide medically-related social services to attain or maintain the highest practicable physical, mental and psychosocial well-being of each resident.

Intent §483.15(g)

To assure that sufficient and appropriate social services are provided to meet the resident's needs.

Guidelines: §483.15(g)(1)

Regardless of size, all facilities are required to provide for the medically related social services needs of each resident. This requirement specifies that facilities aggressively identify the need for medically-related social services and pursue the provision of these services. It is not required that a qualified social worker necessarily provide all of these services. Rather, it is the responsibility of the facility to identify the medically-related social services needs of the resident and assure that the needs are met by the appropriate disciplines.

"Medically-related social services" means services provided by the facility's staff to assist residents in maintaining or improving their ability to manage their everyday physical, mental and psychosocial needs. These services might include, for example:
- Making arrangements for obtaining needed adaptive equipment, clothing and personal items;
- Maintaining contact with family (with resident's permission) to report on changes in health, current goals, discharge planning and encouragement to participate in care planning;
- Assisting staff to inform residents and those they designate about the resident's health status and health care choices and their ramifications;
- Making referrals and obtaining services from outside entities (e.g., talking books, absentee ballots, community wheelchair transportation);
- Assisting residents with financial and legal matters (e.g., applying for pensions, referrals to lawyers, referrals to funeral homes for preplanning arrangements);
- Discharge planning services (e.g., helping to place a resident on a waiting list for community congregate living, arranging intake for home care services for residents returning home, assisting with transfer arrangements to other facilities);
- Providing or arranging provision of needed counseling services;
- Through the assessment and care planning process, identifying and seeking ways to support resident's individual needs and preferences, customary routines, concerns and choices;
- Building relationships between residents and staff and teaching staff how to understand and support resident's individual needs;
- Promoting actions by staff that maintain or enhance each resident's dignity in full recognition of each resident's individuality;
- Assisting residents to determine how they would like to make decisions about their health care and whether or not they would like anyone else to be involved in those decisions;
- Finding options that most meet the physical and emotional needs of each resident;
- Providing alternatives to drug therapy or restraints by understanding and communicating to staff why residents act as they do, what they are attempting to communicate and what needs the staff must meet;
- Meeting the needs of residents who are grieving; and
- Finding options which most meet their physical and emotional needs.

Factors with a potentially negative effect on physical, mental and psychosocial well-being include an unmet need for:
- Dental/denture care;
- Podiatric care;
- Eye care;
- Hearing services;
- Equipment for mobility or assistive eating devices; and

- Need for homelike environment, control, dignity, privacy.

Where needed services are not covered by the Medicaid State Plan, nursing facilities are still required to attempt to obtain these services. For example, if a resident requires transportation services that are not covered under a Medicaid State Plan, the facility is required to provide these services. This could be achieved, for example, through obtaining volunteer assistance.

Types of conditions to which the facility should respond with social services by staff or referral include:
- Lack of an effective family/social support system;
- Behavioral symptoms;
- If a resident with dementia strikes out at another resident, the facility should evaluate the resident's behavior. (For example, a resident may be re-enacting an activity he or she used to perform at the same time everyday. If that resident senses that another is in the way of his or her re-enactment, the resident may strike out at the resident impeding his or her progress. The facility is responsible for the safety of any potential resident victims while it assesses the circumstances of the resident's behavior);
- Presence of a chronic disabling medical or psychological condition (e.g., multiple sclerosis, chronic obstructive pulmonary disease, Alzheimer's disease, schizophrenia);
- Depression;
- Chronic or acute pain;
- Difficulty with personal interaction and socialization skills;
- Presence of legal or financial problems;
- Abuse of alcohol or other drugs;
- Inability to cope with loss of function;
- Need for emotional support;
- Changes in family relationships, living arrangements and/or resident's condition or functioning; and
- A physical or chemical restraint.

For residents with or who develop mental disorders as defined by the *Diagnostic and Statistical Manual for Mental Disorders (DSM-IV)*, see §483.45, F406.

Probes: §483.15(g)(1)

For residents selected for a comprehensive or focused review, as appropriate:
- How do facility staff implement social services interventions to assist the resident in meeting treatment goals?
- How do staff responsible for social work monitor the resident's progress in improving physical, mental and psychosocial functioning? Has goal attainment been evaluated and the care plan changed accordingly?
- How does the care plan link goals to psychosocial functioning/well-being?
- Have the staff responsible for social work established and maintained relationships with the resident's family or legal representative?
- (NFs) What attempts does the facility make to access services for Medicaid recipients when those services are not covered by a Medicaid State Plan?

Look for evidence that social services interventions successfully address residents' needs and link social supports, physical care and physical environment with residents' needs and individuality.

For sampled residents review MDS, Section H.

Tag F251 This tag specifies the qualifications of the individuals providing social services and the requirement for one full time social services professional for any facility with 120 beds or more.

Tag F252 All areas of the facility must provide a homelike environment. The resident has the right to keep some of his/her personal possessions in his/her room (including furniture) as long as its presence does not jeopardize the health and safety of the other residents.

Tags F253 – F258 These six tags provide guidelines for the quality and comfort level of the living space for the residents. For a more in-depth review of these tags the reader should review the OBRA Environmental Review Form in this book.

Tag F272 The facility is required to conduct a comprehensive assessment on each resident when s/he is admitted and then at intervals during his/her stay. This assessment must done using a standardized assessment (the MDS), the findings must be accurate, the staff who do the assessment must be qualified to do the assessment and a variety of staff must be able to get substantially similar results (reliability). This tag also explains that the testing tools that the staff use (i.e., the nursing assessment, the social services assessment, the activity assessment) must, when put together, measure everything that is required to be written into the MDS. Each facility must use the RAI (which includes both the MDS and the RAPs). The areas measured include:
- medically defined conditions and prior medical history
- medical status measurement
- physical and mental functional status
- sensory and physical impairments
- nutritional status and requirements
- special treatments and procedures
- mental and psychosocial status
- discharge potential
- dental condition
- activities potential (The resident's ability and desire to take part in activities that maintain or improve physical, mental and psychosocial well-being. Activity pursuits refer to any activity outside of ADLs that a person pursues in order to obtain a sense of well-being. Also included are activities that provide benefits in the areas of self-esteem, pleasure, comfort, health education, creativity, success and financial or emotional independence. The assessment should consider the resident's normal everyday routines and lifetime preferences.)
- rehabilitation potential
- cognitive status, including the resident's ability to problem solve, decide, remember and be aware of and respond to safety hazards
- drug therapy

Tags F273 – F276 These four tags specify the timing associated with assessing and reassessing the resident. By Federal law, the first MDS must be completed within 14 days of admission, reassessed quarterly and redone at least once every 12 months. These tags also specify what kind of medical and social events would trigger a complete reassessment before 12 months are up.

Tag F278 Assessments must be done accurately and signed by each person who completes a portion of the assessment.

Tags F279 – F280 Each resident is required to have a comprehensive care plan based on his/her needs that were identified in the assessment process. This care plan must be developed no later than 7 days after the completion of the MDS. This care plan must be developed by the resident (and/or his/her legal guardian or family) working along with the treatment team and must be reviewed periodically to ensure that it is still appropriate.

Tags F281 – F282 These two tags state that each professional within the facility must provide his/her services in a way that will meet or exceed the standards of practice published by his/her professional group, as well as any other governmental or accrediting standards that apply. For facilities who are surveyed by either the Joint Commission or CARF: the Rehabilitation Accreditation Commission, the professional will want to comply with the standards of those groups to also comply with this tag.

Tags F283 – F284 These two tags outline the requirements for discharge summaries.

Tags F308 – F309 These two tags state that the resident must receive the types and quality of care indicated as needed by the assessment and outlined in the care plan. If the facility has some difficulty meeting this requirement, Tag F309 will be cited. If the facility has significant difficulty meeting this requirement, Tag F308 will be cited.

Tags F310 – F318 These tags specify the facilities responsibilities related to the resident's activities of daily living, vision and hearing, pressure sores, urinary incontinence and range of motion.

Tags F319 – F320 These two tags provide the facility with a detailed explanation of the scope and depth of services and treatment expected for the mental and psychosocial functioning of each resident.

Tags F323 – F324 These tags sets the expectation that the environment will be free of accident hazards and that each resident will receive adequate supervision and assistance to be able to avoid accidental injury.

Tag F330 This tag sets forth a very rigid set of standards and steps required before any resident admitted to a nursing home is given antipsychotic drugs for the first time. The entire treatment team should be familiar with the steps they are required to take before a resident may receive an antipsychotic medication. The physician, who is seldom in the facility, will need to rely on input from many of the professionals (not just nursing) working with the resident before prescribing such medications.

Tags F410 – F412 This requirement concerns dental care. The rest of the tags in this section outline the types of dental care that should be available to the resident as well as the kind of help the staff needs to provide to meet the resident's dental needs. The book, *Dental First Aid for Families* (Diamond, 2000, Idyll Arbor) includes information on taking care of dentures. This book will be a helpful addition to each facility.

Tag F464 The facility must provide one or more rooms designed for resident dining and activities. These rooms must be well lighted. Carole B. Lewis in her book *Improving Mobility In Older Persons* (Aspen Publications, 1989) states: "The lens of the eye becomes thicker with age and the person needs more light to see correctly. Treatment suggestion: use a lot of light (200 watts) especially in functional areas (e.g., reading spots, kitchens and bathrooms." (page 95)). The facility must have adequate ventilation and if a room is a non-smoking area, the signage indicating such must meet state requirements. The facility's rooms must be adequately furnished. Furnishings are structurally sound and functional (e.g., chairs of varying sizes to meet varying needs of residents, wheelchairs can fit under the dining room table). The activity room must have sufficient space to accommodate all activities. Space should be adaptable to a variety of uses and resident needs. Residents and staff have maximum flexibility in arranging furniture to accommodate residents who use walkers, wheelchairs and other mobility aids. No crowding evident. Space does not limit resident access.

Tag F514 How often should the professional write in the progress notes? The questions surveyors are instructed to ask themselves is: Is there enough recorded documentation for staff to conduct a care program and to revise the program as necessary to respond to the changing status of the resident as a result of interventions? How is the clinical record used in managing the resident's progress in maintaining or improving functional abilities and psychosocial status?

Tags F520 – F521 The facility must have a functioning quality assurance committee , which meets at least quarterly and develops and implements appropriate plans of action to correct quality deficiencies.

Surveys

Each of the settings providing treatment services and health care to elderly, psychiatric and DD clients are governed by federal and state regulations.

CMS (Centers for Medicare and Medicaid Services) is responsible for issuing the Federal Register (federal regulations). Each state then reviews these federal guidelines and interprets them for state regulations, which will be in compliance with the federal government standards. In some cases the state may add regulations. It may not remove regulations.

In order to be a participant in the Medicare/Medicaid program, long term care facilities and other agencies, are reviewed and certified. Also, to receive a license by the state to operate as a business, the facilities need to be reviewed and re-licensed annually.

Every aspect of the facility is reviewed for compliance with both federal and state regulations. Because activities and social services are required and extremely important to the well-being of the resident, they are reviewed yearly in this process. The department heads need to be very clear on what the requirements are for these departments. Documentation needs to be presented to the surveyors upon request. You will also have the opportunity to share with them the special programs that you have implemented. The table below outlines some important considerations that will help you do well in the survey process.

Things To Remember About Survey

1. Know your regulations.

2. Be friendly and welcome conversation about what you do. Surveyors play an important role in assuring quality of care and quality of life.

3. Have records of participation, calendars from the past three months, bedside logs, resident council information (member list and minutes of meetings) and PR available for review. Present a packet of information (approved by your administrator) to the surveyors when they first get to the facility.

4. Have your office and supplies neatly organized and labeled.

5. Be responsible for your department but do not involve yourself in issues related to the other departments. They are better trained to do this themselves, just as you are for the service your department provides.

6. Discussion and clarity are important in communicating what and why you do something. If your treatments follow from your assessments and you have made sure that the treatments are carried out according to the resident care plans, there should be no problem during survey.

7. Be yourself.

Compliance with Regulations

Compliance with health care regulations is required. The goal of the federal government is for every health care facility to be in **substantial compliance** with all regulations. Substantial compliance means that the facility is providing a reasonable quality of care to its residents. There can be no deficiencies (services or equipment that do not meet standards) that cause actual harm to any resident and no more than the potential for minimal harm.

Prior to the implementation of the OBRA Final Rule in July 1995, there were instances of facilities not caring if one or two tags were out. For repeated minor deficiencies, there were no penalties. The facilities knew that they could implement a plan of correction and stay in business. If they were out of compliance again by the next survey, there was still no penalty.

The OBRA Final Rule changed that. Now there are required penalties for every facility that is out of substantial compliance. The intent of the new process is to have facilities stay in compliance year round and not experience the previous "yo-yo" compliance at survey time.

When deciding on the penalties, the surveyors look at the severity of the deficiency and its scope for deficiencies found in **Quality of Care**, **Quality of Life** or **Resident Behavior and Facility Practices**. Severity measures the level of harm being caused by the deficiency as shown below:

Level 1: No actual harm with potential for minimal harm	Nothing has happened to a resident and the worst that can happen is a minor negative impact.
Level 2: No actual harm with potential for more than minimal harm that is not immediate jeopardy.	The resident has been impacted in a minor negative way and/or there is a potential for significant harm that has not actually happened yet.
Level 3: Actual harm that is not immediate jeopardy	The resident has been significantly harmed by some practice at the facility and has been prevented from reaching his/her highest practicable level of well-being.
Level 4: Immediate jeopardy	Immediate jeopardy is a situation where immediate corrective action is necessary because what the facility is doing either has caused or may cause serious injury, serious harm or death to a resident in the facility.

Scope refers to the number of residents who are affected by the deficiency. See the table below:

Isolated	One or a very limited number of residents, staff or locations are involved.
Pattern	More than a limited number of residents, staff or locations are involved or the same resident has been affected by the deficiency on repeated occasions.
Widespread	The problems causing the deficiency exist throughout the facility and large portions of the residents have been affected or might be affected.

The surveyors look at the cause of the deficiency as well as the number of deficiencies to determine the scope. If the deficiencies are because the facility does not have a policy or system, the deficiency will probably be widespread. If the deficiency results from inadequate implementation, there will probably be a pattern of deficiency. If only one or a very limited number of residents are affected, the scope is isolated.

If the deficiencies are serious enough or widespread enough, the surveyors will find that the facility is providing a Substandard Quality of Care. This is an official term that means a certain level of deficiency is found during survey. Any Immediate Jeopardy is Substandard Quality of Care. Any pattern of Actual Harm or widespread Actual Harm (Level 3) or Potential for More Than Minimal Harm (Level 2) that is widespread is also considered Substandard Quality of Care. In the chart below the white areas are areas of Substantial Compliance, the light gray areas are out of Substantial Compliance, but not considered Substandard Care. The dark gray areas are Substandard Care. The boldface letters in the bottom right corner of each box are used by CMS to label the boxes in the chart. Refer to them if you are given a letter to describe the results of a survey. The chart also shows the level of penalty required for facilities that are out of substantial compliance.

	ISOLATED	PATTERN	WIDESPREAD
Level 4. Immediate jeopardy to resident health/safety	Plan of Correction Required: Cat. 3 Optional: Cat. 2 Optional: Cat. 1 **J**	Plan of Correction Required: Cat 3 Optional: Cat 2 Optional: Cat 1 **K**	Plan of Correction Required: Cat 3 Optional: Cat 2 Optional: Cat 1 **L**
Level 3. Actual harm that is not Immediate Jeopardy	Plan of Correction Required*: Cat. 2 Optional: Cat. 1 **G**	Plan of Correction Required*: Cat. 2 Optional: Cat. 1 **H**	Plan of Correction Required*: Cat 2 Optional: Temporary Management. Optional: Cat. 1 **I**
Level 2. No actual harm with potential for more than minimal harm that is not immediate jeopardy	Plan of Correction Required*: Cat. 1 Optional: Cat. 2 **D**	Plan of Correction Required*: Cat. 1 Optional: Cat. 2 **E**	Plan of Correction Required*: Cat. 2 Optional: Cat. 1 **F**
Level 1. No actual harm with potential for minimal harm	No remedies No Plan of Correction Commitment to correct **A**	Plan of Correction **B**	Plan of Correction **C**

*It is possible to terminate the operation of the facility instead of imposing these penalties. If termination is not chosen, these penalties are required.

The penalties in the chart above increase depending on the category of penalties.

Category 1 penalties include:
- Directed plan of correction;
- State monitor and/or
- Directed inservice training

Category 2 penalties include:
- Denial of payment for new admissions;
- Denial of payment for all residents and/or
- Civil penalties of $50 to $3000 per day

Category 3 penalties include:
- Temporary management
- Termination
- Optional civil money penalties of $3050 to $10,000 per day

There are two more conditions for compliance in addition to these penalties. They state that:
- Denial of payment for new admissions must be imposed when a facility is not in substantial compliance within three months after being found out of compliance.
- Denial of payment and state monitoring must be imposed when a facility has been found to have provided substandard quality of care on three consecutive standard surveys.

The new penalty structure makes it more important than ever for a facility to be in compliance with regulations. One of the best ways for professionals to do their part is to participate in the quality assurance process at their facility and to regularly check the compliance of their department using the Survey Checklist forms at the end of this section.

Professionals will be asked to give input to the plan of corrections. This is the plan that the facility creates to "fix" the identified problem. It is a response to the CMS form known as the *Statement of Deficiencies* or #2567 form.

The plan of corrections must include the following areas of information:
- How the corrective action will be accomplished for residents found to have been affected by the deficient practice.
- How the facility will identify other residents having the potential to be affected by the same deficient practice.
- What measures will be put into place or systemic changes made to ensure that the deficient practice will not recur.
- How the facility will monitor its corrective actions to ensure that the deficient practice is being corrected and will not recur. (This will be the Quality Assurance/Continuous Quality Indicators program that the facility is mandated to have in place.)

Survey Groups

There are several different survey groups that may be responsible for looking at your facility. The major ones are in the following list:

CMS
Centers for Medicare and Medicaid Services: Responsible for ensuring that minimal federal standards are met. Required of all long term care facilities. Usually sub-contract with state to do their surveys.

State Department of Health, Licensing & Certification Division
State surveys are required at least every twelve months unless the state requests an extension. The surveyors may also survey specific state regulations concerning long term care services.

JCAHO
Joint Commission on Accreditation of Healthcare Organizations: This is a private credentialing body that conducts voluntary surveys. Standards are usually more stringent with a different focus than state and federal regulations. The intent of this survey process is to acknowledge a higher level of standards above federal, state and corporate standards. There is a charge to the facility for this survey process. More and more nursing facilities are requesting this accreditation as the services being provided in many facilities are more specialized and resident based.

CARF: The Rehabilitation Accreditation Commission

CARF: The Rehabilitation Accreditation Commission: This is a private credentialing body that conducts voluntary surveys. CARF Standards apply to rehab services. There is a charge for this survey.

Peer Review
The peer review survey process is a voluntary process requested by the facility. The team may be comprised of management staff from the corporation that owns the facility, a peer review team of a sister facility or a survey team comprised of staff members from a professional long term care organization or community group. There are usually no fees associated with this process, as it is an assurance review process in preparation for any of the above reviews.

Federal Regulations

The federal regulations are standard to all states. In 1987 the Omnibus Budget Reconciliation Act (discussed earlier in the chapter) was enacted. All nursing facilities or "long term care facilities" participating in Medicare and Medicaid are subject to the Act. The regulations serve as the basis for survey activities for the purpose of determining whether a facility meets the requirements for participation in Medicare and Medicaid.

State Regulations

Each state also has regulations for licensing and certification of long term care facilities. These regulations may be stricter than the federal regulations but not more lenient. They will be used in addition to the federal regulations for survey purposes. It is not possible in the scope of this book to review each state's requirements. A copy of the state regulations should be available in the facility. If not, a copy can be reviewed at the county law library.

Corporate or Facility Policy

Many corporations standardize policies and procedures in all of their facilities across the United States. Others allow facilities to adopt their own policies and procedures. Independently owned facilities adopt standardized procedures or create their own. Again, these policies and procedures can be stricter than federal and state law but may not be more lenient. A copy should be available in the facility and in the activity and social services departments.

If a policy is no longer applicable or needs to be revised, this should be brought to the attention of the administrator. Facility policy and procedures must be followed, just as state and federal law must be followed. It is in the best interest of the professional to follow all laws, regulations and policies. They serve as a protection and provide a rationale for any action that may be taken in the care and treatment of the resident.

Survey Checklists

You should use the survey checklists on the following pages to see if your program will pass survey.

OBRA

Quality of Life Review Form

F240 A – Quality of Life
"A facility must care for its residents in a manner and in an environment that promotes maintenance or enhancement of each resident's quality of life."

Facility:_____   **Date:**_____

		+ = Met - = Not Met
Requirement	**Interpretation**	
F241 Dignity	Focus on a resident as an individual Respect for space and property Treating residents respectfully as adults Promoting independence and dignity in dining	

<u>Self-Determination and Participation.</u> The resident has the right to —		
F242 Choose activities, schedules and health care consistent with his or her interests, assessment and plans of care	Accommodating individual schedules and needs according to resident's requests and previous lifestyle and interests	
F242 Interact with members of the community both inside and outside the facility	Facilitating involvement in community groups and matters which were important to resident before admission	
F242 Make choices about aspects of his or her life in the facility *that are significant to the resident*	Providing smoking areas for residents who smoke Working around the resident's schedule (including television programs)	

F243-244 Participation in resident and family groups in the facility	Provide a private space for family and resident groups upon requests	
F243 Facility must provide a designated staff person responsible for providing assistance and responding to written requests that result from group meetings	This staff person listens, records and assists administration with following through with grievances and recommendations	
F246 Accommodation of Needs (1)…adaptations of the facility's physical environment and staff behaviors to assist residents in maintaining independent functioning, dignity, well-being and self-determination.	Accommodation of Needs pertains to how well the team is enhancing and maintaining independence vs. dependence on staff and environment including: telephone access, personal property, married couples, activities, social services, psychosocial functioning, homelike environment, activities of daily living and accidents & prevention-assistive devices	
F247 (2)…Receive notice before the resident's room or roommate in the facility changes	Resident must have a say in who his/her roommate is and the timing of any change	

OBRA

Environment Review Form

Facility: _____ **Date:** _____

F252 — Environment
"The facility must provide a safe, clean, comfortable and homelike environment, allowing the resident to use his or her personal belongings to the extent possible."

Be sure to review the *Environmental Assessment Form* to begin problem solving.

Requirements	Interpretation	+ = Met - = Not Met
De-emphasize institutional character	Encourage personal belongings.	
Cleanliness	How clean is the facility? Are there odors detected in any of the rooms and halls?	
Individuality	Do you get to know who this person is and what his/her past interests were by observing his/her room and personal things and style?	
Clutter	Are day rooms and private rooms cluttered? Is there space for wheelchair and equipment accessibility?	
F253 Housekeeping and Maintenance Services	Assuring cleanliness and an infection-free environment for resident's equipment and supplies: toothbrush, dentures, denture cups, bed pans, urinals, feeding tubes, leg bags, catheter bags, pads and positioning devices.	
F254 Clean bed and bath linens that are in good condition	Are there adequate linens available? Are they in good condition and without stains?	
F255 Private closet space in each room	Closets must be provided with ample space and accessible shelves for resident use.	
F256 Adequate lighting	Lighting suitable to tasks that residents choose to perform or facility staff must perform. Minimal glare and comfortable to the visually impaired. Is lighting accessible to the resident?	
F257 Comfortable and safe temperature levels	Ambient temperature levels to decrease likelihood of temperature changes that could affect well-being of residents. Are there any rooms that are noticeably cold or too warm?	
F258 Comfortable sound levels	Is conversation easy or do you have to raise your voice to be heard? Are there many distractions during group events? Are TVs and radios on too loud and too early or late at night?	

OBRA

Activities Potential Review Form

F272 (x) Activities Potential
"…The resident's ability and desire to take part in activities which maintain or improve physical, mental and psychosocial well-being."

Requirements	Interpretation	+ = Met - = Not Met
All activities which are not Activities of Daily Living	These would be activity/leisure involvement that a resident pursues for a sense of well-being.	
Self-esteem	Focus on the individual. Meaningful activities that highlight the abilities and uniqueness of each resident.	
Health education	Nutrition related activities, wellness, leisure education, relaxation, understanding medical conditions and treatment plans.	
Pleasurable experiences	These can be social activities that encourage passive or active participation. What brings the pleasure is feeling safe, familiar surroundings, rekindling past interests.	
Opportunities for creative expression	Art, creative writing, oral histories, poetry, music, drama, gardening, cooking.	
Opportunities for achieving success	Can be incorporated in all activities at any level. Activities must be adapted and segmented into tasks for success at each level.	
Opportunities for achieving financial independence	Money management. Involvement in previous interests such as the stock market, investments and banking.	
Opportunities for achieving emotional independence	Problem solving activities and situations. Creative and expressive outlets. Activities that promote self-respect and individuality. Life review. Activities that assist others so that the resident has the chance to continue giving to others.	

Medications in the Elderly[62]

In the United States, the use of medications by those who are elderly is far too common. They consume over 30% of all prescription drugs and 40% of all non-prescription drugs. Those who are living in long term care facilities average more than six drugs per resident. All medications cause a change in the body. Because of the normal changes in how the body functions as one ages, the additional changes caused by medications may have a significant effect on the person's overall well-being. The chart below outlines some of the typical changes in one's body as one ages which help increase the impact of medications.

Common Body Changes Associated with Aging

Cardiovascular Function: Congestive Heart Failure	a.	Decreased organ perfusion: as the heart weakens, it is less able to supply blood to the various vital organs.
	b.	Decreased metabolism: decreased blood flow to the liver or to the kidneys may result in decreased drug metabolism and excretion and, in turn, greater drug activity.
Central Nervous System: Degenerative Changes	a.	Over time, the central nervous system (CNS) may exhibit degeneration and also the tissues in the CNS often have an enhanced response to medications.
Kidney and Liver Function	a.	Decreased functional ability: may be a result of decreases in blood perfusion or a long-term disease process such as diabetes mellitus or high blood pressure.
	b.	Decreases in metabolism and excretion.
Body Composition Changes	a.	Decreased lean body mass: decreases in muscle mass and protein stores may influence the response to a medication.
	b.	Contributes to changes in drug activity.
Sensitivity to Drugs	a.	The tissues in the body and various receptor sites where medications exert their pharmaceutical activity may show increased sensitivity resulting in a greater response to a particular drug. This may result in an increased number of side effects.

Adverse Drug Reactions

All drugs have the potential to cause a side effect or adverse reaction. The elderly are more likely to experience an adverse effect and are more likely to be hospitalized as a result. Adverse drug reactions fall into three categories: 1. they are as a result of an allergic reaction to the medication, 2. they are as a result of a non-allergic reaction to a medication or 3. they are considered to be an unusual or idiosyncratic reaction to a medication. There are six general risk factors considered to increase the risk of an adverse drug reaction. Generally, individuals who are elderly have many of these risk factors present, which increase the likelihood of experiencing a side effect to a medication. The risk factors are

1. Age   3. Duration of Treatment   5. Dosage
2. Number of Drugs   4. Gender (Female)   6. Underlying Condition

Medications are frequently grouped together by "types" because they are prescribed for similar disorders, they change the body in similar ways and they frequently share common side effects.

---

[62] Written by Gina C. Johnson, Pharm.D.

The chart below shows some of the medication types that are most frequently prescribed for those who are older and common side effects.

Frequently Prescribed Medications and Their Side Effects		
Type	**Medications**	**Potential Side Effects**
Cardiovascular Medications	Digoxin Verapamil	a. Dizziness, weakness, syncope due to low blood pressure. b. Abnormal heart rhythm c. Confusion, depression
Diuretics	Lasix Hydrochlorothiazide	a. Dehydration b. Headache c. Weakness, fatigue d. Nausea, vomiting
Potassium Products		a. Stomach distress
Pain Medications	Tylenol with Codeine Vicodin	a. Stomach: bleeding, nausea, pain b. Dizziness, drowsiness, confusion, depression c. Narcotics: physical and psychological dependence
Antidiabetic Agents	Insulin Micronase	a. Low blood sugar (Hypoglycemia) b. Chills c. Nausea d. Nervousness e. Confusion f. Hunger g. Rapid, shallow breathing h. Fast heartbeat i. Fatigue
Stomach-Intestinal Medications	Tagamet Reglan Lomotil	a. Diarrhea b. Confusion c. Dizziness d. Depression
Psychoactive Medications: Antipsychotic Medications	Haldol Mellaril Thorazine Navane Risperdal Zyprexa	a. Drowsiness b. Low blood pressure c. Tremors, shaking d. Inability to sit still (akathesia) e. Tardive dyskinesia— irreversible abnormal movements of the mouth and tongue
Psychoactive Medications: Antidepressants	Elavil Desyrel Imipramine	a. Low blood pressure b. Fast heart rate c. Dry mouth, blurred vision, constipation d. Lethargy
Psychoactive Medications: Antidepressants	Prozac Paxil Zoloft	a. Insomnia b. Anxiety, nervousness c. Tremors
Psychoactive Medications: Anti-Anxiety and Sleeping Medications	Valium, BuSpar Ativan, Librium Xanax Klonopin Restoril Dalmane	a. Lethargy, tiredness b. Clumsiness, drunken walk c. Confusion d. Depression

Summary

The responsibilities and challenges of activity, social services and recreational therapy professionals keep growing in direct proportion to the increased needs of the people they serve.

Increased emphasis has been placed on quality of care — regardless of where it is received. The type of staff performance once expected only in hospitals has now worked its way into standards of nursing homes, assisted living and adult day centers. Federal regulations and voluntary accreditation standards have changed the face of long term care forever. These changes have added to the work responsibilities for all staff members. The beauty of the change is that the focus is on the individual and how we as a team can assist each one in meeting goals and projecting outcomes. The medical model focused on the diagnosis and now our functional/holistic model focuses on how a person heals, what gives him/her the resilience to meet new challenges, how the environment either enhances or negatively impacts his/her ability to improve and have a high quality of life.

As you have seen in the flow of information in this book, the authors have attempted to bring you full circle with why the services are important, who the people we serve might be, what the environment offers and how we, as staff, make a profound difference in individual lives — regardless of cognitive and functional abilities and/or limitations.

The impact of quality programming and teamwork are inspirational and do make a difference in both our lives and the lives of the very special individuals who find themselves in need of our services.

Many things change but, as Socrates observed far back in history, much remains the same:

> *I consider the old who have gone before us along a road which we must all travel in our turn and it is good we should ask them of the nature of that road.*

The work that you put your spirit and soul into will not only make an impact on the people we serve living today in long term care settings, but create increasingly higher standards for the generations in the future.

Appendix A
Abbreviations

c̄	with
s̄	without
AC	Activity Coordinator
ADL	activities of daily living
aka	also known as
am	morning
amt	amount
ASHD	arterial sclerotic heart disease
B&C	board and care
bid	2x daily
bp	blood pressure
BRP	bath room privileges
c/o	complain of
CHF	congestive heart failure
COPD	chronic obstructive pulmonary disease
CPR	cardiopulmonary resuscitation
CTRS	Certified Therapeutic Recreation Specialist
CVA	cerebral vascular accident
d/c	discontinue
DD	developmentally disabled
dme	durable medical equipment
DON	Director of Nursing
dx	diagnosis
ETOH	alcohol
fx	fracture
GI	gastrointestinal
gm	gram
H&P	history and physical
HBV	Hepatitis B Virus
HIV	Human Immunodeficiency Virus
HOH	hard of hearing
I	independent
IDT	interdisciplinary team

IM	intramuscular
IV	intravenous
L	left
lb	pound
LE	lower extremity
MDS	Minimum Data Set
mg	milligram
MI	mentally ill: myocardial infarction;
MS	multiple sclerosis
noc	night
NPO	nothing by mouth
∅	no/none
OBRA	Omnibus Budget Reconciliation Act
OOB	out of bed
OT	Occupational Therapy
pm	afternoon, evening
PO	by mouth
PoC	Plan of Correction
PPS	Prospective Payment System
prn	as necessary
Pt	patient
PT	Physical Therapy
q	every
qd	every day
qh	every hour
R	right
r/t	related to
RA	rheumatoid arthritis; restorative aide
RAP	Resident Assessment Protocol
rehab	rehabilitation
res.	resident
ROM	range of motion

RT	Respiratory Therapist; Recreational Therapist
s/p	status post (after)
SNF	skilled nursing facility
SOB	shortness of breath
SP/ST	Speech Pathologist, Therapist
SSC/SSD	Social Services Coordinator/Director
Stat	immediately
T-22	Title 22 (California)
THR	total hip replacement
TIA	transient ischemic attack
tid	3x daily
tx	treatment
UE	upper extremity
URI	upper respiratory infection
UTI	urinary tract infection
w/c	wheel chair
WFL	within functional limits
wk	week
WNL	within normal limits
wt	weight
X	times

Appendix B
Minimum Data Set and the Resident Assessment System

Facilities in the United States that receive Medicare funds are required to use a specific, standardized assessment on every resident admitted to the facility. This standardized assessment, called the Minimum Data Set (MDS), is an interdisciplinary assessment. Each member of the interdisciplinary team is required to conduct his/her own assessment of the resident, analyze the resident's status and then summarize that information on the MDS form within 14 days of the resident's admission to the facility.

The MDS provides health care workers in long term care settings with two advantages: 1. it standardizes medical vocabulary across the nation and 2. it provides the mechanism for the collection of information: demographic information, mortality and morbidity statistics and treatment outcomes. The MDS has been used long enough for us to be able to recognize when a "score" on the MDS indicates health or when it indicates the need to provide some kind of treatment. A book that is used with the MDS, called *Resident Assessment System for Long Term Care*, outlines which scores or combination of scores point up the need for specific interventions.

A "slang" term has arisen called "RAPs." RAPs (Resident Assessment Protocols) refers to the system of deciding which types of interventions will be needed by scoring the MDS and reviewing the results in the book *Resident Assessment System for Long Term Care*. By reviewing the RAPs each health care professional will be able to determine if there is a specific treatment required for the resident. The treatment interventions "triggered" by using RAPs indicate the basic, minimum standard of treatment for residents in long term care facilities. Not implementing a RAPs treatment intervention (unless otherwise medically indicated) would be providing substandard care.

There are 18 identified RAPs:

- Delirium
- Cognitive Loss/Dementia
- Visual Function
- Communication
- ADL Functional/Rehab Potential
- Urinary Incontinence and Indwelling Catheter
- Psychosocial Well-Being
- Mood State
- Behavior Problem
- Activities
- Falls
- Nutritional Status
- Feeding Tubes
- Dehydration/Fluid Maintenance
- Dental Care
- Pressure Ulcers
- Psychoactive Drug Use
- Physical Restraints

All professionals should be familiar with the MDS, the *Resident Assessment System for Long Term Care*, RAPs and how to decide if a treatment intervention is indicated. *Chapter 12: Resident Assessment Instrument* provides an overview of many of the RAPs that may "trigger" the need for action by the professional. To help the reader develop a fuller understanding of the MDS and RAPs process, a copy of the MDS, the basic instructions for using RAPs and two specific protocols have been included in this appendix. The RAPs in this book are from *Resident Assessment System for Long Term Care* published by the US Department of Commerce, National Technical Information Service, Springfield, VA.

Numeric Identifier_____

MINIMUM DATA SET (MDS) — *VERSION 2.0*
FOR NURSING HOME RESIDENT ASSESSMENT AND CARE SCREENING

BASIC ASSESSMENT TRACKING FORM

SECTION AA. IDENTIFICATION INFORMATION

1.	RESIDENT NAME⊙	
		a. (First) b. (Middle Initial) c. (Last) d. (Jr/Sr)
2.	GENDER⊙	1. Male 2. Female
3.	BIRTHDATE⊙	☐☐ — ☐☐ — ☐☐☐☐ Month Day Year
4.	RACE/⊙ ETHNICITY	1. American Indian/Alaskan Native 4. Hispanic 2. Asian/Pacific Islander 5. White, not of 3. Black, not of Hispanic origin Hispanic origin
5.	SOCIAL SECURITY⊙ AND MEDICARE NUMBERS⊙ [C in 1st box if non med. no.]	a. Social Security Number ☐☐☐ — ☐☐ — ☐☐☐☐ b. Medicare number (or comparable railroad insurance number)
6.	FACILITY PROVIDER NO.⊙	a. State No. b. Federal No.
7.	MEDICAID NO. ["+" if pending, "N" if not a Medicaid recipient]⊙	

8.	REASONS FOR ASSESS-MENT	[Note—Other codes do not apply to this form]
		a. Primary reason for assessment
		  1. Admission assessment (required by day 14)
		  2. Annual assessment
		  3. Significant change in status assessment
		  4. Significant correction of prior full assessment
		  5. Quarterly review assessment
		  10. Significant correction of prior quarterly assessment
		  0. *NONE OF ABOVE*
		
		b. *Codes for assessments required for Medicare PPS or the State*
		  1. *Medicare 5 day assessment*
		  2. *Medicare 30 day assessment*
		  3. *Medicare 60 day assessment*
		  4. *Medicare 90 day assessment*
		  5. *Medicare readmission/return assessment*
		  6. *Other state required assessment*
		  7. *Medicare 14 day assessment*
		  8. *Other Medicare required assessment*

9. Signatures of Persons who Completed a Portion of the Accompanying Assessment or Tracking Form

I certify that the accompanying information accurately reflects resident assessment or tracking information for this resident and that I collected or coordinated collection of this information on the dates specified. To the best of my knowledge, this information was collected in accordance with applicable Medicare and Medicaid requirements. I understand that this information is used as a basis for ensuring that residents receive appropriate and quality care, and as a basis for payment from federal funds. I further understand that payment of such federal funds and continued participation in the government-funded health care programs is conditioned on the accuracy and truthfulness of this information, and that I may be personally subject to or may subject my organization to substantial criminal, civil, and/or administrative penalties for submitting false information. I also certify that I am authorized to submit this information by this facility on its behalf.

	Signature and Title	Sections	Date
a.			
b.			
c.			
d.			
e.			
f.			
g.			
h.			
i.			
j.			
k.			
l.			

GENERAL INSTRUCTIONS

Complete this information for submission with all full and quarterly assessments (Admission, Annual, Significant Change, State or Medicare required assessments, or Quarterly Reviews, etc.)

⊙ = Key items for computerized resident tracking

☐ = When box blank, must enter number or letter   ☐a. = When letter in box, check if condition applies

MDS 2.0 September, 2000

Resident _____   Numeric Identifier_____

MINIMUM DATA SET (MDS) — *VERSION 2.0*
FOR NURSING HOME RESIDENT ASSESSMENT AND CARE SCREENING

BACKGROUND (FACE SHEET) INFORMATION AT ADMISSION

SECTION AB. DEMOGRAPHIC INFORMATION

1.	DATE OF ENTRY	*Date the stay began. Note — Does not include readmission if record was closed at time of temporary discharge to hospital, etc. In such cases, use prior admission date*

     ☐☐ — ☐☐ — ☐☐☐☐
     Month   Day   Year

2.	ADMITTED FROM (AT ENTRY)	1. Private home/apt. with no home health services 2. Private home/apt. with home health services 3. Board and care/assisted living/group home 4. Nursing home 5. Acute care hospital 6. Psychiatric hospital, MR/DD facility 7. Rehabilitation hospital 8. Other
3.	LIVED ALONE (PRIOR TO ENTRY)	0. No 1. Yes 2. In other facility
4.	ZIP CODE OF PRIOR PRIMARY RESIDENCE	☐☐☐☐☐
5.	RESIDEN-TIAL HISTORY 5 YEARS PRIOR TO ENTRY	(***Check all settings** resident **lived in** during 5 years prior to date of entry given in item AB1 above)*

Prior stay at this nursing home		a.
Stay in other nursing home		b.
Other residential facility—board and care home, assisted living, group home		c.
MH/psychiatric setting		d.
MR/DD setting		e.
NONE OF ABOVE		f.

6.	LIFETIME OCCUPA-TION(S) [Put "/" between two occupations]	☐☐☐☐☐☐☐☐☐☐☐☐☐☐
7.	EDUCATION (*Highest Level Completed*)	1. No schooling 5. Technical or trade school 2. 8th grade/less 6. Some college 3. 9-11 grades 7. Bachelor's degree 4. High school 8. Graduate degree
8.	LANGUAGE	*(Code for correct response)* **a.** Primary Language 0. English 1. Spanish 2. French 3. Other **b. If other, specify**
9.	MENTAL HEALTH HISTORY	Does resident's RECORD indicate any history of mental retardation, mental illness, or developmental disability problem? 0. No 1. Yes
10.	CONDITIONS RELATED TO MR/DD STATUS	(***Check all conditions** that are related to MR/DD status that were manifested before age 22, and are likely to continue indefinitely)*

Not applicable—no MR/DD (Skip to AB11)		a.
MR/DD with organic condition		
Down's syndrome		b.
Autism		c.
Epilepsy		d.
Other organic condition related to MR/DD		e.
MR/DD with no organic condition		f.

11.	DATE BACK-GROUND INFORMA-TION COMPLETED	☐☐ — ☐☐ — ☐☐☐☐ Month Day Year

SECTION AC. CUSTOMARY ROUTINE

1.	CUSTOMARY ROUTINE	(*Check all that apply. If all information UNKNOWN, check last box only.*)
	(*In year prior to DATE OF ENTRY to this nursing home, or year last in community if now being admitted from another nursing home*)	

CYCLE OF DAILY EVENTS

Stays up late at night (e.g., after 9 pm)	a.
Naps regularly during day (at least 1 hour)	b.
Goes out 1+ days a week	c.
Stays busy with hobbies, reading, or fixed daily routine	d.
Spends most of time alone or watching TV	e.
Moves independently indoors (with appliances, if used)	f.
Use of tobacco products at least daily	g.
NONE OF ABOVE	h.

EATING PATTERNS

Distinct food preferences	i.
Eats between meals all or most days	j.
Use of alcoholic beverage(s) at least weekly	k.
NONE OF ABOVE	l.

ADL PATTERNS

In bedclothes much of day	m.
Wakens to toilet all or most nights	n.
Has irregular bowel movement pattern	o.
Showers for bathing	p.
Bathing in PM	q.
NONE OF ABOVE	r.

INVOLVEMENT PATTERNS

Daily contact with relatives/close friends	s.
Usually attends church, temple, synagogue (etc.)	t.
Finds strength in faith	u.
Daily animal companion/presence	v.
Involved in group activities	w.
NONE OF ABOVE	x.
UNKNOWN—Resident/family unable to provide information	y.

SECTION AD. FACE SHEET SIGNATURES

SIGNATURES OF PERSONS COMPLETING FACE SHEET:

a. Signature of RN Assessment Coordinator   Date

I certify that the accompanying information accurately reflects resident assessment or tracking information for this resident and that I collected or coordinated collection of this information on the dates specified. To the best of my knowledge, this information was collected in accordance with applicable Medicare and Medicaid requirements. I understand that this information is used as a basis for ensuring that residents receive appropriate and quality care, and as a basis for payment from federal funds. I further understand that payment of such federal funds and continued partici-pation in the government-funded health care programs is conditioned on the accuracy and truthful-ness of this information, and that I may be personally subject to or may subject my organization to substantial criminal, civil, and/or administrative penalties for submitting false information. I also certify that I am authorized to submit this information by this facility on its behalf.

Signature and Title	Sections	Date
b.		
c.		
d.		
e.		
f.		
g.		

☐ = When box blank, must enter number or letter   ☐a. = When letter in box, check if condition applies

Resident _____ Numeric Identifier _____

MINIMUM DATA SET (MDS) — *VERSION 2.0*
FOR NURSING HOME RESIDENT ASSESSMENT AND CARE SCREENING
FULL ASSESSMENT FORM
(Status in last 7 days, unless other time frame indicated)

SECTION A. IDENTIFICATION AND BACKGROUND INFORMATION

1.	RESIDENT NAME				
		a. (First)	b. (Middle Initial)	c. (Last)	d. (Jr/Sr)

2.	ROOM NUMBER	

3.	ASSESS-MENT REFERENCE DATE	a. Last day of MDS observation period

Month — Day — Year

b. Original (0) or corrected copy of form (enter number of correction)

4a.	DATE OF REENTRY	Date of reentry from most recent temporary discharge to a hospital in last 90 days (or since last assessment or admission if less than 90 days)

Month — Day — Year

5.	MARITAL STATUS	1. Never married 3. Widowed 5. Divorced
		2. Married 4. Separated

6.	MEDICAL RECORD NO.	

7.	CURRENT PAYMENT SOURCES FOR N.H. STAY	(Billing Office to indicate; check all that apply in last 30 days)		
		Medicaid per diem	a.	VA per diem	f.
		Medicare per diem	b.	Self or family pays for full per diem	g.
		Medicare ancillary part A	c.	Medicaid resident liability or Medicare co-payment	h.
		Medicare ancillary part B	d.	Private insurance per diem (including co-payment)	i.
		CHAMPUS per diem	e.	Other per diem	j.

8.	REASONS FOR ASSESS-MENT	a. Primary reason for assessment
	[Note—If this is a discharge or reentry assessment, only a limited subset of MDS items need be completed]	1. Admission assessment (required by day 14)
		2. Annual assessment
		3. Significant change in status assessment
		4. Significant correction of prior full assessment
		5. Quarterly review assessment
		6. Discharged—return not anticipated
		7. Discharged—return anticipated
		8. Discharged prior to completing initial assessment
		9. Reentry
		10. Significant correction of prior quarterly assessment
		0. NONE OF ABOVE
		b. Codes for assessments required for Medicare PPS or the State
		1. Medicare 5 day assessment
		2. Medicare 30 day assessment
		3. Medicare 60 day assessment
		4. Medicare 90 day assessment
		5. Medicare readmission/return assessment
		6. Other state required assessment
		7. Medicare 14 day assessment
		8. Other Medicare required assessment

9.	RESPONSI-BILITY/ LEGAL GUARDIAN	(Check all that apply)		Durable power attorney/financial	d.
		Legal guardian	a.	Family member responsible	e.
		Other legal oversight	b.	Patient responsible for self	f.
		Durable power of attorney/health care	c.	NONE OF ABOVE	g.

10.	ADVANCED DIRECTIVES	(For those items with supporting documentation in the medical record, check all that apply)		
		Living will	a.	Feeding restrictions	f.
		Do not resuscitate	b.	Medication restrictions	g.
		Do not hospitalize	c.	Other treatment restrictions	h.
		Organ donation	d.	NONE OF ABOVE	i.
		Autopsy request	e.		

SECTION B. COGNITIVE PATTERNS

1.	COMATOSE	(Persistent vegetative state/no discernible consciousness)
		0. No 1. Yes (If yes, skip to Section G)

2.	MEMORY	(Recall of what was learned or known)
		a. Short-term memory OK—seems/appears to recall after 5 minutes 0. Memory OK 1. Memory problem
		b. Long-term memory OK—seems/appears to recall long past 0. Memory OK 1. Memory problem

3.	MEMORY/ RECALL ABILITY	(Check all that resident was normally able to recall during last 7 days)		
		Current season	a.	That he/she is in a nursing home	d.
		Location of own room	b.		
		Staff names/faces	c.	NONE OF ABOVE are recalled	e.

4.	COGNITIVE SKILLS FOR DAILY DECISION-MAKING	(Made decisions regarding tasks of daily life)
		0. INDEPENDENT—decisions consistent/reasonable
		1. MODIFIED INDEPENDENCE—some difficulty in new situations only
		2. MODERATELY IMPAIRED—decisions poor; cues/supervision required
		3. SEVERELY IMPAIRED—never/rarely made decisions

5.	INDICATORS OF DELIRIUM— PERIODIC DISOR-DERED THINKING/ AWARENESS	(Code for behavior in the last 7 days.) [Note: Accurate assessment requires conversations with staff and family who have direct knowledge of resident's behavior over this time].
		0. Behavior not present
		1. Behavior present, not of recent onset
		2. Behavior present, over last 7 days appears different from resident's usual functioning (e.g., new onset or worsening)
		a. EASILY DISTRACTED—(e.g., difficulty paying attention; gets sidetracked)
		b. PERIODS OF ALTERED PERCEPTION OR AWARENESS OF SURROUNDINGS—(e.g., moves lips or talks to someone not present; believes he/she is somewhere else; confuses night and day)
		c. EPISODES OF DISORGANIZED SPEECH—(e.g., speech is incoherent, nonsensical, irrelevant, or rambling from subject to subject; loses train of thought)
		d. PERIODS OF RESTLESSNESS—(e.g., fidgeting or picking at skin, clothing, napkins, etc; frequent position changes; repetitive physical movements or calling out)
		e. PERIODS OF LETHARGY—(e.g., sluggishness; staring into space; difficult to arouse; little body movement)
		f. MENTAL FUNCTION VARIES OVER THE COURSE OF THE DAY—(e.g., sometimes better, sometimes worse; behaviors sometimes present, sometimes not)

6.	CHANGE IN COGNITIVE STATUS	Resident's cognitive status, skills, or abilities have changed as compared to status of 90 days ago (or since last assessment if less than 90 days)
		0. No change 1. Improved 2. Deteriorated

SECTION C. COMMUNICATION/HEARING PATTERNS

1.	HEARING	(With hearing appliance, if used)
		0. HEARS ADEQUATELY—normal talk, TV, phone
		1. MINIMAL DIFFICULTY when not in quiet setting
		2. HEARS IN SPECIAL SITUATIONS ONLY—speaker has to adjust tonal quality and speak distinctly
		3. HIGHLY IMPAIRED/absence of useful hearing

2.	COMMUNI-CATION DEVICES/ TECH-NIQUES	(Check all that apply during last 7 days)	
		Hearing aid, present and used	a.
		Hearing aid, present and not used regularly	b.
		Other receptive comm. techniques used (e.g., lip reading)	c.
		NONE OF ABOVE	d.

3.	MODES OF EXPRESSION	(Check all used by resident to make needs known)		
		Speech	a.	Signs/gestures/sounds	d.
		Writing messages to express or clarify needs	b.	Communication board	e.
		American sign language or Braille	c.	Other	f.
				NONE OF ABOVE	g.

4.	MAKING SELF UNDER-STOOD	(Expressing information content—however able)
		0. UNDERSTOOD
		1. USUALLY UNDERSTOOD—difficulty finding words or finishing thoughts
		2. SOMETIMES UNDERSTOOD—ability is limited to making concrete requests
		3. RARELY/NEVER UNDERSTOOD

5.	SPEECH CLARITY	(Code for speech in the last 7 days)
		0. CLEAR SPEECH—distinct, intelligible words
		1. UNCLEAR SPEECH—slurred, mumbled words
		2. NO SPEECH—absence of spoken words

6.	ABILITY TO UNDER-STAND OTHERS	(Understanding verbal information content—however able)
		0. UNDERSTANDS
		1. USUALLY UNDERSTANDS—may miss some part/intent of message
		2. SOMETIMES UNDERSTANDS—responds adequately to simple, direct communication
		3. RARELY/NEVER UNDERSTANDS

7.	CHANGE IN COMMUNI-CATION/ HEARING	Resident's ability to express, understand, or hear information has changed as compared to status of 90 days ago (or since last assessment if less than 90 days)
		0. No change 1. Improved 2. Deteriorated

[ ] = When box blank, must enter number or letter [a.] = When letter in box, check if condition applies

MDS 2.0 September, 2000

Resident _____   Numeric Identifier _____

SECTION D. VISION PATTERNS

1.	VISION	(Ability to see in adequate light and with glasses if used) 0. *ADEQUATE*—sees fine detail, including regular print in newspapers/books 1. *IMPAIRED*—sees large print, but not regular print in newspapers/books 2. *MODERATELY IMPAIRED*—limited vision; not able to see newspaper headlines, but can identify objects 3. *HIGHLY IMPAIRED*—object identification in question, but eyes appear to follow objects 4. *SEVERELY IMPAIRED*—no vision or sees only light, colors, or shapes; eyes do not appear to follow objects	
2.	VISUAL LIMITATIONS/ DIFFICULTIES	Side vision problems—decreased peripheral vision (e.g., leaves food on one side of tray, difficulty traveling, bumps into people and objects, misjudges placement of chair when seating self)	a.
		Experiences any of following: sees halos or rings around lights; sees flashes of light; sees "curtains" over eyes	b.
		NONE OF ABOVE	c.
3.	VISUAL APPLIANCES	Glasses; contact lenses; magnifying glass 0. No 1. Yes	

SECTION E. MOOD AND BEHAVIOR PATTERNS

1.	INDICATORS OF DEPRES- SION, ANXIETY, SAD MOOD	(Code for indicators observed in last 30 days, irrespective of the assumed cause) 0. Indicator not exhibited in last 30 days 1. Indicator of this type exhibited up to five days a week 2. Indicator of this type exhibited daily or almost daily (6, 7 days a week)	

VERBAL EXPRESSIONS OF DISTRESS

a. Resident made negative statements—e.g., "*Nothing matters; Would rather be dead; What's the use; Regrets having lived so long; Let me die*"

b. Repetitive questions—e.g., "*Where do I go; What do I do?*"

c. Repetitive verbalizations— e.g., calling out for help, ("*God help me*")

d. Persistent anger with self or others—e.g., easily annoyed, anger at placement in nursing home; anger at care received

e. Self deprecation—e.g., "*I am nothing; I am of no use to anyone*"

f. Expressions of what appear to be unrealistic fears—e.g., fear of being abandoned, left alone, being with others

g. Recurrent statements that something terrible is about to happen—e.g., believes he or she is about to die, have a heart attack

h. Repetitive health complaints—e.g., persistently seeks medical attention, obsessive concern with body functions

i. Repetitive anxious complaints/concerns (non-health related) e.g., persistently seeks attention/ reassurance regarding schedules, meals, laundry, clothing, relationship issues

SLEEP-CYCLE ISSUES

j. Unpleasant mood in morning

k. Insomnia/change in usual sleep pattern

SAD, APATHETIC, ANXIOUS APPEARANCE

l. Sad, pained, worried facial expressions—e.g., furrowed brows

m. Crying, tearfulness

n. Repetitive physical movements—e.g., pacing, hand wringing, restlessness, fidgeting, picking

LOSS OF INTEREST

o. Withdrawal from activities of interest—e.g., no interest in long standing activities or being with family/friends

p. Reduced social interaction

2.	MOOD PERSIS- TENCE	One or more indicators of depressed, sad or anxious mood **were not easily altered by attempts to "cheer up", console, or reassure the resident over last 7 days** 0. No mood 1. Indicators present, 2. Indicators present, indicators easily altered not easily altered	
3.	CHANGE IN MOOD	Resident's mood status has changed as compared to status of 90 **days ago** (or since last assessment if less than 90 days) 0. No change 1. Improved 2. Deteriorated	

4.	BEHAVIORAL SYMPTOMS	(A) *Behavioral symptom* **frequency in last 7 days** 0. Behavior not exhibited in last 7 days 1. Behavior of this type occurred 1 to 3 days in last 7 days 2. Behavior of this type occurred 4 to 6 days, but less than daily 3. Behavior of this type occurred daily (B) *Behavioral symptom* **alterability in last 7 days** 0. Behavior not present OR behavior was easily altered 1. Behavior was not easily altered	(A) (B)

a. WANDERING (moved with no rational purpose, seemingly oblivious to needs or safety)

b. VERBALLY ABUSIVE BEHAVIORAL SYMPTOMS (others were threatened, screamed at, cursed at)

c. PHYSICALLY ABUSIVE BEHAVIORAL SYMPTOMS (others were hit, shoved, scratched, sexually abused)

d. SOCIALLY INAPPROPRIATE/DISRUPTIVE BEHAVIORAL SYMPTOMS (made disruptive sounds, noisiness, screaming, self-abusive acts, sexual behavior or disrobing in public, smeared/threw food/feces, hoarding, rummaged through others' belongings)

e. RESISTS CARE (resisted taking medications/ injections, ADL assistance, or eating)

5.	CHANGE IN BEHAVIORAL SYMPTOMS	Resident's behavior status has changed as compared to **status of 90 days ago** (or since last assessment if less than 90 days) 0. No change 1. Improved 2. Deteriorated	

SECTION F. PSYCHOSOCIAL WELL-BEING

1.	SENSE OF INITIATIVE/ INVOLVE- MENT	At ease interacting with others	a.
		At ease doing planned or structured activities	b.
		At ease doing self-initiated activities	c.
		Establishes own goals	d.
		Pursues involvement in life of facility (e.g., makes/keeps friends; involved in group activities; responds positively to new activities; assists at religious services)	e.
		Accepts invitations into most group activities	f.
		NONE OF ABOVE	g.
2.	UNSETTLED RELATION- SHIPS	Covert/open conflict with or repeated criticism of staff	a.
		Unhappy with roommate	b.
		Unhappy with residents other than roommate	c.
		Openly expresses conflict/anger with family/friends	d.
		Absence of personal contact with family/friends	e.
		Recent loss of close family member/friend	f.
		Does not adjust easily to change in routines	g.
		NONE OF ABOVE	h.
3.	PAST ROLES	Strong identification with past roles and life status	a.
		Expresses sadness/anger/empty feeling over lost roles/status	b.
		Resident perceives that daily routine (customary routine, activities) is very different from prior pattern in the community	c.
		NONE OF ABOVE	d.

SECTION G. PHYSICAL FUNCTIONING AND STRUCTURAL PROBLEMS

1. (A) ADL SELF-PERFORMANCE—(*Code for resident's PERFORMANCE OVER ALL SHIFTS during last 7 days—Not including setup*)

0. *INDEPENDENT*—No help or oversight —OR— Help/oversight provided only 1 or 2 times during last 7 days

1. *SUPERVISION*—Oversight, encouragement or cueing provided 3 or more times during last 7 days —OR— Supervision (3 or more times) plus physical assistance provided only 1 or 2 times during last 7 days

2. *LIMITED ASSISTANCE*—Resident highly involved in activity; received physical help in guided maneuvering of limbs or other nonweight bearing assistance 3 or more times — OR—More help provided only 1 or 2 times during last 7 days

3. *EXTENSIVE ASSISTANCE*—While resident performed part of activity, over last 7-day period, help of following type(s) provided 3 or more times:
—Weight-bearing support
—Full staff performance during part (but not all) of last 7 days

4. *TOTAL DEPENDENCE*—Full staff performance of activity during entire 7 days

8. *ACTIVITY DID NOT OCCUR* during entire 7 days

(B) ADL SUPPORT PROVIDED—(*Code for MOST SUPPORT PROVIDED OVER ALL SHIFTS during last 7 days; code regardless of resident's self-performance classification*)

0. No setup or physical help from staff
1. Setup help only
2. One person physical assist
3. Two+ persons physical assist
8. ADL activity itself did not occur during entire 7 days

			(A) SELF-PERF	(B) SUPPORT
a.	BED MOBILITY	How resident moves to and from lying position, turns side to side, and positions body while in bed		
b.	TRANSFER	How resident moves between surfaces—to/from: bed, chair, wheelchair, standing position (EXCLUDE to/from bath/toilet)		
c.	WALK IN ROOM	How resident walks between locations in his/her room		
d.	WALK IN CORRIDOR	How resident walks in corridor on unit		
e.	LOCOMO- TION ON UNIT	How resident moves between locations in his/her room and adjacent corridor on same floor. If in wheelchair, self-sufficiency once in chair		
f.	LOCOMO- TION OFF UNIT	How resident moves to and returns from off unit locations (e.g., areas set aside for dining, activities, or treatments). **If facility has only one floor,** how resident moves to and from distant areas on the floor. If in wheelchair, self-sufficiency once in chair		
g.	DRESSING	How resident puts on, fastens, and takes off all items of **street clothing**, including donning/removing prosthesis		
h.	EATING	How resident eats and drinks (regardless of skill). Includes intake of nourishment by other means (e.g., tube feeding, total parenteral nutrition)		
i.	TOILET USE	How resident uses the toilet room (or commode, bedpan, urinal); transfer on/off toilet, cleanses, changes pad, manages ostomy or catheter, adjusts clothes		
j.	PERSONAL HYGIENE	How resident maintains personal hygiene, including combing hair, brushing teeth, shaving, applying makeup, washing/drying face, hands, and perineum (EXCLUDE baths and showers)		

MDS 2.0 September, 2000

Resident _____　　　　Numeric Identifier _____

2.	BATHING	How resident takes full-body bath/shower, sponge bath, and transfers in/out of tub/shower (EXCLUDE washing of back and hair.) *Code for most dependent in self-performance and support.* (A) BATHING SELF-PERFORMANCE codes appear below	(A)	(B)
		0. Independent—No help provided		
		1. Supervision—Oversight help only		
		2. Physical help limited to transfer only		
		3. Physical help in part of bathing activity		
		4. Total dependence		
		8. Activity itself did not occur during entire 7 days		
		(Bathing support codes are as defined in **Item 1, code B above***)*		

3.	TEST FOR BALANCE (see training manual)	*(Code for ability during test in the last 7 days)* 0. Maintained position as required in test 1. Unsteady, but able to rebalance self without physical support 2. Partial physical support during test; or stands (sits) but does not follow directions for test 3. Not able to attempt test without physical help	
		a. Balance while standing	
		b. Balance while sitting—position, trunk control	

4.	FUNCTIONAL LIMITATION IN RANGE OF MOTION (see training manual)	*(Code for limitations during last 7 days that interfered with daily functions or placed resident at risk of injury)* (A) *RANGE OF MOTION*　　　(B) *VOLUNTARY MOVEMENT* 0. No limitation　　　　　0. No loss 1. Limitation on one side　　1. Partial loss 2. Limitation on both sides　2. Full loss	(A)	(B)
		a. Neck		
		b. Arm—Including shoulder or elbow		
		c. Hand—Including wrist or fingers		
		d. Leg—Including hip or knee		
		e. Foot—Including ankle or toes		
		f. Other limitation or loss		

5.	MODES OF LOCOMOTION	*(Check all that apply during last 7 days)*		
		Cane/walker/crutch	a.	
		Wheeled self	b.	Wheelchair primary mode of locomotion	d.
		Other person wheeled	c.	NONE OF ABOVE	e.

6.	MODES OF TRANSFER	*(Check all that apply during last 7 days)*		
		Bedfast all or most of time	a.	Lifted mechanically	d.
		Bed rails used for bed mobility or transfer	b.	Transfer aid (e.g., slide board, trapeze, cane, walker, brace)	e.
		Lifted manually	c.	NONE OF ABOVE	f.

7.	TASK SEGMENTATION	Some or all of ADL activities were broken into subtasks during **last 7 days** so that resident could perform them 0. No　　1. Yes	

8.	ADL FUNCTIONAL REHABILITATION POTENTIAL	Resident believes he/she is capable of increased independence in at least some ADLs	a.
		Direct care staff believe resident is capable of increased independence in at least some ADLs	b.
		Resident able to perform tasks/activity but is very slow	c.
		Difference in ADL Self-Performance or ADL Support, comparing mornings to evenings	d.
		NONE OF ABOVE	e.

9.	CHANGE IN ADL FUNCTION	Resident's ADL self-performance status has changed as compared to status of **90 days ago** (or since last assessment if less than 90 days) 0. No change　　1. Improved　　2. Deteriorated	

SECTION H. CONTINENCE IN LAST 14 DAYS

1.	CONTINENCE SELF-CONTROL CATEGORIES *(Code for resident's PERFORMANCE OVER ALL SHIFTS)*
	0. *CONTINENT*—Complete control *[includes use of indwelling urinary catheter or ostomy device that does not leak urine or stool]*
	1. *USUALLY CONTINENT*—BLADDER, incontinent episodes once a week or less; BOWEL, less than weekly
	2. *OCCASIONALLY INCONTINENT*—BLADDER, 2 or more times a week but not daily; BOWEL, once a week
	3. *FREQUENTLY INCONTINENT*—BLADDER, tended to be incontinent daily, but some control present (e.g., on day shift); BOWEL, 2-3 times a week
	4. *INCONTINENT*—Had inadequate control BLADDER, multiple daily episodes; BOWEL, all (or almost all) of the time

a.	BOWEL CONTINENCE	Control of bowel movement, with appliance or bowel continence programs, if employed	
b.	BLADDER CONTINENCE	Control of urinary bladder function (if dribbles, volume insufficient to soak through underpants), with appliances (e.g., foley) or continence programs, if employed	

2.	BOWEL ELIMINATION PATTERN	Bowel elimination pattern regular—at least one movement every three days	a.	Diarrhea	c.
				Fecal impaction	d.
		Constipation	b.	NONE OF ABOVE	e.

MDS 2.0 September, 2000

3.	APPLIANCES AND PROGRAMS	Any scheduled toileting plan	a.	Did not use toilet room/ commode/urinal	f.
		Bladder retraining program	b.	Pads/briefs used	g.
		External (condom) catheter	c.	Enemas/irrigation	h.
		Indwelling catheter	d.	Ostomy present	i.
		Intermittent catheter	e.	NONE OF ABOVE	j.

4.	CHANGE IN URINARY CONTINENCE	Resident's urinary continence has changed as compared to status of **90 days ago** (or since last assessment if less than 90 days) 0. No change　　1. Improved　　2. Deteriorated	

SECTION I. DISEASE DIAGNOSES

Check only those diseases that have a relationship to current ADL status, cognitive status, mood and behavior status, medical treatments, nursing monitoring, or risk of death. (Do not list inactive diagnoses)

1.	DISEASES	*(If none apply, CHECK the NONE OF ABOVE box)*				
		ENDOCRINE/METABOLIC/ NUTRITIONAL		Hemiplegia/Hemiparesis	v.
		Diabetes mellitus	a.	Multiple sclerosis	w.
		Hyperthyroidism	b.	Paraplegia	x.
		Hypothyroidism	c.	Parkinson's disease	y.
		HEART/CIRCULATION		Quadriplegia	z.
		Arteriosclerotic heart disease (ASHD)	d.	Seizure disorder	aa.
		Cardiac dysrhythmias	e.	Transient ischemic attack (TIA)	bb.
		Congestive heart failure	f.	Traumatic brain injury	cc.
		Deep vein thrombosis	g.	**PSYCHIATRIC/MOOD**	
		Hypertension	h.	Anxiety disorder	dd.
		Hypotension	i.	Depression	ee.
		Peripheral vascular disease	j.	Manic depression (bipolar disease)	ff.
		Other cardiovascular disease	k.	Schizophrenia	gg.
		MUSCULOSKELETAL		**PULMONARY**	
		Arthritis	l.	Asthma	hh.
		Hip fracture	m.	Emphysema/COPD	ii.
		Missing limb (e.g., amputation)	n.	**SENSORY**	
		Osteoporosis	o.	Cataracts	jj.
		Pathological bone fracture	p.	Diabetic retinopathy	kk.
		NEUROLOGICAL		Glaucoma	ll.
		Alzheimer's disease	q.	Macular degeneration	mm.
		Aphasia	r.	**OTHER**	
		Cerebral palsy	s.	Allergies	nn.
		Cerebrovascular accident (stroke)	t.	Anemia	oo.
				Cancer	pp.
		Dementia other than Alzheimer's disease	u.	Renal failure	qq.
				NONE OF ABOVE	rr.

2.	INFECTIONS	*(If none apply, CHECK the NONE OF ABOVE box)*				
		Antibiotic resistant infection (e.g., Methicillin resistant staph)	a.	Septicemia	g.
				Sexually transmitted diseases	h.
		Clostridium difficile (c. diff.)	b.	Tuberculosis	i.
		Conjunctivitis	c.	Urinary tract infection **in last 30 days**	j.
		HIV infection	d.	Viral hepatitis	k.
		Pneumonia	e.	Wound infection	l.
		Respiratory infection	f.	NONE OF ABOVE	m.

3.	OTHER CURRENT OR MORE DETAILED DIAGNOSES AND ICD-9 CODES	a. _____	| | | • |
		b. _____	| | | • |
		c. _____	| | | • |
		d. _____	| | | • |
		e. _____	| | | • |

SECTION J. HEALTH CONDITIONS

1.	PROBLEM CONDITIONS	*(Check all problems present in last 7 days unless other time frame is indicated)*				
		INDICATORS OF FLUID STATUS		Dizziness/Vertigo	f.
		Weight gain or loss of 3 or more pounds within a 7 day period	a.	Edema	g.
				Fever	h.
				Hallucinations	i.
		Inability to lie flat due to shortness of breath	b.	Internal bleeding	j.
				Recurrent lung aspirations in **last 90 days**	k.
		Dehydrated; output exceeds input	c.	Shortness of breath	l.
				Syncope (fainting)	m.
		Insufficient fluid; did **NOT** consume all/almost all liquids provided during **last 3 days**	d.	Unsteady gait	n.
				Vomiting	o.
		OTHER		NONE OF ABOVE	p.
		Delusions	e.		

Resident _____

Numeric Identifier _____

2.	PAIN SYMPTOMS	(Code the **highest level of pain** present in the last 7 days)
		a. FREQUENCY with which resident complains or shows evidence of pain 0. No pain (**skip to J4**) 1. Pain less than daily 2. Pain daily	**b. INTENSITY** of pain 1. Mild pain 2. Moderate pain 3. Times when pain is horrible or excruciating

3.	PAIN SITE	(If pain present, **check all sites** that apply in **last 7 days**)				
		Back pain		a.	Incisional pain	f.
		Bone pain		b.	Joint pain (other than hip)	g.
		Chest pain while doing usual activities		c.	Soft tissue pain (e.g., lesion, muscle)	h.
		Headache		d.	Stomach pain	i.
		Hip pain		e.	Other	j.

4.	ACCIDENTS	(**Check all that apply**)				
		Fell in **past 30 days**	a.	Hip fracture in **last 180 days**	c.
		Fell in **past 31-180 days**	b.	Other fracture in **last 180 days**	d.
				NONE OF ABOVE	e.

5.	STABILITY OF CONDITIONS	Conditions/diseases make resident's cognitive, ADL, mood or behavior patterns unstable—(fluctuating, precarious, or deteriorating)	a.
		Resident experiencing an acute episode or a flare-up of a recurrent or chronic problem	b.
		End-stage disease, 6 or fewer months to live	c.
		NONE OF ABOVE	d.

SECTION K. ORAL/NUTRITIONAL STATUS

1.	ORAL PROBLEMS	Chewing problem	a.
		Swallowing problem	b.
		Mouth pain	c.
		NONE OF ABOVE	d.

2.	HEIGHT AND WEIGHT	Record (**a.**) **height in inches** and (**b.**) **weight in pounds**. Base weight on most recent measure in **last 30 days**; measure weight consistently in accord with standard facility practice—e.g., in a.m. after voiding, before meal, with shoes off, and in nightclothes
		a. HT (in.) [ ][ ][ ] **b.** WT (lb.) [ ][ ][ ][ ]

3.	WEIGHT CHANGE	**a. Weight loss**—5 % or more in **last 30 days**; or 10 % or more in **last 180 days** 0. No 1. Yes
		b. Weight gain—5 % or more in **last 30 days**; or 10 % or more in **last 180 days** 0. No 1. Yes

4.	NUTRITIONAL PROBLEMS	Complains about the taste of many foods	a.	Leaves 25% or more of food uneaten at most meals	c.
		Regular or repetitive complaints of hunger	b.	NONE OF ABOVE	d.

5.	NUTRITIONAL APPROACHES	(**Check all that apply in last 7 days**)				
		Parenteral/IV	a.	Dietary supplement between meals	f.
		Feeding tube	b.		
		Mechanically altered diet	c.	Plate guard, stabilized built-up utensil, etc.	g.
		Syringe (oral feeding)	d.	On a planned weight change program	h.
		Therapeutic diet	e.		
				NONE OF ABOVE	i.

6.	PARENTERAL OR ENTERAL INTAKE	(**Skip to Section L if neither 5a nor 5b is checked**)
		a. Code the proportion of **total calories** the resident received through parenteral or tube feedings in the **last 7 days** 0. None 3. 51% to 75% 1. 1% to 25% 4. 76% to 100% 2. 26% to 50%
		b. Code the average **fluid intake** per day by IV or tube in **last 7 days** 0. None 3. 1001 to 1500 cc/day 1. 1 to 500 cc/day 4. 1501 to 2000 cc/day 2. 501 to 1000 cc/day 5. 2001 or more cc/day

SECTION L. ORAL/DENTAL STATUS

1.	ORAL STATUS AND DISEASE PREVENTION	Debris (soft, easily movable substances) present in mouth prior to going to bed at night	a.
		Has dentures or removable bridge	b.
		Some/all natural teeth lost—does not have or does not use dentures (or partial plates)	c.
		Broken, loose, or carious teeth	d.
		Inflamed gums (gingiva); swollen or bleeding gums; oral abcesses; ulcers or rashes	e.
		Daily cleaning of teeth/dentures or daily mouth care—by resident or staff	f.
		NONE OF ABOVE	g.

SECTION M. SKIN CONDITION

1.	ULCERS (Due to any cause)	(Record the number of ulcers at each ulcer stage—regardless of cause. If none present at a stage, record "0" (zero). Code all that apply during **last 7 days**. Code 9 = 9 or more.) [**Requires full body exam.**]	Number at Stage
		a. Stage 1. A persistent area of skin redness (without a break in the skin) that does not disappear when pressure is relieved.	
		b. Stage 2. A partial thickness loss of skin layers that presents clinically as an abrasion, blister, or shallow crater.	
		c. Stage 3. A full thickness of skin is lost, exposing the subcutaneous tissues - presents as a deep crater with or without undermining adjacent tissue.	
		d. Stage 4. A full thickness of skin and subcutaneous tissue is lost, exposing muscle or bone.	

2.	TYPE OF ULCER	(For each type of ulcer, **code for the highest stage in the last 7 days** using scale in item M1—i.e., 0=none; stages 1, 2, 3, 4)	
		a. Pressure ulcer—any lesion caused by pressure resulting in damage of underlying tissue	
		b. Stasis ulcer—open lesion caused by poor circulation in the lower extremities	

3.	HISTORY OF RESOLVED ULCERS	Resident had an ulcer that was resolved or cured in LAST 90 DAYS 0. No 1. Yes	

4.	OTHER SKIN PROBLEMS OR LESIONS PRESENT	(**Check all that apply** during **last 7 days**)	
		Abrasions, bruises	a.
		Burns (second or third degree)	b.
		Open lesions other than ulcers, rashes, cuts (e.g., cancer lesions)	c.
		Rashes—e.g., intertrigo, eczema, drug rash, heat rash, herpes zoster	d.
		Skin desensitized to pain or pressure	e.
		Skin tears or cuts (other than surgery)	f.
		Surgical wounds	g.
		NONE OF ABOVE	h.

5.	SKIN TREATMENTS	(**Check all that apply** during **last 7 days**)	
		Pressure relieving device(s) for chair	a.
		Pressure relieving device(s) for bed	b.
		Turning/repositioning program	c.
		Nutrition or hydration intervention to manage skin problems	d.
		Ulcer care	e.
		Surgical wound care	f.
		Application of dressings (with or without topical medications) other than to feet	g.
		Application of ointments/medications (other than to feet)	h.
		Other preventative or protective skin care (other than to feet)	i.
		NONE OF ABOVE	j.

6.	FOOT PROBLEMS AND CARE	(**Check all that apply** during **last 7 days**)	
		Resident has one or more foot problems—e.g., corns, callouses, bunions, hammer toes, overlapping toes, pain, structural problems	a.
		Infection of the foot—e.g., cellulitis, purulent drainage	b.
		Open lesions on the foot	c.
		Nails/calluses trimmed during **last 90 days**	d.
		Received preventative or protective foot care (e.g., used special shoes, inserts, pads, toe separators)	e.
		Application of dressings (with or without topical medications)	f.
		NONE OF ABOVE	g.

SECTION N. ACTIVITY PURSUIT PATTERNS

1.	TIME AWAKE	(**Check appropriate time periods over last 7 days**) Resident awake all or most of time (i.e., naps no more than one hour per time period) in the:		
		Morning	a.	Evening	c.
		Afternoon	b.	NONE OF ABOVE	d.

(If resident is comatose, skip to Section O)

2.	AVERAGE TIME INVOLVED IN ACTIVITIES	(When awake and not receiving treatments or ADL care) 0. Most—more than 2/3 of time 2. Little—less than 1/3 of time 1. Some—from 1/3 to 2/3 of time 3. None	

3.	PREFERRED ACTIVITY SETTINGS	(**Check all settings** in which activities are **preferred**)				
		Own room	a.		
		Day/activity room	b.	Outside facility	d.
		Inside NH/off unit	c.	NONE OF ABOVE	e.

4.	GENERAL ACTIVITY PREFERENCES (adapted to resident's current abilities)	(**Check all PREFERENCES** whether or not activity is currently available to resident)				
		Cards/other games	a.	Trips/shopping	g.
		Crafts/arts	b.	Walking/wheeling outdoors	h.
		Exercise/sports	c.	Watching TV	i.
		Music	d.	Gardening or plants	j.
		Reading/writing	e.	Talking or conversing	k.
		Spiritual/religious activities	f.	Helping others	l.
				NONE OF ABOVE	m.

Resident_____ Numeric Identifier_____

5.	PREFERS CHANGE IN DAILY ROUTINE	Code for resident preferences in daily routines 0. No change 1. Slight change 2. Major change	
		a. Type of activities in which resident is currently involved	
		b. Extent of resident involvement in activities	

SECTION O. MEDICATIONS

1.	NUMBER OF MEDICA-TIONS	(**Record the number of different** medications used in the **last 7 days**; enter "0" if none used)	
2.	NEW MEDICA-TIONS	(Resident currently receiving medications that were initiated during the **last 90 days**) 0. No 1. Yes	
3.	INJECTIONS	(**Record the number of DAYS** injections of any type received during the **last 7 days**; enter "0" if none used)	
4.	DAYS RECEIVED THE FOLLOWING MEDICATION	(**Record the number of DAYS** during **last 7 days**; enter "0" if not used. Note—enter "1" for long-acting meds used less than weekly)	

a. Antipsychotic		d. Hypnotic	
b. Antianxiety		e. Diuretic	
c. Antidepressant			

SECTION P. SPECIAL TREATMENTS AND PROCEDURES

1.	SPECIAL TREAT-MENTS, PROCE-DURES, AND PROGRAMS	a. SPECIAL CARE—**Check** treatments or programs received during the **last 14 days**	

TREATMENTS		Ventilator or respirator	l.
Chemotherapy	a.	**PROGRAMS**	
Dialysis	b.	Alcohol/drug treatment program	m.
IV medication	c.		
Intake/output	d.	Alzheimer's/dementia special care unit	n.
Monitoring acute medical condition	e.	Hospice care	o.
Ostomy care	f.	Pediatric unit	p.
Oxygen therapy	g.	Respite care	q.
Radiation	h.	Training in skills required to return to the community (e.g., taking medications, house work, shopping, transportation, ADLs)	r.
Suctioning	i.		
Tracheostomy care	j.		
Transfusions	k.	NONE OF ABOVE	s.

b. THERAPIES - Record the number of days and total minutes each of the following therapies was administered (for at least 15 minutes a day) in the **last 7 calendar days** (Enter 0 if none or less than 15 min. daily) [Note—count only post admission therapies] (A) = # of days administered for **15 minutes or more** (B) = total # of minutes provided in **last 7 days**	DAYS (A)	MIN (B)
a. Speech - language pathology and audiology services		
b. Occupational therapy		
c. Physical therapy		
d. Respiratory therapy		
e. Psychological therapy (by any licensed mental health professional)		

2.	INTERVEN-TION PROGRAMS FOR MOOD, BEHAVIOR, COGNITIVE LOSS	(**Check all** interventions or strategies used in last 7 days—no matter where received)	
		Special behavior symptom evaluation program	a.
		Evaluation by a licensed mental health specialist in **last 90 days**	b.
		Group therapy	c.
		Resident-specific deliberate changes in the environment to address mood/behavior patterns—e.g., providing bureau in which to rummage	d.
		Reorientation—e.g., cueing	e.
		NONE OF ABOVE	f.

3.	NURSING REHABILITA-TION/ RESTOR-ATIVE CARE	Record the NUMBER OF DAYS each of the following rehabilitation or restorative techniques or practices was **provided to the resident for more than or equal to 15 minutes per day in the last 7 days** (Enter 0 if none or less than 15 min. daily.)	

a. Range of motion (passive)		f. Walking	
b. Range of motion (active)		g. Dressing or grooming	
c. Splint or brace assistance		h. Eating or swallowing	
TRAINING AND SKILL PRACTICE IN:		i. Amputation/prosthesis care	
d. Bed mobility		j. Communication	
e. Transfer		k. Other	

4.	DEVICES AND RESTRAINTS	(Use the following codes for **last 7 days**:) 0. Not used 1. Used less than daily 2. Used daily	
		Bed rails	
		a. — Full bed rails on all open sides of bed	
		b. — Other types of side rails used (e.g., half rail, one side)	
		c. Trunk restraint	
		d. Limb restraint	
		e. Chair prevents rising	
5.	HOSPITAL STAY(S)	Record number of times resident was admitted to hospital with an overnight stay **in last 90 days** (or since last assessment if less than 90 days). (Enter 0 if no hospital admissions)	
6.	EMERGENCY ROOM (ER) VISIT(S)	Record number of times resident visited ER without an overnight stay **in last 90 days** (or since last assessment if less than 90 days). (Enter 0 if no ER visits)	
7.	PHYSICIAN VISITS	In the **LAST 14 DAYS** (or since admission if less than 14 days in facility) how many days has the physician (or authorized assistant or practitioner) examined the resident? (Enter 0 if none)	
8.	PHYSICIAN ORDERS	In the **LAST 14 DAYS** (or since admission if less than 14 days in facility) how many days has the physician (or authorized assistant or practitioner) changed the resident's orders? Do not include order renewals without change. (Enter 0 if none)	
9.	ABNORMAL LAB VALUES	Has the resident had any abnormal lab values during the **last 90 days** (or since admission)? 0. No 1. Yes	

SECTION Q. DISCHARGE POTENTIAL AND OVERALL STATUS

1.	DISCHARGE POTENTIAL	a. Resident expresses/indicates preference to return to the community 0. No 1. Yes	
		b. Resident has a support person who is positive towards discharge 0. No 1. Yes	
		c. Stay projected to be of a short duration— discharge projected **within 90 days** (do not include expected discharge due to death) 0. No 2. Within 31-90 days 1. Within 30 days 3. Discharge status uncertain	

2.	OVERALL CHANGE IN CARE NEEDS	Resident's overall self sufficiency has changed significantly as compared to status of **90 days ago** (or since last assessment if less than 90 days)
		0. No change 1. Improved—receives fewer 2. Deteriorated—receives
		                  supports, needs less more support
		                  restrictive level of care	

SECTION R. ASSESSMENT INFORMATION

1.	PARTICIPA-TION IN ASSESS-MENT	a. Resident: 0. No 1. Yes	
		b. Family: 0. No 1. Yes 2. No family	
		c. Significant other: 0. No 1. Yes 2. None	
2.	SIGNATURE OF PERSON COORDINATING THE ASSESSMENT:		

a. Signature of RN Assessment Coordinator (sign on above line)

b. Date RN Assessment Coordinator signed as complete			
Month	Day	Year	

Resident _____   Numeric Identifier _____

SECTION T. THERAPY SUPPLEMENT FOR MEDICARE PPS

1.	SPECIAL TREAT-MENTS AND PROCE-DURES	**a. RECREATION THERAPY**—*Enter number of days and total minutes of recreation therapy administered* (**for at least 15 minutes a day**) *in the last 7 days* (*Enter 0 if none*)		
			DAYS (A)	MIN (B)
		(A) = # of days administered for 15 minutes or more **(B) = total # of minutes** provided in last 7 days		
		Skip unless this is a Medicare 5 day or Medicare readmission/return assessment.		
		b. ORDERED THERAPIES—*Has physician ordered any of following therapies to begin in FIRST 14 days of stay—physical therapy, occupational therapy, or speech pathology service?* 0. No 1. Yes		
		If not ordered, skip to item 2		
		c. Through day 15, provide an estimate of the number of days when at least 1 therapy service can be expected to have been delivered.		
		d. Through day 15, provide an estimate of the number of therapy minutes (across the therapies) that can be expected to be delivered?		
2.	WALKING WHEN MOST SELF SUFFICIENT	*Complete item 2 if ADL self-performance score for TRANSFER (G.1.b.A) is 0,1,2, or 3 AND at least one of the following are present:* • Resident received physical therapy involving gait training (P.1.b.c) • Physical therapy was ordered for the resident involving gait training (T.1.b) • Resident received nursing rehabilitation for walking (P.3.f) • Physical therapy involving walking has been discontinued within the past 180 days		
		Skip to item 3 if resident did not walk in last 7 days		
		(FOR FOLLOWING FIVE ITEMS, BASE CODING ON THE EPISODE WHEN THE RESIDENT WALKED THE FARTHEST WITHOUT SITTING DOWN. INCLUDE WALKING DURING REHABILITATION SESSIONS.)		
		a. Furthest distance walked without sitting down during this episode. 0. 150+ feet 3. 10-25 feet 1. 51-149 feet 4. Less than 10 feet 2. 26-50 feet		
		b. Time walked without sitting down during this episode. 0. 1-2 minutes 3. 11-15 minutes 1. 3-4 minutes 4. 16-30 minutes 2. 5-10 minutes 5. 31+ minutes		
		c. Self-Performance in walking during this episode. 0. *INDEPENDENT*—No help or oversight 1. *SUPERVISION*—Oversight, encouragement or cueing provided 2. *LIMITED ASSISTANCE*—Resident highly involved in walking; received physical help in guided maneuvering of limbs or other nonweight bearing assistance 3. *EXTENSIVE ASSISTANCE*—Resident received weight bearing assistance while walking		
		d. Walking support provided associated with this episode (code regardless of resident's self-performance classification). 0. No setup or physical help from staff 1. Setup help only 2. One person physical assist 3. Two+ persons physical assist		
		e. Parallel bars used by resident in association with this episode. 0. No 1. Yes		
3.	CASE MIX GROUP	Medicare [ ][ ][ ][ ][ ] State [ ][ ][ ][ ][ ]		

SECTION V. RESIDENT ASSESSMENT PROTOCOL SUMMARY   Numeric Identifier _____

Resident's Name:	Medical Record No.:

1. Check if RAP is triggered.

2. For each triggered RAP, use the RAP guidelines to identify areas needing further assessment. Document relevant assessment information regarding the resident's status.

- Describe:
  — Nature of the condition (may include presence or lack of objective data and subjective complaints).
  — Complications and risk factors that affect your decision to proceed to care planning.
  — Factors that must be considered in developing individualized care plan interventions.
  — Need for referrals/further evaluation by appropriate health professionals.

- Documentation should support your decision-making regarding whether to proceed with a care plan for a triggered RAP and the type(s) of care plan interventions that are appropriate for a particular resident.

- Documentation may appear anywhere in the clinical record (e.g., progress notes, consults, flowsheets, etc.).

3. Indicate under the <u>Location of RAP Assessment Documentation</u> column where information related to the RAP assessment can be found.

4. For each triggered RAP, indicate whether a new care plan, care plan revision, or continuation of current care plan is necessary to address the problem(s) identified in your assessment. The Care Planning Decision column must be completed within 7 days of completing the RAI (MDS and RAPs).

A. RAP PROBLEM AREA	(a) Check if triggered	Location and Date of RAP Assessment Documentation	(b) Care Planning Decision—check if addressed in care plan
1. DELIRIUM			
2. COGNITIVE LOSS			
3. VISUAL FUNCTION			
4. COMMUNICATION			
5. ADL FUNCTIONAL/ REHABILITATION POTENTIAL			
6. URINARY INCONTINENCE AND INDWELLING CATHETER			
7. PSYCHOSOCIAL WELL-BEING			
8. MOOD STATE			
9. BEHAVIORAL SYMPTOMS			
10. ACTIVITIES			
11. FALLS			
12. NUTRITIONAL STATUS			
13. FEEDING TUBES			
14. DEHYDRATION/FLUID MAINTENANCE			
15. DENTAL CARE			
16. PRESSURE ULCERS			
17. PSYCHOTROPIC DRUG USE			
18. PHYSICAL RESTRAINTS			

B. _____   2. ☐☐–☐☐–☐☐☐☐
1. Signature of RN Coordinator for RAP Assessment Process   Month   Day   Year

_____   4. ☐☐–☐☐–☐☐☐☐
3. Signature of Person Completing Care Planning Decision   Month   Day   Year

MDS 2.0 September, 2000

Resident Assessment Protocols

Each of the 18 resident assessment protocols (RAPs) organizes comprehensively clinical information to assist long term care facility staff in thinking about care planning and treatment decisions. A RAP has two parts: 1. a RAP KEY that summarizes all MDS elements applicable to thinking about assessment and care planning in that particular clinical area; and 2. instructions, including clinical background information and suggested approaches to additional assessment. Upon completing a RAP, staff will have:

- Identified the unique problems the resident has that may affect adversely his/her highest practicable physical, mental and psychosocial functioning.
- Identified factors that place the resident's highest practicable physical, mental and psychosocial functioning at risk.
- Considered whether the identified problems and risk factors could be prevented or reversed and evaluated the extent to which the resident is able to attain a higher level of well-being and functional independence.
- Evaluated ongoing care practices for that resident by, for example, considering alternative therapies and the need for medical consultation or consultation(s) by other health professionals such as occupational or physical therapists.

To use RAPs, long term care facility staff shall follow these steps:

- As specified in the utilization guidelines, complete MDS elements, using common definitions.
- Review MDS information. Use the Resident Assessment Protocol Trigger Legend Worksheet that shows which MDS elements serve as triggers for each RAP.
- If MDS items and codes trigger a RAP, circle the RAP that has been triggered.
- Complete triggered RAPs following instructions for each RAP. Delegate completion of a particular RAP to the facility staff who can address that care area most knowledgeably, whether it be nursing personnel, therapists, social workers, activity specialist or physicians. Whenever possible, get the person(s) who completed the MDS trigger(s) for that RAP to apply the full RAP.
- After competing a RAP, use the Resident Assessment Protocol Summary to document decisions about care planning and to specify where in the resident's record summary information gained from the assessment has been noted, for example, progress note or care plan.
- This summary information must include, as appropriate to the individual resident, documentation of problems, complications and risk factors, the need for referral to appropriate health professionals and the reasons for deciding to proceed or not to proceed to care planning for the specific problems identified.
- The registered nurse coordinating the assessment must sign and date the Resident Assessment Protocol Summary verifying that the triggered RAPs have been applied.

Resident Assessment Protocol: Psychosocial Well-Being

I. Problem

Well-being refers to feelings about self and social relationships. Positive attributes include initiative and involvement in life; negative attributes include distressing relationships and concern about loss of status. On average, 30% of residents in a typical nursing facility will experience problems in this area, two-thirds of whom will also have serious behavior and/or mood problems. When such problems coexist, initial treatment is often focused on mood and behavior manifestations. In such situations, treatment for psychosocial distress is dependent on how the resident responds to the primary mood/behavior treatment regimen.

II. Triggers

Well-being problem or need to maintain psychosocial strengths suggested if one or more of the following present:

- Withdrawal from activities of interest (problem)* [E1o = 1,2]
- Conflict with staff (problem) [F2a = checked]
- Unhappy with roommate (problem) [F2b = checked]
- Unhappy with other resident (problem) [F2c = checked]
- Conflict with family or friends (problem) [F2d = checked]
- Grief over lost status or roles (problem) [F3b = checked]
- Daily routine is very different from prior pattern in the community (problem) [F3c = checked]
- Establishes own goals (strength) [F1d = checked]
- Strong identification with past (strength) [F3a = checked]

Note: This item also triggers on the Mood State RAP.

III. Guidelines

Sequentially review the items found on the RAP key.

Confounding Problems

Treatments for mood or behavior problems are often immediately beneficial to well-being.

> - Does the resident have an increasing or persistently sad mood?
> - Does the resident have increasing frequency or daily disturbing behavior?
> - Did the mood or behavior problems appear before the reduced sense of well-being?
> - Has the resident's condition deteriorated since last assessment?
> - Have ongoing treatment programs been effective?

Situational Factors That May Impede Ability to Interact with Others

Environmental and situational problems are often amenable to staff intervention without the burden of staff having to "change the resident."

> - Have key social relationships been altered or terminated (e.g., loss of family member, friend or staff)?
> - Have changes in the resident's environment altered access to others or to routine activities — for example, room assignment, use of physical restraints, assignment to new dining area?

Resident Characteristics That May Impede Ability to Interact with Others

These items focus on areas where the resident may lack the ability to enter freely into satisfying social relationships. They represent substantial impediments to easy interaction with others and highlight areas where staff intervention may be crucial.

- Do cognitive or communication deficits or a lack of interest in activities impeded interactions with others?
- Does resident indicate unease in social relationships?

Lifestyles Issues

Residents can withdraw or become distressed because they feel life lacks meaning.

- Was life more satisfactory prior to entering the nursing facility?
- Is resident preoccupied with the past, unwilling to respond to the needs of the present?
- Has the facility focused on a daily schedule that resembles the resident's prior lifestyle?

Additional Information to Clarify the Nature of the Problem

Supplemental assessment items can be used to specify the nature of the well-being problem for residents for whom a well-being care plan is anticipated. These items represent topics around which to phrase questions and to establish a trusting exchange with the resident. Each item includes the positive and negative end of a continuum, representing the possible range that staff can use in thinking about these issues. Staff can use or not use the items in this list. For those items selected, the following issues should be considered:

- How do staff or resident perceive the severity of the problem?
- Has the resident ever demonstrated (while in the facility) strengths in the area under review?
- Are corrective strategies now being used? Have they been used in the past? To what effect?
- Is this an area that might be improved?

PSYCHOSOCIAL WELL-BEING RAP KEY *(for MDS Version 2.0)*

Triggers

Well-being problem or need to maintain psychosocial strengths suggested if one or more of the following present:

- Withdrawal from activities of interest (problem)* [E1o = 1,2]
- Conflict with staff (problem) [F2a = checked]
- Unhappy with roommate (problem) [F2b = checked]
- Unhappy with other resident (problem) [F2c = checked]
- Conflict with family or friends (problem) [F2d = checked]
- Grief over lost status or roles (problem) [F3b = checked]
- Daily routine is very different from prior pattern in the community (problem) [F3c = checked]
- Establishes own goals (strength) [F1d = checked]
- Strong identification with past (strength) [F3a = checked]

Note: This item also triggers on the Mood State RAP.

Guidelines

Confounding Problems:
- Increasing/persistent sad mood [E2, E3]
- Increasing or daily disturbing behavior [E4, E5]
- Resident's condition deteriorated since last assessment [Q2]

Situational Factors That May Impede Ability To Interact With Others:
- Loss of family member, friend or staff close to resident [F2f; from record]
- Initial use of physical restraints [P4]
- New admission [AB1, A4a], change in room assignment [A2] or change in dining location or table mates [from record]

Resident Characteristics That May Impeded Ability To Interact With Others:
- Delirium or cognitive decline [B5, B6]
- Communication deficit or decline [C4, C5, C6, C7]
- Not at ease interacting with others [F1a]
- Locomotion deficit or use of wheelchair [G1c, G1d, G1f, G5b, G5c, G5d]
- Diseases that impede communication — mental retardation [AB10], Alzheimer's [I1q], aphasia [I1r], other dementia [I1u], depression [I1ee]
- Uninvolved in activities [N2, N4]

Lifestyle Issues:
- Incongruence of current and prior style of life [AC, F3c]
- Strong identification with past roles or status [F3a]
- Length of time problem existed [from record]

Supplemental Problem Clarification Issues [from resident or family if necessary]:
- ***Ability to relate to others.*** Skill or unease in dealing with others; reaches out or distances self; friendly or unapproachable; flexible or ridiculed by others.
- ***Relationships resident could draw on.*** Supported or isolated; many friends or friendless.
- ***Dealing with grief.*** Moving through grief or bitter and inconsolable; religious faith or feels punished.

Resident Assessment Protocol: Activities

I. Problem

The Activities RAP targets residents for whom a revised activity care plan may be required to identify those residents whose inactivity may be a major complication in their lives. Resident capabilities may not be fully recognized: the resident may have recently moved into the facility or staff may have focused too heavily on the instrumental needs of the resident and may have lost sight of complications in the institutional environment.

Resident involvement in passive as well as active activities can be as important in the nursing home as it was in the community. The capabilities of the average resident have obviously been altered as abilities and expectations change, disease intervenes, situational opportunities become less frequent and extended social relationships less common. But something that should never be overlooked is the great variability within the resident population: many will have ADL deficits, but few will be totally dependent; impaired cognition will be widespread, but so will the ability to apply old skills and learn new ones; and senses may be impaired, but some type of two-way communication is almost always possible.

For the nursing home, activity planning is a universal need. For this RAP, the focus is on cases where the system may have failed the resident, or where the resident has distressing conditions that warrant review of the activity care plan. The types of cases that will be triggered are: (1) residents who have indicated a desire for additional activity choices; (2) cognitively intact, distressed residents who may benefit from an enriched activity program; (3) cognitively deficient, distressed residents whose activity levels should be evaluated; and (4) highly involved residents whose health may be in jeopardy because of their failure to slow down,

In evaluating triggered cases, the following general questions may be helpful:

- Is inactivity disproportionate to the resident's physical/cognitive abilities or limitations?
- Have decreased demands of nursing home life removed the need to make decisions, to set schedules, to meet challenges? Have these changes contributed to resident apathy?
- What is the nature of the naturally occurring physical and mental challenges the resident experiences in everyday life?
- In what activities is the resident involved? Is he/she normally an active participant in the life of the unit? Is the resident reserved, but actively aware of what is going on around him/her? Or is he/she unaware of surroundings and activities that take place?
- Are there proven ways to extend the resident's inquisitive/active engagement in activities?
- Might simple staff actions expedite resident involvement in activities? For example: Can equipment be modified to permit greater resident access of the unit? Can the resident's location or position be changed to permit greater access to people, views or programs? Can time and/or distance limitations for activities be made less demanding without destroying the challenge? Can staff modes of interacting with the resident be more accommodating, possibly less threatening, to resident deficits?

II. Triggers

ACTIVITIES TRIGGER A (Revise)

Consider revising activity plan if one or more of following present:

Involved in activities little or none of time
$[N2 = 2, 3]$
Prefers change in daily routine
$[N5a = 1, 2][N5b = 1, 2]$

ACTIVITIES TRIGGERS B (Review)

Review of activity plan suggested if both of following present:

Awake all or most of time in morning
    [Nla = checked]
involved in activities most of time
    [N2 = 0]

III.   Guidelines

The follow up review looks for factors that may impede resident involvement in activities. Although many factors can play a role, age as a valid impediment to participation can normally be ruled out. If age continues to be linked as a major cause of lack of participation, a staff education program may prove effective in remedying what may be overprotective staff behavior.

Issues to be Considered as Activity Plan is Developed.

Is Resident Suitably Challenged, Overstimulated? To some extent, competence depends on environmental demands. When the challenge is not sufficiently demanding, a resident can become bored, perhaps withdrawn, may resort to fault-finding and perhaps even behave mischievously to relieve the boredom. Eventually, such a resident may become less competent because of the lack of challenge. In contrast, when the resident lacks the competence to meet challenges presented by the surroundings, he or she may react with anger and aggressiveness.

- *Do available activities correspond to resident lifetime values, attitudes and expectations?*
- *Does resident consider leisure activities a waste of time — he/she never really learned to play or to do things just for enjoyment?*
- *Have the resident's wishes and prior activity patterns been considered by activity and nursing professionals?*
- *Have staff considered how activities requiring lower energy levels may be of interest to the resident — e.g., reading a book, talking with family and friends, watching the world go by, knitting?*
- *Does the resident have cognitive/functional deficits that either reduce options or preclude involvement in all/most activities that would otherwise have been of interest to him/her?*

Confounding Problems to be Considered

Health-related factors that may affect participation in activities. Diminished cardiac output, an acute illness, reduced energy reserves and impaired respiratory function are some of the many reasons that activity level may decline. Most of these conditions need not necessarily incapacitate the resident. All too often, disease-induced reduction of activity may lead to progressive decline through disuse and further decrease in activity levels. However, this pattern can be broken: many activities can be continued if they are adapted to require less exertion or if the resident is helped in adapting to a lost limb, decreased communication skills, new appliances and so forth.

- *Is the resident suffering from an acute health problem?*
- *Is resident hindered because of embarrassment/unease due to presence of health-related equipment (tubes, oxygen tank, colostomy bag, wheelchair)?*
- *Has the resident recovered from an illness? Is the capacity for participation in activities greater?*
- *Has an illness left the resident with some disability (e.g., slurred speech, necessity for use of cane/walker/wheelchair, limited use of hands)?*
- *Does resident's treatment regimen allow little time or energy for participation in preferred activities?*

Other Issues to be Considered

Recent decline in resident status — cognition, communication, function, mood or behavior. When pathologic changes occur in any aspect of the resident's competence, the pleasurable challenge of activities may narrow. Of special interest are problematic changes that may be related to the use of psychoactive medications. When residents or staff overreact to such losses, compensatory strategies may be helpful — e.g., impaired residents may benefit from periods of both activity and rest; task segmentation can be considered; or available resident energies can be reserved for pleasurable activities (e.g., using usual stamina reserves to walk to the card room, rather than the bathroom) or activities that have individual significance (e.g., sitting unattended at a daily prayer service rather than at group activity programs).

* *Has staff or the resident been overprotective? Or have they misread the seriousness of resident cognitive/functional decline? In what ways?*
* *Has the resident retained skills, or the capacity to learn new skills, sufficient to permit greater activity involvement?*
* *Does staff know what the resident was like prior to the most recent decline? Has the physician/other staff offered a prognosis for the resident's future recovery, or chance of continued decline?*
* *Is there any substantial reason to believe that the resident cannot tolerate or would be harmed by increased activity levels? What reasons support a counter opinion?*
* *Does resident retain any desire to learn or master a specific new activity? Is this realistic?*
* *Has there been a lack of participation in the majority of activities which he/she stated as preference, even though these types of activities are provided?*

Environmental factors. Environmental factors include recent changes in resident location, facility rules, season of the year and physical space limitations that hinder effective resident involvement.

* *Does the interplay of personal, social and physical aspects of the facility's environment hamper involvement in activities? How might this be addressed?*
* *Are current activity levels affected by the season of the year or the nature of the weather during the MDS assessment period?*
* *Can the resident choose to participate in or to create an activity? How is this influenced by facility rules?*
* *Does resident prefer to be with others, but the physical layout of the unit gets in the way? Do other features in the physical plant frustrate the resident's desire to be involved in the life of the facility? What corrective actions are possible? Have any been taken?*

Changes in availability of family/friends/staff support. Many residents will experience not only a change in residence but also a loss of relationships. When this occurs, staff may wish to consider ways for resident to develop a supportive relationship with another resident, staff member or volunteer that may increase the desire to socialize with others and/or to participate in activities with this new friend.

* *Has a staff person who has been instrumental in involving a resident in activities left the facility/been reassigned?*
* *Is a new member in a group activity viewed by a resident as taking over?*
* *Has another resident who was a leader on the unit died or left the unit?*
* *Is resident shy, unable to make new friends?*
* *Does resident's expression of dissatisfaction with fellow residents indicate he/she does not want to be a part of an activities group?*

Possible Confounding Problems to be Considered for Those Now Actively Involved in Activities. Of special interest are cardiac and other diseases that might suggest a need to slow down.

ACTIVITIES RAP KEY *(For MDS Version 2.0)*

TRIGGERS - REVISION

ACTIVITIES TRIGGER A (Revise)

Consider revising activity plan if one or more of the following present.

- Involved in activities little or none of time [N2 = 2,3]

- Prefers change in daily routine [N5a = 1,2] [N5b = 1,2]

ACTIVITIES TRIGGERS B (Review)

Review of activity plan suggested if both of following present.

Awake all or most of time in morning [N1a = checked]

Involved in activities most of time [N2 = 0]

GUIDELINES

Issues to be considered as activity plan is developed.

- Time in facility [AB1]
- Cognitive status [B2, B4]
- Walking/locomotion pattern [G1c, d, e, f]
- Unstable/acute health conditions [J5a, b]
- Number of treatments received [P1]
- Use of Psychoactive medications [O4a, b, c, d]

Confounding problems to be considered.

- Performs tasks slowly and at different levels (reduced energy reserves) [G8c, d]
- Cardiac dysrhythmias [I1e]
- Hypertension [I1h]
- CVA [I1t]
- Respiratory diseases [I1hh, I1ii]
- Pain [J2]

Other issues to be considered.

- Customary routines [AC]
- Mood [E1, E2] and Behavioral Symptoms [E4]
- Recent loss of close family member/friend or staff [F2f, from record]
- Whether daily routine is very different from prior pattern in the community [F3c]

Appendix C
Standards of Practice

One of the best ways to determine if your department or facility is providing quality services is to compare your services to your professional organization's standards of practice. Standards of practice are written statements that outline the minimum level and scope of services that a professionally trained individual will perform. While each professional organization has its own set of standards, common threads weave through each. Below are the National Association for Activity Professional's Scope of Practice, Standards of Practice and Ethical Standards. There are two standards of practice for recreational therapy. Contact each organization for a copy of its standards (National Therapeutic Recreation Society, 22377 Belmont Ridge Road, Ashburn, VA 20148-4501, 703-858-2151 www.nrpa.org/branches/ntrs.htm and American Therapeutic Recreation Association, 1414 Prince Street, Suite 204, Alexandria, VA 22314, 703-683-9420 www.atra.org.)

National Association of Activity Professionals

Scope of Practice

The Activity Professional provides activity services and programs, which enable the client/resident to maximize their potential in activity participation. The provisions of activity services are primarily for geriatric populations, who are in a variety of settings that may include other populations with special needs. Activity practice is based on assessment, development, implementation, documentation, and evaluation of the programs provided and of the unique needs and interests of the individuals served. Activity services are directed and provided by professionals who are trained and certified to provide activity services for geriatric populations.

National Association of Activity Professionals

Standards of Practice[63]

PROVISION OF ACTIVITY SERVICES

1. ACTIVITY ASSESSMENT/PROFILE:

The Activity Professional shall conduct an activity assessment/profile for each client/resident to determine his/her activity needs, interests, preferences and abilities.

2. ACTIVITY PLAN:

The Activity Professional shall develop an individual, interdisciplinary activity plan with each client/resident. The activity plan shall be based on the resident's/client's activity assessment/profile and shall be designed to enable each resident/client to achieve and/or maintain his/her highest level of well-being.

3. IMPLEMENTATION OF ACTIVITY PLAN:

The Activity Professional shall direct the activity plan and shall involve the interdisciplinary team in the implementation of the individualized therapeutic interventions.

4. EVALUATION OF THE ACTIVITY PLAN:

The Activity Professional shall continuously evaluate and document the resident's/ client's response to each activity. The revision of the activity plan shall be based on the resident's/client's response to the therapeutic interventions.

5. ACTIVITY PROGRAM:

The Activity Professional shall be resident/client centered and enable the resident/ client to maximize his/her potential in the activity program.

MANAGEMENT OF ACTIVITY SERVICES

6. STAFF CREDENTIALS/EDUCATION:

The Activity Department shall establish a plan to ensure each activity employee is qualified to perform his/her assigned tasks, maintains appropriate credentials and is provided with opportunities for professional development.

7. PLAN OF OPERATION:

The Activity Department shall have written policies and procedures based on the National Association of Activity Professionals (NAAP) *Standards of Practice* and *Scope of Practice*; regulatory requirements; facility/corporate requirements and the standards established by accrediting agencies.

8. RESOURCE UTILIZATION:

The Activity Department shall develop and maintain a plan for identifying, acquiring and utilizing resources to achieve the department's goals.

9. QUALITY IMPROVEMENT/PROGRAM EVALUATION:

The Activity Department shall develop and implement a systematic and ongoing plan to evaluate the quality, effectiveness and integrity of the activity services.

10. ETHICAL CONDUCT:

The Activity Professional shall adhere to the NAAP *Code of Ethics*.

Ethical Aspects of Practice

An "ethic" is a belief that is shared by members of an occupational group. Ethics statements let us know which behaviors are considered appropriate and which behaviors are considered unacceptable. They are formalized and approved by professional organizations. Ethical statements are developed by the organizations through past experiences with behaviors on the part of individual professionals. These behaviors either made the profession proud or disturbed the profession as a group. In essence, these standards for professional behaviors are developed along with, and because of, information about practice that came to light because of quality assurance programs and the developing body of knowledge.

The code of ethics statement below is from the National Association for Activity Professionals.

National Association of Activity Professionals[64]

Code of Ethics

Preamble:

The National Association of Activity Professionals and its members are dedicated to providing activity services and programs which meet the unique needs and interests of the individuals we serve.

Principles:

I.	Conduct	The Activity Professional shall maintain high standards of personal conduct and professional integrity on the job site at all times. The Activity Professional shall treat colleagues with professional courtesy and ensure that credit is given to others for use of their ideas, materials and programs.
II.	Dignity/Rights	The Activity Professional shall treat the client/resident with a regard towards personal dignity at all times. The Activity Professional shall respect and protect the rights, civil, legal and human, of the residents at all times. The Activity Professional shall report abuse, exploitation and work through appropriate channels to protect the rights of clients/residents.
III.	Confidentiality	The Activity Professional shall treat as confidential any information about the client/resident. Information which must be shared in the course of care to other staff and volunteers shall be exchanged in a professional manner.
IV.	Empowerment	The Activity Professional shall enable clients/residents to participate in the planning and implementation of their care, as well as to make independent medical, legal and financial decisions.
V.	Participation	The Activity Professional shall enable clients/residents to maximize their potential in activity participation through adaptation, cues/prompts, protection from undue interruption and assistance in the rescheduling of other events which may interfere with the client/resident's ability to participate in activities of their choice.
VI.	Record Keeping	The Activity Professional shall maintain client/records in an accurate, confidential and timely manner. The Activity Professional shall follow facility policies and procedures in the formatting of such records. In the absence of facility policy, the appropriate state and/or federal guidelines shall be followed.

---

[64] ©1996, National Association of Activity Professionals, *Code of Ethics* adopted April 1996. Used with permission. May not be reproduced without written permission from the National Association of Activity Professionals.

VII.	Professional	The Activity Professional shall participate in continuing education opportunities, strive for professional competence, ensure accurate resumes and differentiate between personal comments/actions and official NAAP positions.
VIII.	Supervisory	The Activity Professional shall treat persons supervised with dignity and respect, protect their rights and provide accurate and fair evaluations.
IX.	Communication	The Activity Professional shall strive to maintain open channels of communication with other departments, with administration and with families and clients/residents.
X.	Provision of Services	The Activity Professional shall provide programs, regardless of race, religion or absence thereof, ethnic origin, social or marital status, sex or sexual orientation, age, health status or payment source, which assist the client/resident in achieving and maintaining the highest practicable level of physical, intellectual, psychosocial, emotional and spiritual well-being.
XI.	Legal	The Activity Professional shall comply with all applicable Federal, State and Local laws regarding the provision of services.

Appendix D
References and Further Reading

Allen-Burket, Gayle. (1988). *Time Well-Spent: A Manual for Visiting Older Adults.* Madison, WI: BiFolkal Productions, Inc.

American Occupational Therapy Association. (1989). *Uniform Terminology for Reporting Occupational Therapy, 2nd Ed.* Bethesda, MD.

American Psychiatric Association. (1994). *Diagnostic and Statistical Manual of Mental Disorders Fourth Edition.* Washington, DC.

Armstrong, Missy and Lauzen, Sarah. (1994). *Community Integration Program, 2nd Edition.* Ravensdale, WA: Idyll Arbor, Inc.

Atkinson, R. C. and Shiffrin, R. M. (1971). "The control of short-term memory and its control processes." *Scientific American, 225,* 82-90.

Ayres, A. Jean. (1971). *Sensory Integration and Learning Disorders.* Los Angeles, CA: Western Psychological Services.

Blackman, J. A. (1990). *Medical Aspects of Developmental Disabilities in Children Birth to Three.* Gaithersburg, MD: Aspen Publications.

Bond-Howard, Barbara. (1993). *Introduction to Stroke.* Ravensdale, WA: Idyll Arbor, Inc.

Bowlby, Carol. (1993). *Therapeutic Activities with Persons Disabled by Alzheimer's Disease and Related Disorders.* Gaithersburg, MD: Aspen Publishers.

Bradford, Leland P. (1976). *Making Meetings Work: A Guide for Leaders and Group Members.* La Jolla, CA: University Associates.

Brasile, F., Skalko, T. K. and burlingame, j. (1998). *Perspectives in Recreational Therapy: Issues of a Dynamic Profession.* Ravensdale, WA: Idyll Arbor, Inc.

burlingame, j. (1999). Reprint from *Idyll Arbor's Journal of Recreational Therapy Practice.* www.IdyllArbor.com, April 1999.

burlingame, j. and Blaschko, T. M. (1991). *Therapy in Intermediate Care Facilities for the Mentally Retarded.* Ravensdale, WA: Idyll Arbor, Inc.

burlingame, j. and Blaschko, T. M. (2002). *Assessment Tools for Recreational Therapy and Related Fields, Third Edition.* Ravensdale, WA: Idyll Arbor, Inc.

Burnside, Irene Mortenson. (1978). *Working with the Elderly: Group Process and Techniques.* Belmont, CA: Duxbury Press.

Campanelli, Linda and Leviton, Dan. (1989). "Intergenerational health promotion and rehabilitation: The adult health and development program model." *Topics in Geriatric Rehab; 4*(3) 61-69. Gaithersburg, MD: Aspen Publishing, Inc.

Campbell, Joseph with Moyer, Bill. (1988). *The Power of Myth*. New York, NY: Doubleday.

Cunninghis, R. N. and Best Martini, E. (1996). *Quality Assurance for Activity Programs, Second Edition*. Ravensdale, WA: Idyll Arbor, Inc.

Cunninghis, Richelle. (1995). *Reality Activities: A How to Manual for Increasing Orientation, Second Edition*. Ravensdale, WA: Idyll Arbor, Inc.

D'Antonio-Nocera, Anne, DeBolt, Nancy and Touhey, Nadine, Eds. (1996). *The Professional Activity Manager and Consultant*. Ravensdale, WA: Idyll Arbor, Inc.

Eliopoulos, Charlotte. (1993). *Gerontological Nursing, Third Edition*. Philadelphia, PA: J. B. Lippincott Company.

Erikson, Erik H., Erikson, Joan M., and Kivnick, Helen Q. (1994). *Vital Involvement in Old Age*. New York, NY: W. W. Norton.

Feil, Naomi. (1993). *The Validation Breakthrough*. Baltimore, MD: Health Professions Press.

Feldt, K. S. (2000). Checklist of Nonverbal Pain Indicators. *Pain Management Nursing, 1*(1), 13–21.

Geriatric Video Productions. (1998). Treatment of Pain in Cognitively Impaired Compared with Cognitively Intact Older Patients with Hip Fractures. http://www.geriatricvideo.com/cfdocs/archives_titles.cfm?date=01-JAN-98&end_date=01-JAN-99.

Hall, Beth A. and Nolta, Michele M. (2000). *Care Planning Cookbook for Activities and Recreation*. San Diego, CA: Recreation Therapy Consultants.

Harris Lord, Janice. (1988). *Beyond Sympathy: What to Say and Do for Someone Suffering an Injury, Illness or Loss*. CA: Pathfinder Publishing.

Health Care Financing Administration. (1990). *Resident Assessment System For Long Term Care Facilities*. Springfield, VA: US Department of Commerce National Technical Information Service.

Health Care Financing Administration. (1995). *State Operations Manual Provider Certification*. Springfield, VA: US Department of Commerce National Technical Information Service.

Health Care Financing Administration. *RAI Training Manual*. Springfield, VA: US Department of Commerce National Technical Information Service.

Hopkins, H. L. and Smith, H. D. (1983). *Willard and Spackman's Occupational Therapy, Sixth Edition*. New York, NY: J. B. Lippincott Company.

Hospital Service. (1919, June 30). *The Red Cross Bulletin, 3*(27), 2-3. Referenced in James, A. "The conceptual development of recreational therapy" In Brasile, F., Skalko, T. K. and burlingame, j. (1998). *Perspectives in Recreational Therapy: Issues of a Dynamic Profession*. Ravensdale, WA: Idyll Arbor.

Kaplan, H. I., Sadock, B. J. and Grebb, J. A. (1994). *Kaplan and Sadock's Synopsis of Psychiatry, Seventh Edition*. Baltimore, MD: Williams and Wilkins.

Karam, C. (1989). *A Practical Guide to Cardiac Rehabilitation*. Gaithersburg, MD: Aspen Publications.

Kemp, B., Brummel-Smith, K. and Ramsdell, J. W. (1990). *Geriatric Rehabilitation*. Boston, MA: College Hill Publications.

Kisner, C. and Colby, L. A. (1990). *Therapeutic Exercise: Foundations and Techniques, Second Edition*. Philadelphia, PA: F. A. Davis.

Krames Communications. (1898). *Risk Management: Your Role in Providing Quality Care.* Daly City, CA: Krames Communication.

Kübler-Ross, E. (1969). *On Death and Dying.* New York, NY: Macmillan Publishing Co., Inc.

Lewis, C. B. (1989). *Improving Mobility in Older Persons: A Manual for Geriatric Specialists.* Gaithersburg, MD: Aspen Publication.

Lewis, C. S. (1961). *A Grief Observed.* New York, NY: Bantam Books.

Lightner, Candy and Nancy Hathaway. (1990). *Giving Sorrow Words: How to Cope with Grief and Get on with Your Life.* New York, NY: Warner Books.

MacNeil, Richard D. and Teague, Michael L. (1987). *Aging and Leisure Vitality in Later Life.* Englewood Cliffs, NJ: Prentice Hall.

Manning, Doug. (1985). *Comforting Those Who Grieve: A Guide for Helping Others.* New York, NY: Harper and Row.

McKay, M. Davis, M. and Fanning, P. (1983). *Messages: The Communication Skills Book.* Oakland, CA: New Harbinger Publications.

National Center for Assisted Living. (2000). *Assisted Living Move-In/Move Out Profiles.* May 28, 2000 web site. http://www.ncal.org/about/resident.htm

National Center for Assisted Living. (2000). *Assisted Living Resident Profile,* May 28, 2000 web site. http://www.ncal.org/about/resident.htm

National Therapeutic Recreation Society. (1998-1999). *NTRS Report 24*(1) p.17.

Parker, Sandra and Will, Carol. (1993). *Activities for the Elderly Volume 2, A Guide to Working with Residents with Significant Physical and Cognitive Disabilities.* Ravensdale, WA: Idyll Arbor, Inc.

Peabody, Larry. (1982). *Deskbook on Writing.* Olympia, WA: Writing Services.

Randall-David, E. (1989). *Strategies for Working with Culturally Diverse Communities and Clients.* Bethesda, MD: Association for the Care of Children's Health.

Reber, A. S. (1985). *Dictionary of Psychology.* New York, NY: Penguin Books.

Richardson-Brown, C. and Payton, G. (1993). *CompuPlan Guide.* Indianapolis, IN: Med America Corporation.

Rodman, G. P., McEwen, C. and Wallace. S. L. (1973). *Primer on the Rheumatic Diseases.* Reprinted from *The Journal of the American Medical Association 224, no. 5* (April 30, 1973) (Supplement).

Romney, G. O. (1945). *Off the Job Living.* Washington, DC: McGrath Publishing Co. and National Recreation and Park Association. Referenced in James, A. "The conceptual development of recreational therapy" In Brasile, F., Skalko, T. K. and burlingame., j. (1998). *Perspectives in Recreational Therapy: Issues of a Dynamic Profession.* Ravensdale, WA: Idyll Arbor, Inc.

Ross, Mildred and Burdick, Dona. (1981). *Sensory Integration.* Thorofare, NJ: Slack, Inc.

Selye, Hans. (1976). *The Stress of Life, Revised Edition.* New York: McGraw-Hill.

Simon, P. (1971). *Play and Game Theory in Group Work: A Collection of Papers by Neva Leona Boyd.* Referenced in James, A. "The conceptual development of recreational therapy" In Brasile, F., Skalko, T. K. and burlingame, j. (1998). *Perspectives in Recreational Therapy: Issues of a Dynamic Profession.* Ravensdale, WA: Idyll Arbor, Inc.

Toglia, J. P. (1992). "Cognitive Rehabilitation" in Zoltan, 1996. *Vision, Perception and Cognition, Third Edition.* Thorofare, NJ: Slack.

Uniack, Ann. (1996). *Documentation in a SNAP for Activity Programs (with MDS Version 2.0)*. San Anselmo, CA: SNAP.

Uniform Data System for Medical Rehabilitation. (1997). *Guide for the Uniform Data Set for Medical Rehabilitation (including the FIM™ instrument). Version 5.1*. Buffalo, NY: State University at Buffalo.

US Department of Health and Human Services. (1983). *CDC Guidelines for Isolation Precautions in Hospitals and CDC Guidelines for Infection Control in Hospital Personnel*. Atlanta, GA: Centers for Disease Control.

Voelkl, J. E. (1988). *Risk Management in Therapeutic Recreation: A Component of Quality Assurance*. State College, PA: Venture Publishing.

Williams, J. M. (1987). *Cognitive Stimulation in the Home Environment: The Rehabilitation of Cognitive Disabilities*. New York, NY: Center for Applied Psychological Research, Memphis State University. Plenum Press.

Zoltan, Barbara, Siev, Ellen and Freishtat, Brenda. (1986). *The Adult Stroke Patient: A Manual for Evaluation and Treatment of Perceptual and Cognitive Dysfunction*. Thorofare, NJ: Slack.

Zoltan, Barbara. (1996). *Vision, Perception and Cognition: A Manual for Evaluation and Treatment of the Neurologically Impaired Adult, Third Edition*. Thorofare, NJ: Slack.

Index

About the Authors

Elizabeth (Betsy) Best Martini

Elizabeth Best Martini has been a Recreational Therapist Certified (RTC) in California since 1978. She is a nationally Certified Therapeutic Recreation Specialist (CTRS) and also is an Activity Consultant Certified with NAAP (ACC). She received her Master of Science degree in Therapeutic Recreation and Leisure Studies from San Francisco State University. She held the position of Recreation Therapist/Activity Coordinator/Social Services Coordinator for a 99-bed nursing facility.

In 1983, Elizabeth began her private practice under the name of Recreation Consultation. This consulting company provides consultation to long term care settings and other agencies throughout Northern California. Betsy is a well known as a therapist, educator and lecturer, throughout the United States and Canada.

She teaches two Living History classes for elderly clients weekly. Betsy is also a certified fitness instructor with certification through the American Senior Fitness Association. She teaches a Strength Training class with frail elders in a convalescent setting.

She is a qualified instructor for both the NAAP Basic Education and Advanced Management Courses. She currently teaches the BEC Course in three college settings in Northern California.

She is a board member of the National LITA Association. LITA is a volunteer organization that provides one-on-one friends to nursing home residents without family or visitors.

She and her husband live in Marin County, California, with their two pygmy goats, which also visit in long term care settings and appear at National Park Service Visitor Centers.

Mary Anne Weeks

Mary Anne Weeks has worked as a Social Worker (SSC) in nursing facilities since November of 1982. At that time, few facilities in California had yet realized a need for such a discipline so there were no "rules." Fortunately, Mary Anne had long ago, in 1965, worked as a summer intern in a prototype retirement home in Rochester, New York. Her past experience in this setting with various levels of care made the environment in nursing settings more familiar to her.

In the meantime, she had also received an undergraduate degree from the State University of New York, Genesee and pursued graduate work at University of California, Berkeley where she completed her Master Degree in Public Health.

Mary Anne lives in Sonoma, California, with her husband and two children. She is the Social Services Coordinator in a nursing facility, provides consultation in the specialty area of social services and is a lecturer at the community college level.

Priscilla Wirth

Priscilla Wirth is a Health Information Consultant for long term care facilities. She is a Registered Records Administrator, receiving her degree from Seattle University. She has been in the health information profession since 1980.

Her Bachelor of Science degree and Master of Library Sciences were received from Northern Illinois University. Priscilla is currently practicing in Sonoma County, California and is a member of the American Medical Record Association, the California Health Information Association and the Network of Health Record Consultants. She is a lecturer at the community college level.